Pediatric and Adolescent Gynecology
Evidence-Based Clinical Practice
2nd, revised and extended edition

Endocrine Development

Vol. 22

Series Editor

P.-E. Mullis Bern

Pediatric and Adolescent Gynecology

Evidence-Based Clinical Practice

2nd, revised and extended edition

Volume Editor

Charles Sultan Montpellier

65 figures, 4 in color, and 49 tables, 2012

KARGER

Basel · Freiburg · Paris · London · New York · New Delhi · Bangkok · Beijing · Tokyo · Kuala Lumpur · Singapore · Sydney

Endocrine Development
Founded 1999 by Martin O. Savage, London

Prof. Dr. Charles Sultan
Unité d'Endocrinologie –
Gynécologie Pédiatriques
Département de Pédiatrie
Hôpital A. de Villeneuve
Montpellier, France

Library of Congress Cataloging-in-Publication Data

Pediatric and adolescent gynecology : evidence-based clinical practice / volume editor, Charles Sultan. -- 2nd rev. and extended ed.
p. ; cm. -- (Endocrine development, ISSN 1421-7082 ; v. 22)
Includes bibliographical references and index.
ISBN 978-3-8055-9336-6 (hard cover : alk. paper) -- ISBN 978-3-8055-9337-3 (e-ISBN)
I. Sultan, Charles. II. Series: Endocrine development ; v. 22. 1421-7082
[DNLM: 1. Genital Diseases, Female. 2. Adolescent. 3. Child. 4. Evidence-Based Medicine. 5. Gonadal Disorders. 6. Gynecology--methods. 7. Pregnancy in Adolescence. 8. Sexual Behavior. W1 EN3635 v.22 2012 / WS 360]

618.100835--dc23

2012007737

Bibliographic Indices. This publication is listed in bibliographic services, including Current Contents®.

Disclaimer. The statements, opinions and data contained in this publication are solely those of the individual authors and contributors and not of the publisher and the editor(s). The appearance of advertisements in the book is not a warranty, endorsement, or approval of the products or services advertised or of their effectiveness, quality or safety. The publisher and the editor(s) disclaim responsibility for any injury to persons or property resulting from any ideas, methods, instructions or products referred to in the content or advertisements.

Drug Dosage. The authors and the publisher have exerted every effort to ensure that drug selection and dosage set forth in this text are in accord with current recommendations and practice at the time of publication. However, in view of ongoing research, changes in government regulations, and the constant flow of information relating to drug therapy and drug reactions, the reader is urged to check the package insert for each drug for any change in indications and dosage and for added warnings and precautions. This is particularly important when the recommended agent is a new and/or infrequently employed drug.

www.karger.com
Printed in Germany on acid-free and non-aging paper (ISO 9706) by Kraft Druck GmbH, Ettlingen
ISSN 1421–7082
e-ISSN 1662–2979
ISBN 978–3–8055–9336–6
e-ISBN 978–3–8055–9337–3

Contents

The Adolescent Girl

Foreword

Pediatric and adolescent gynecology is now a well-recognized field in medicine and surgery. It is also a very unique approach to care of the female child from birth until adulthood, and it is not simply by chance that pediatric endocrinology has played a central role in its development. It happened to be at the crossroads of most of the specific problems of developmental and reproductive issues.

The first edition has been so successful, under the leadership of Professor Charles Sultan, that a second edition is now being presented. It is the witness of a specific demand to again fill the gap in pre-adult gynecology, a practice involving a large number of topics examining the most recent technology, relevant scientific basis as well as sensitive public health issues.

This second edition has been a challenge for both editor and authors alike. Medical progress in this area has grown tremendously in recent years. Solid traditional practice, more often called evidence-based medicine, is always needed. However, new topics are also presented in a critical way in this unique book. It is well updated on the technological side: use of ultrasound, molecular genetics as performed in most laboratories, and surgery in sex disorders. New problems in relation to reproductive medicine in cancer survivors, patients with genital malformations, or those with expected sterility are also presented.

Adolescent girls are more than ever before being exposed to new problems and risks in their sexual life. Some of these problems are related to transmissible diseases, others are critical social problems related to reproduction and contraception. A comprehensive and prudent approach is needed and is presented here in this edition. The teenage girl deserves the new chapters that have been devoted to her in this book. Pediatricians should be aware of the complexity and importance of female adolescent health care.

I have no doubt that this, the second edition, will be well received and soon be on the desks of many pediatricians, general practitioners and public health specialists. Its content sets a sound basis for clinical practice.

A needed acquisition in girls' and women's health, to which I wish great success.

Raphaël Rappaport, Paris

Preface

The field of pediatric and adolescent gynecology (PAG) has always been of particular interest to physicians. Long at the interface of Pediatrics, Gynecology, Endocrinology, Surgery and Psychiatry, PAG has expanded to now include such fields as Genetics, Legal Medicine, Sport Medicine, Public Health and Sociology.

In response to the growing impact of PAG, a European Post-Graduate Diploma is now being prepared that will equip physicians with the ability to address these many aspects in a comprehensive manner.

I hope this second edition, written by specialists from all over the world and covering a broad range of topics, will be as successful as the first edition.

In my 30 years of clinical practice, I have seen the various disorders of young girls either being minimized and neglected or overdramatized and overtreated.

I am convinced that this book will be an indispensable tool for all physicians caring for the gynecological health of children and adolescents.

Charles Sultan, Montpellier

Sultan C (ed): Pediatric and Adolescent Gynecology. Evidence-Based Clinical Practice. 2nd, revised and extended edition. Endocr Dev. Basel, Karger, 2012, vol 22, pp 1–10

Gynecologic Clinical Examination of the Child and Adolescent

Alaa Cheikhelard[b,c] · Zeina Chaktoura[c,d] · Elisabeth Thibaud[a,c]

[a]Unité de Endocrinologie et Gynécologie Pédatrique, [b]Service de Chirurgie Pédiatrique et [c]Centre de Référence des Pathologies Gynecologiques Rares, Hôpital Necker-Enfants Malades, et [d]Service d'Endocrinologie et Médecine de la Reproduction, Hôpital Pitié-Salpétrière, Paris, France

Abstract

Pediatric gynecological examination is very simple, but usually unrecognized by physicians without a specific experience in pediatric gynecology. It is always necessary and most of the time sufficient in children and adolescents consulting for gynecological complaints, endocrine problems, or sexual abuse. However, accurate evidence-based data on its normality is poor in the literature, because of bias represented by the inclusion of abused patients in these studies. Our aim was to describe the preparation to a full gynecological examination, the adequate positions, and the sequence and technique required for a well-accepted and nontraumatic clinical examination. Normal findings are described depending on the age of the patient (child, newborn, adolescent), and are based on evidence from the literature. Indications for vaginoscopy and bacterial sampling are discussed according to the age of the patient. The most important factors in the achievement of a full gynecological examination and a trusting patient-physician relationship are a good anatomical and physiological knowledge of the genital system in children, and the learning of nonaggressive examination technical skills associated with good communication skills. Clinical examination is always necessary and most of the time is sufficient together with the medical history to diagnose and treat the child's gynecological problems. Evidence-based data on normal genital findings is poor in the literature, because many studies include abused children or present bias in the methods of recruitment and assessment of normal girls [1].

Evidence Leading to Gynecological Examination in Children and Adolescents

Reasons for undertaking a gynecological examination include:

- Gynecological complaints: Vaginal discharge or bleeding, pruritus, vulvar or abdominal pain, indicating that there may be underlying infection, tumor or malformation.
- Endocrine reasons: Abnormal course of puberty, abnormal signs of virilization, abnormal menstrual cycle, evaluation of abnormal genitalia in the context of a disorder of sexual development.

- Suspected or confirmed sexual abuse: The physician may be asked to look for and describe objective evidence of abuse.

Preparation for the Examination

A gynecological examination of the child is very simple and painless if performed properly, but is not trivial and needs the child's confidence. The gynecologist must be very familiar with the anatomy and physiology of genitalia before and during puberty. The child must be reassured to be calm and cooperative, which is usually possible with a good preparation of the examination and attention focused on both her and her mother [2–4]. When old enough to answer, the child should be asked to explain in her own words the reason of the visit. If, as in most cases, the mother or the accompanying adult begins to speak in the child's place, the physician must make sure the child listens, understands and nods to what is being said regarding her problem. The prerequisite for a well-accepted, nontraumatic and even therapeutic gynecological examination is the respect shown to the child by choosing her as the privileged and active interlocutor. During the examination, the mother is usually asked to stay when the child is very young. Between the ages of 10 and 13 the child's wish should be respected. Beyond 13 years of age, the teenager is usually seen firstly with her mother, then alone, and her approach should in the first place be nonjudgmental and supportive to respect her autonomy and modesty. This private consultation (sometimes with a nurse attending) is also essential to detect hidden information that is important for medical evaluation, and that the adolescent will be reluctant to provide in front of her parents [5].

Clinical Examination

Complete pediatric assessment must precede the gynecologic examination itself. Care should be given to assess height and weight, puberty course using Tanner stages [6], pilosity examination, and palpation of the breasts and the abdomen.

Gynecological Examination of a Prepubertal Child

A full gynecologic examination of the child mainly includes inspection of external genitalia and in some cases rectal examination. Performing vaginoscopy and obtaining samples are limited to certain cases [2].

The child must be comfortable. Many positions were described, but the best one is the 'frog-leg' position: the child is in a supine position, her legs flexed, with her knees apart and her feet touching (fig. 1). The physician is sitting facing the child, a lamp

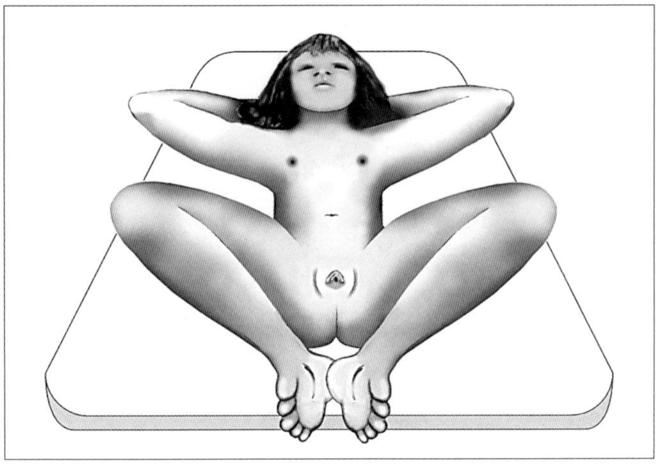

Fig. 1. Child position for gynecological examination.

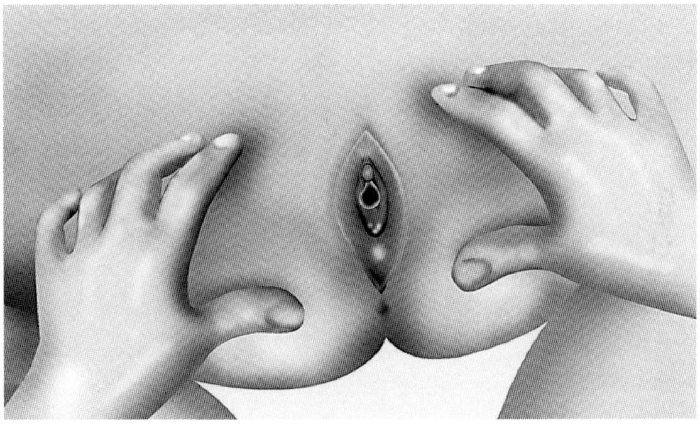

Fig. 2. Vulva examination: separation of labia majora by pulling the inferior part downward and laterally.

providing ample light from behind his/her shoulder. Children under 2 years of age may sometimes be frightened by the table and may instead be examined in the same position on the mother's lap.

The inguinal areas and labia majora are first inspected. Existence of pubic hair is assessed. The labia are then gently separated either by pulling their inferior part downward and laterally (fig. 2) or by pulling them anteriorly (fig. 3). The clinician must absolutely avoid a solely lateral maneuver, which puts a painful strain on the posterior fourchette and may split it, thus provoking a defensive reaction from the child hindering further examination. The size of the clitoris is measured by inspecting and pulling up the clitoral hood. This will help differentiate a true clitoromegaly from a hood skin redundancy. In the prepubertal child, a normal clitoris glans is on average 5 mm in length and 3 mm in transverse diameter and shows little variation after puberty [7] (fig. 4). The labia minora are usually thin and sometimes short. They edge the vulva vestibulum at the bottom of which the urethra and vagina open. On

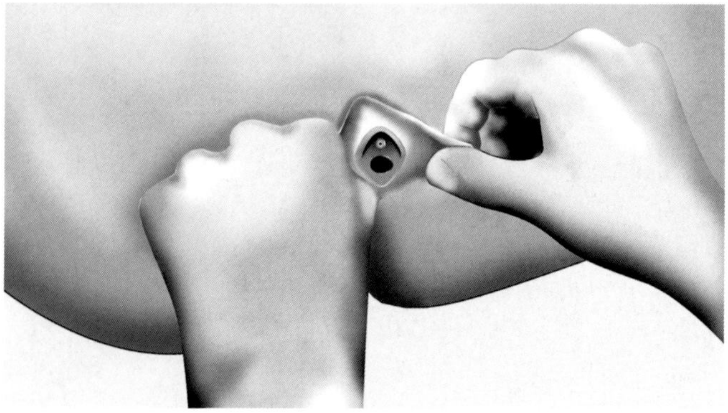

Fig. 3. Vulva examination: separation of labia majora by pulling them anteriorly.

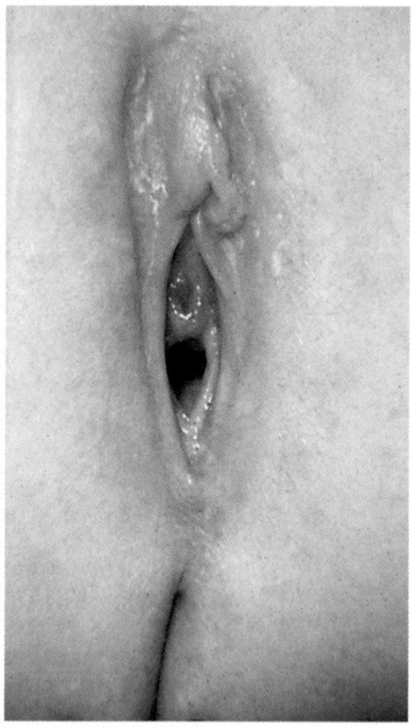

Fig. 4. Prepubertal vulva.

each side of the urethra a Skene's duct can be seen. Without estrogenization the vulvar mucosa appears thin and red and the perihymeneal tissue may look erythematous [2]. The white thick substance noted in the anterior labia folds is called smegma, not to be mistaken for leucorrhea.

The vaginal orifice is edged by the hymen, which varies in size and shape. The hymen will often gape open if the child is asked to take a deep breath or cough, and will allow visualization of the distal vagina. If not, the best maneuver consists of gently pulling the labia anteriorly and laterally. The most often observed types of hymens are as follows [8] (fig. 5):

- The annular hymen with a hymeneal edge varying in size, and a regular annular orifice.

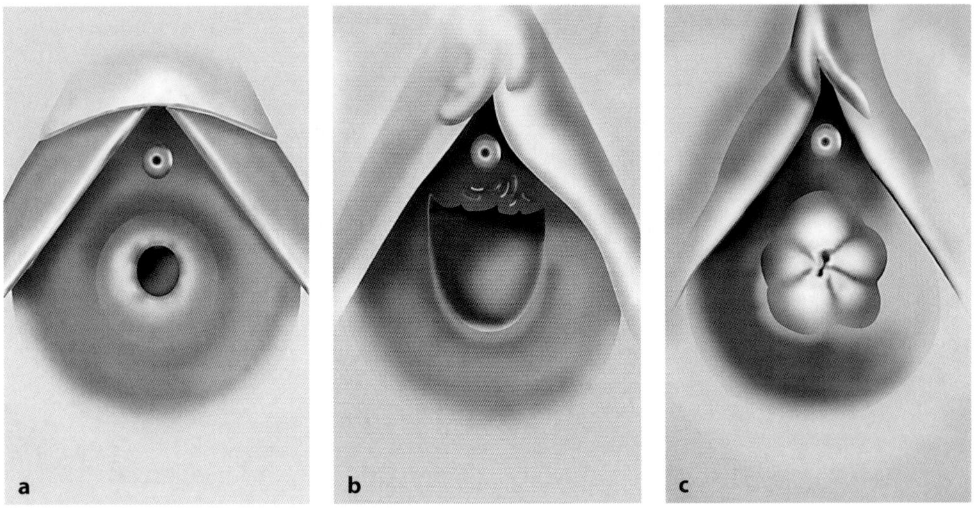

Fig. 5. Configuration of hymen in prepubertal girls. **a** Annular hymen. **b** Crescendic hymen. **c** Redundant hymen. According to Pokorny and Kozinetz [8].

- The crescentic hymen which posterior rim looks like a crescent, and which ends are attached on the lateral vaginal wall, without any hymeneal suburethral tissue.
- The redundant hymen has large and fimbriated hymeneal edges.

The first two types of hymens are the most common from the age of 3 years to the beginning of puberty, while the third is most commonly found below the age of 3 years. Superficial notches are normal findings, but not a complete transection in the inferior rim [1].

On average, the vaginal orifice measures 4–5 mm in girls until the age of 5 and remains under 10 mm until the beginning of puberty. These figures are given as an indication, as the diameter of the vaginal orifice varies a lot with the position of the child, the degree of perineal relaxation, shape of the hymen and the level of estrogenization [9, 10]. It is important to note that the hymen opening size is not a good indicator for trauma, and unhelpful in the diagnosis of abuse, as normal hymens sometimes allow a wide visualization of the vagina, and also because in case of trauma, hymen healing is rapid and sometimes complete without scarring [1].

A narrow and thin hymen does not completely cover the vaginal orifice enabling visualization of the distal half or two-thirds of the vagina without resorting to endoscopy. The most appropriate maneuver is the one described above, which consists of gently pulling the labia majora anteriorly and laterally: the hymen opens and the vaginal axis is corrected. This maneuver is painless and usually easily accepted by the child. It may sometimes be difficult to visualize the free edge of the hymen and the vagina with certain types of hymens, e.g. redundant hymens, microperforate hymens with a suburethral orifice, or septated hymens. The physician can then use a small

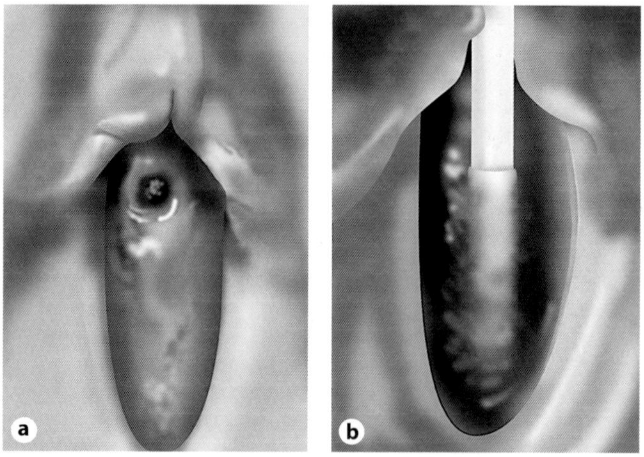

Fig. 6. a Microperforate hymen. **b** Unfold opening with a small catheter.

supple urethral catheter (No. 4–6) to unfold the hymeneal edge and assess hymeneal integrity as the existence of an opening (fig. 6).

The genupectoral position allows good visualization of the vagina, sometimes up to the cervix, and can be useful in case of vulvovaginitis or if a foreign body is present [11]. However, in our personal experience, we do favor the frog-leg position.

Rectal examination is the following and last but not systematic step. It is performed with the little finger until the age of 6 years. It may be used to determine the existence and volume of the cervix that can be palpated on a small midline structure. A normal cervix measures 5 mm in transverse diameter on the average. The ovaries are too small to be felt, thus, any pelvic mass must evoke a cyst or a tumor. The vagina can also be palpated through this rectal exam, allowing to note any foreign body (or tumor) or any vaginal discharge.

Normal vaginal length in prepubertal girls is 3–6 cm at birth, 4–7 cm at age 4 years, and 5.5–8 cm at age 10 years [12]. The vaginal mucosa appears red, thin and folded. It is very sensitive, and petechial lesions may be caused if a vaginoscope is used. The cervix is small, with a centered opening and flush with the vaginal vault, thus making it difficult to visualize.

When the rest of the perineum and rectum are inspected, the clinical examination is complete.

Gynecologic Examination of a Newborn

The examination is conducted as described above. The genitalia are submitted to maternal estrogen effects. Estrogenization signs start to decrease from the 2nd week of life and usually disappear within 6–8 weeks. However, they can persist physiologically until the age of 2 years [10]. The vulva is edematous, and the labia minora are thick and protruding, sometimes beyond the labia majora. The mucosa is pink and covered with physiologic leukorrhea. The clitoral hood may also be relatively thick and the size of the clitoris must be assessed by palpation, after pulling up the clitoral hood. The hymen is frequently thick, pouting out of the introits, and fimbriated. The vaginal orifice is sometimes difficult to visualize, and the physician should then use a small urethral catheter to assert the existence of an opening. The vagina measures between 3 and 6 cm in length [12]. The vaginal mucosa is thick, covered with pH-acid white physiologic secretions including *Lactobacilli*. Over the first 10 days of life (seldom later), there may be neonatal vaginal bleeding.

Gynecologic Clinical Examination of the Adolescent

The gynecologic examination of an adolescent has a three aims:
- Clinical assessment.
- Diagnosis and therapy.
- Establishment of an interpersonal confident relationship as the basis for support to those teenage girls who may be facing deeply emotional problems such as puberty, sexuality and fertility. For this purpose, the physician may remind the patient that he/she is bound to medical secret [13].

A gynecological examination is never a routine examination, despite other author's opinion [4, 5]. The clinician should be prepared to spend time listening to the adolescent's concerns and gathering information on the personal and family background. The consultation should be simple and interactive when the teenager is healthy, well-informed, and coming for birth control advice or simple menstrual dysfunctions. On the contrary, when the adolescent shows serious chronic pathology, DSD, or has been sexually abused, the consultation will be difficult, critical and fraught with consequences, all the more when these situations are not spoken of, which is often the case.

In any case, the examination principles remain identical:
- It must be preceded by a full medical assessment.
- It must be conducted only after the patient has been given a thorough explanation of the examination as well as of its objectives, and after obtaining her consent.
- Only the least-invasive examination that will be sufficient to assess the problem should be performed.
- The examinations should not be omitted solely because of the age of the patient. However, in some cases, the examination may be postponed to the next appointment if the patient is not comfortable enough to accept it.
- The physician must recognize cultural issues and respect them.

For an adolescent who is not sexually active, the examination is identical to that of a prepubertal child. Vaginoscopy and pelvic examination should not be performed systematically. The vulva is estrogenized and there are physiologic secretions. The vulva axis has become horizontal, the labia minora have developed and may sometimes have become browner, and the labia majora usually cover the vulva. As in adults, the vagina measures on average 9.6 cm in length (range 6.5–12.5) [14]. Upon rectal examination the uterus is often laterally oriented to the left. One-finger pelvic exam is possible if the teenager is relaxed and her hymen is yielding. A small 'virgin' speculum may be used if necessary.

For a sexually active patient, pelvic examination and vaginoscopy with a speculum (with samples if necessary) are also required to look for potential genital infections.

Breast examination is part of the gynecological examination. At the beginning of its development the breast is tender, and the breast bud may be palpated before being seen. It appears as a small, hard mound beneath an enlarged areola. Physiologic breast development is sometimes unequal and asymmetric in its early stage, as there may be a 3- to 12-month difference between the beginnings of the development of each breast. The breast reaches its fully developed size in 2–4 years, but this period may vary. During the development phase, the breast is often firm upon palpation but rarely sensitive. Skin marks are frequent. They are red when they first appear and turn progressively white after a few months. They have no pathological meaning.

Once the examination is over, the physician should sit down with the adolescent to discuss the potential therapy with the help, if necessary, of an anatomical chart. As we said earlier, parents or caregivers should stay in the waiting room during the examination. Information will be subsequently related to them by the adolescent herself or by the physician with her agreement and in her presence. She may ask that some elements of the examination remain confidential and her wish must be respected. A trusty relationship between the physician and the adolescent is absolutely necessary in case of long-term treatment, especially concerning chronic diseases.

Indications for Vaginoscopy and Bacteriological Sampling

In postpubertal sexually active adolescents, indications for vaginoscopy and sampling are the same as in the adult population.

In prepubertal children and nonactive adolescents, vaginoscopy must be limited to the identification of a tumor or foreign body if the clinical examination and ultrasound were not able to provide the origin of a vaginal bleeding (in case of a tumor for example). This examination may need general anesthesia in some cases.

Visualization of a foreign body is not always easy, particularly when important leukorrhea coexist. In this case, vaginal inspection can be facilitated by flushing it with the help of a small urethral catheter and 10–20 ml of saline by manual irrigation.

Samples for bacteriological cultures are sometimes necessary, but limited to cases of true vaginal leukorrhea that are not caused by a foreign body. They are rarely necessary in the case of vulvitis (unless specific and infrequent infections are suspected such as yeast or streptococcus). They can be performed by only touching the fragile mucosa with a cotton swab without rubbing it to avoid any pain, the swab being impregnated with the leukorrhea by capillarization. Another technique has been described using a small angiocatheter (with the needle removed) introduced into a No. 12 red rubber catheter connected to a small syringe containing saline, slowly introduced through the vaginal opening. The vagina is delicately flushed and the liquid drawn up in the syringe to collect sufficient secretions [15]. In all cases, results need to be interpreted according to the clinical context since the vaginal mucosa and the vulva are the homes of normal flora.

Conclusion

Few evidence-based data exist on the normal findings in gynecological examination of children and adolescents. Many established findings that were considered suspicious of abuse are in fact normal. Most important is a deep anatomical and physiological knowledge of the genital system in the child, including the learning of nonaggressive examination technical skills. The training for communication skills is also important [13]. It involves a nonjudgmental approach to the child and adolescent gynecological patient, which will allow the development of a trusting relationship between a confident patient and a supportive physician.

References

1 Pillai M: Genital findings in prepubertal girls: what can be concluded from an examination? J Pediatr Adolesc Gynecol 2008;21:177–185.
2 Emans J: Office evaluation of the child and adolescent; in Emans J, Laufer MM, Goldstein DP (eds): Pediatric and Adolescent Gynecology. Philadelphia, Lippincott, 2005.
3 Cowell CA: The gynecologic examination of infants, children, and young adolescents. Pediatr Clin North Am 1981;28:247–266.
4 Rey-Stocker I : Principes généraux d'examen gynécologique; in Salomon-Bernard Y, Thibaud E, Rappaport R (eds): Traité médico-chirurgical de gynécologie de l'enfant et de l'adolescente. Paris, Doin, 1992.
5 Beyth Y, Hardoff D, Rom E, Ziv A: A simulated patient-based program for training gynecologists in communication with adolescent girls presenting with gynecological problems. J Pediatr Adolesc Gynecol 2009;22:79–84.
6 Marshall WA, Tanner JM: Variations in pattern of pubertal changes in girls. Arch Dis Child 1969;44: 291–303.
7 Sane K, Pescovitz OH: The clitoral index: a determination of clitoral size in normal girls and in girls with abnormal sexual development. J Pediatr 1992; 120:264–266.
8 Pokorny SF, Kozinetz CA: Configuration and another anatomic details of the prepubertal hymen. Adolesc Pediatr Gynecol 1988;1:97—103.
9 Gardner JJ: Descriptive study of genitalia variation in healthy, non abused premenarchal girls. J Pediatr 1992;120:251–257.
10 McCann J, Voris J, Simon M, Wells R: Comparison of genital examination techniques in prepubertal girls. Pediatrics 1990;85:182–187.
11 Emans SJ, Goldstein DP: The gynecologic examination of the prepubertal child with vulvovaginitis: use of the knee-chest position. Pediatrics 1980; 65:758–760.
12 Sarpel U, Palmer SK, Dolgin SE: The incidence of complete androgen insensitivity in girls with inguinal hernias and assessment of screening by vaginal length measurement. J Pediatr Surg 2005;40:133–136; discussion 136–137.

13 Ventegodt S: Every contact with the patient should be therapeutic. J Pediatr Adolesc Gynecol 2007;20: 323–324.
14 Lloyd J, Crouch NS, Minto CL, Liao LM, Creighton SM: Female genital appearance: 'normality' unfolds. BJOG 2005;112:643–646.
15 Pokorny SF, Stormer J: Atraumatic removal of secretions from the prepubertal vagina. Am J Obstet Gynecol 1987;156:581–582.

Elisabeth Thibaud
Hôpital Necker-Enfants Malades
149, rue de Sèvres
FR–75743 Paris Cédex (France)
Tel. +33 1 44 49 48 01, Fax +33 1 44 49 48 00, E-Mail elisabeth.thibaud@nck.aphp.fr

Sultan C (ed): Pediatric and Adolescent Gynecology. Evidence-Based Clinical Practice. 2nd, revised and extended edition. Endocr Dev. Basel, Karger, 2012, vol 22, pp 11–23

Normal Female Puberty in a Developmental Perspective

Jean-Pierre Bourguignon[a] · Anders Juul[b]

[a]Department of Pediatrics and GIGA Neurosciences, CHU de Liège, University of Liège, Liège, Belgium,
[b]Department of Growth and Reproduction, Rigshospitalet, University of Copenhagen, Copenhagen, Denmark

Abstract

Puberty is unique in the sense that its onset shows an extraordinary individual variability of about 5 years, the basis of which being still elusive despite research efforts to understand the reason why. Continuing changes in environmental influences and interaction with genetic determinants are suggested by the still evolving pattern of the pubertal process both clinically and mechanistically. For instance, secular trends towards earlier breast development have been observed during the two past decades in some countries, resulting in possible skewing of the age distribution of that pubertal sign with less obvious changes in menarcheal age. Conceptually, puberty and subsequent reproduction appear now to be influenced by conditions not only at the time when they occur, but also during fetal and perinatal life. In addition, these influences can be apparently opposing since early maturation follows fetal malnourishment and postnatal overfeeding. In this review, the semiology and pathophysiology of puberty are discussed in a lifelong developmental perspective.

Puberty is a transition period between childhood and adulthood that is characterized by the development of sex characteristics and attainment of reproductive capacity. The pioneering work of Tanner [1] provided detailed clinical description of the pubertal process. Since then, several contributions unraveled the critical role of fetal life events in determining some aspects of the pubertal process beyond sex differentiation. For instance, fetal GnRH neurons and olfactory neurons were shown to originate in the olfactory placode of the rostral brain before they migrate to the hypothalamic area [2]. These observations provided a key to the pathogenesis of Kallmann syndrome resulting from impairment of an X-linked gene (KAL) involved in the control of migration of those neurons and accounting for associated anosmia-hyposmia and central hypogonadism [3]. Also, the first activation of the hypothalamic-pituitary-gonadal system was shown to occur in fetal life around mid-gestation. It is followed by a second activation early postnatally and a third one at puberty [4]. Recently, further emphasis on fetal life came from the interpretation of variations in pubertal timing as an adaptive mechanism determined by fetal life conditions [5]. This concept integrated puberty into the 'developmental origin of health and disease' consistent with the so-called Barker hypothesis [6]. Here, our option is to discuss normal female pubertal development in the light of fetal determinants, considering that puberty and its timing reflect interactions between genetic and environmental factors early in life.

Clinical Aspects

Parameters of Puberty

Age at first menstrual bleeding (menarche) is the most commonly used marker of puberty in population based studies, as information on this dichotomized variable (yes/no) can be obtained from questionnaires without pubertal evaluation. It is a rather late pubertal marker occurring 2–2.5 years after breast budding in the average girl. However, the duration from stage B2 to menarche may be longer in early maturing girls, and shorter in late maturing girls. Typically, the first menstrual bleedings are anovulatory, and highly irregular menstrual bleeding patterns are to be expected in the years following menarche. The time from menarche to regular cycling is approximately 3 years, but large interpersonal variability exists [7].

The onset of the pubertal growth spurt (OGS) can be used as an indirect marker of start of puberty, and age at peak height velocity (PHV) as a late pubertal marker. The average girl will growth another 6–7 cm after menarche. Ideally, precise estimation of age at OGS and PHV requires 3-monthly growth measurements, but in many cases 6-monthly measurements may suffice [8]. Bone age can be determined by different manual (Greulich-Pyle, Tanner-Whitehouse) or computerized (BoneXpert) methods [9] from X-ray of the left hand and wrist and indicate the biological age depending on the degree of estrogenization of the epiphyses. Adult height predictions can be derived from actual height and bone age according to different algorithms.

Physiological Variations in Age at Pubertal Development around the World

Traditionally, mean ages at B2 and menarche in European and American populations have been reported to be approximately 11 and 13 years, respectively (fig. 1). These ages at sexual maturation depend on socioeconomic status. In the 19th century, mean age at menarche was around 17 years in European countries, but has declined to approximately 13 years until the 1960s presumably due to improved living conditions and hygiene. Hereafter, age at menarche has stabilized around 13 years for the last 4–5 decades.

Girls from developing countries with poor living standards have later mean age at menarche as compared to girls from well-off countries. This is illustrated by the high mean menarcheal ages of 15.4 and 16.0 years which have been reported from an underprivileged part of India and from Senegal, respectively [for review, see 10].

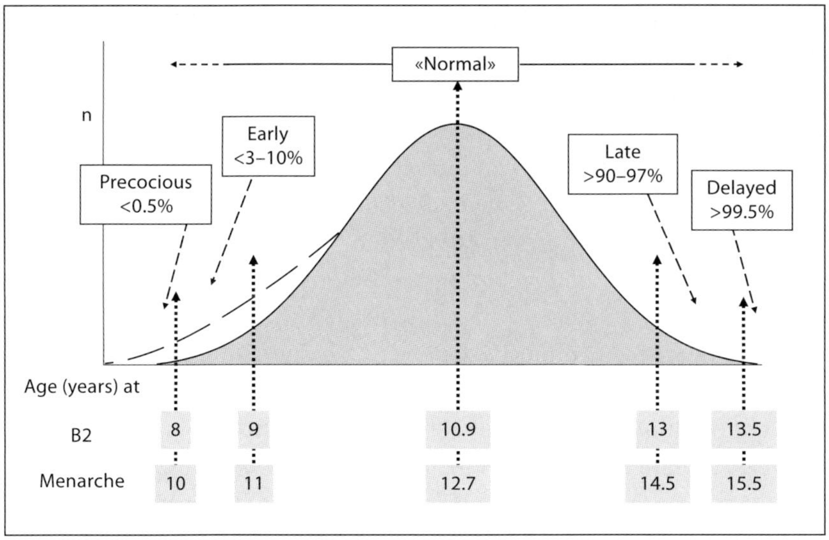

Fig. 1. Distribution of age at onset of breast development (B2) and menarcheal age indicating limits for abnormal timing of puberty and borderline normal conditions as well as possible skewing towards early ages.

Secular Changes in Pubertal Timing

During the past 15–20 years, studies from the US (Pediatric Research in Office Settings, PROS and National Health and Nutrition Examination Survey III, NHANES III) and Europe reported earlier breast development in girls [8, 11–13], as compared to historical data. The NHANES III and the PROS studies both reported a lower average age at entering Tanner breast stage 2 (B2) and Tanner pubic hair stage 2 (PH2) than earlier investigations. Both studies clearly suggested an earlier age at puberty onset in American girls in the 1980–1990s compared to the 1930s and 1940s. However, age at menarche occurred at the same time or slightly earlier compared to the previous studies. Thus, the time span from breast development to menarche seemed to have increased. The findings could reflect that the observed breast development and appearance of pubic hair at an earlier age may be induced by exogenous or lifestyle factors, which may influence the typical sequence of pubertal events. In fact, the earlier thelarche seen among contemporary Danish girls did not seem to be associated with activation of the pituitary-gonadal axis. The mean age at B2 was 9.88 years in Denmark [8] and even lower (9.2 years) in another recent study from China [14]. However, another recent European study from Belgium found only marginally lower age at B2 (10.7 years) but the age distribution was skewed so that 3% of the girls have started breast by 7.7 years [15]. Differences in statistical approaches (parametric versus non-parametric models) may account for some of the differences in the more recent studies. Due to the uneven changes in age at B2 and menarche seen industrialized countries, it is possible that the mean age at sexual maturation may no longer follow a normal Gaussian distribution, and that the distribution may be skewed to the left towards sexual precocity (fig. 1).

Particular Conditions (International Adoption, SGA)
Children adopted from foreign countries mature earlier than in their country of origin, and also earlier than their peers in their new foster country. This has been demonstrated in several independent reports from Sweden, Denmark, The Netherlands, France and the USA [10]. The risk of developing precocious puberty was significantly increased 10–20 times in adopted girls compared with girls with Danish background. The risk of developing precocious puberty depended on the country of origin and older age at adoption significantly increased the risk of precocious puberty in adoptees independent of region of origin [16]. Theoretically, several etiological factors may be involved in this phenomenon. An insufficient intrauterine environment resulting in a low birth weight for gestational age could play a role, as being born SGA has been associated with earlier maturation in some studies of nonadopted children [17]. Postnatal catch-up growth following adoption per se could also induce premature sexual maturation. However, adopted children with no evidence of pre- or postnatal growth restriction also seem to experience early puberty making this a less likely theory. It has also been hypothesized that relief from stressful conditions or from exposure to endocrine disrupting chemicals in the country of origin following adoption to another country may induce premature activation of the pituitary-gonadal axis [10]. Altogether, some factors, as yet to be determined, related to migration and change of environment must be involved in this phenomenon.

Mechanistic Aspects

Hypothalamic-Pituitary-Ovarian System
Some of the components of the hypothalamic-pituitary-ovarian system and their interactions at the time of puberty are schematically represented in figure 2. The central role of the hypothalamus in the onset of puberty has been highlighted by Knobil and coworkers who administered synthetic GnRH intermittently to monkeys with lesioned hypothalamus. Based on changes in gonadotropin secretion, they introduced the concept of GnRH pulse generator and showed its increased frequency and amplitude of activity at onset of puberty [18, 19]. Such a concept was further substantiated using ultrasensitive gonadotropin assays in clinical conditions.

In essence, the onset of puberty could result from either disappearance of inhibitory inputs or occurrence of stimulatory inputs or both. During the past decades, key hypothalamic mediators involved in trans-synaptic regulation of GnRH neurons were identified. Among the numerous hypothalamic modulators shown to possibly account for the developmental inhibition in GnRH secretion, GABA appeared to be a key component of the prepubertal inhibition in primates [20]. Data obtained in the rat

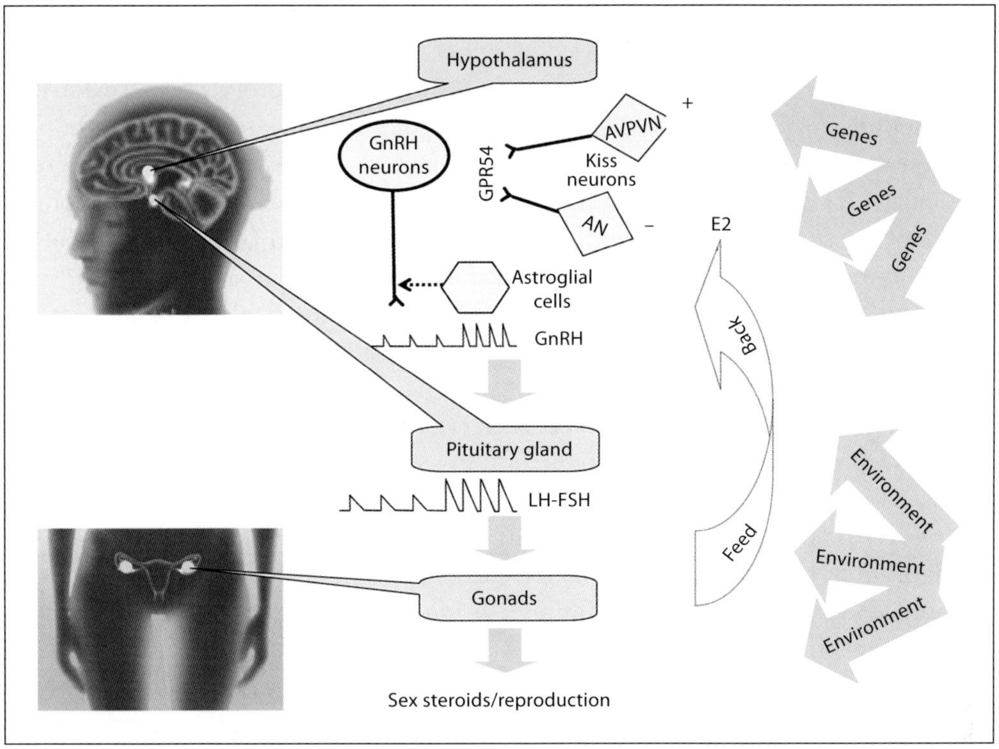

Fig. 2. Schematic representation of the hypothalamic-pituitary-ovarian system with the developmental changes in GnRH and LH secretion; some changes can be seen among the hypothalamic regulators as well as feedback and environmental factors.

and evidence from a patient with nonketotic hyperglycinemia [21] indicated the role of GABA in the prepubertal restraint in rodents and humans as well. Several inhibitory neuromodulators such as beta-endorphin and melatonin were shown to display reduced activity at the time of sexual maturation [22]. Their causal involvement in puberty was however debated since they were dependent on sex steroids for their effects and their action was more obvious during than before puberty. Therefore, their role in mediating the prepubertal restraint remained uncertain. Among the modulators with dual effects on GnRH/LH secretion, Neuropeptide Y was shown to have either stimulatory or inhibitory effects, the latter being developmentally regulated in the monkey [23]. As opposed to GABA, glutamate is a central excitatory component of puberty through the N-methyl-D-aspartate (NMDA) subtype of receptors in primates and rodents with some evidence of involvement in humans [21]. Recently, the permissive role of a G-protein coupled receptor (GPR54) was demonstrated both in rodents and humans [24, 25]. Mutations or deletions in the gene encoding GPR54/Kiss1R, the specific receptor binding kisspeptin, were found in patients with hypogonadotropic hypogonadism. Conversely, an activating GPR54 mutation was reported in a girl with precocious puberty [26]. The expression of kisspeptin in the rodent and primate hypothalamus increased at puberty while estradiol positive feedback appeared to be a prequisite to kisspeptin expression in the anteroventral periventricular area of the hypothalamus [27]. Astroglial regulation appeared to play an important role at puberty through the production of factors such as PGE_2, growth factors, particularly TGFα, and adhesion molecules [28]. Among their effects, they control plasticity, i.e. structural aspects influencing contacts between GnRH neurons, other regulatory neurons, astroglial cells and blood capillaries.

Among the above mechanisms, few were studied during fetal life. In the fetal rat hypothalamus, we found that increase in activity of glutaminase, an enzyme critical for glutamate biosynthesis, contributed to perinatal occurrence of pulsatile GnRH secretion [29]. Sex steroid negative feedback is also an important component of maturation through a developmental reduction in sensitivity that was conceptualized as the gonadostat [4]. The effects of sex steroids are complex due to several dual aspects: central versus peripheral, estrogenic versus androgenic or secondarily estrogenic after aromatization, negative versus positive feedback, and immediate versus differed and possibly linked with early programming. During fetal life, sex steroids are crucial for sexual differentiation of the hypothalamus since exposure to aromatizable androgens or estrogens disrupted the central drive of the preovulatory LH surge in many species [30]. Data obtained in the lamb exposed to testosterone in utero suggested that pubertal timing was programmed in utero since virilization of fetal lambs was associated with a shift from the female to the male pattern of pubertal timing together with disturbed cyclicity [31, 32].

The Adrenals

In girls, androgenic steroids of adrenal origin, chiefly dehydroepiandrosterone (DHEA), provide a significant contribution to the development of pubic hair (pubarche). The secretion of adrenal androgens increases around puberty following a maturational process in the adrenals (adrenarche) which occurs independently of gonadarche i.e. pituitary-gonadal maturation, as shown in different conditions [4]. In physiological conditions, adrenarche does not influence the onset of puberty. In pathological conditions such as congenital adrenal hyperplasia, however, the excess of sex steroids can secondarily lead to sexual precocity, such as in other forms of peripheral precocious puberty. It is possible that central puberty becomes manifest in those conditions after treatment of the primary condition has reduced the level of sex steroids and, consequently, their central negative feedback effect [10].

Genetic Factors

Based on twin and family studies, the variance in pubertal timing appeared to be predominantly (50–80%) explained by genetic factors [33]. However, the likely polygenic control of physiological variations in pubertal timing remains not elucidated. Polymorphism of genes involved in sex steroid metabolism could play some role

[34]. Besides the KAL gene and kisspeptin-GPR 54 genes already mentioned, other genes were shown to be implicated in hypogonadotrophic hypogonadism: FGFR1, leptin and leptin receptor, GnRH receptor. Genetic alterations of transcription factors (HESX1, PROP1, LHX3) accounted for hypogonadism associated with other pituitary deficiencies. The upstream genomic control of puberty in rodents and primates also involves transcription factors such as Oct-2 that activates transforming growth factor alpha, a glial factor involved that we discussed already [35]. More recently, a new gene 'Enhanced at puberty-1' (EAP-1) was identified that encoded a transcription factor expressed in neurons involved in the hypothalamic control of reproduction [36]. In a recent GWAS study, a correlation between pubertal timing and genetic variation in the gene LIN28B, a potent and specific regulator of microRNA processing, was observed [37]. It appears, however, that such a gene would only account for a few percent of the variability in pubertal timing per major allele [32]. Also, recent studies indicate that epigenetic mechanisms could take place early in life in the hypothalamus as shown for sexual differentiation [38].

Environmental Factors

Nutrition

Since the 'critical fat mass' hypothesis proposed by Frisch and Revelle four decades ago, the role of postnatal nutrition in the regulation of pubertal development has been confirmed, particularly in the female. However, the influence of energy balance was not univoqual probably due to the many other interfering factors and differences between physiological variations and abnormally insufficient or excessive adiposity [10]. Further insight into the role of nutrition came after the discovery of leptin, a crucial link between the status of peripheral energy stores and the homeostasis of energy balance and reproduction. We provided direct evidence that leptin and ghrelin which are, respectively, anorectic and orexigenic, also had opposing effects on pulsatile GnRH secretion [39]. As already mentioned, the permissive role of leptin was confirmed by the hypogonadism in leptin deficiency and its reversal after leptin treatment.

As shown in figure 3, nutritional conditions during both fetal life, as reflected in birth weight for gestational age, and early postnatal life were shown to be possible determinants of different physiological and disordered events throughout life [5, 6]. The severity of leanness at birth was shown to be correlated with the likelihood of subsequent disorders including premature adrenarche and pubarche, ovarian hyperandrogenism and insulin resistance [17]. While the correlation between birthweight and menarcheal age was controversial [10], the velocity in weight increase during first year of life was found to predict age at menarche [40]. We recently reviewed some of the many neuroendocrine connections between homeostasis of reproduction and homeostasis of energy balance, during both prenatal/neonatal and postnatal life [41]. Fetal malnourishment was shown to possibly result in low birth weight and early

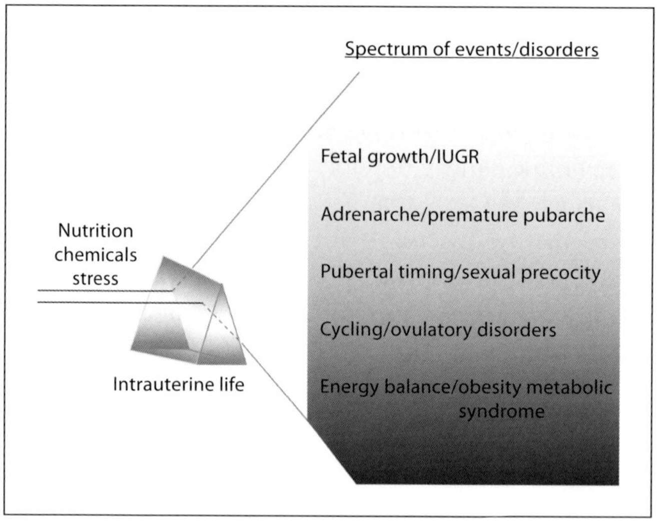

Fig. 3. Schematic representation of pubertal issues integrated into the 'developmental origin of health and disease'. Intrauterine life works like a prism translating early conditions including nutrition quantitatively and qualitatively, exposure to chemicals, and stress into a spectrum of influenced or disordered events throughout postnatal life.

puberty in the female rat [42]. Moreover, the consequences of fetal malnourishment on adult adiposity excess and metabolic syndrome could be prevented by neonatal or early postnatal leptin treatment indicating the critical role of this peripheral peptide in fetal/neonatal programming [43].

Physical Activity and Stress

While chronic or severe diseases and physical or mental critical illnesses are known to impair pituitary-gonadal function, the mechanisms are complex with intricated nutritional and stress factors. Exemplifying conditions are adolescent dancers or gymnasts involved together in strenuous activity and strict control of weight increase [10]. In the female monkey, amenorrhea in conditions of strenuous physical activity seemed to be more dependent on energy availability than stress since food supplementation resulted in restoration of menarche [44]. In contrast, among anorexia nervosa patients who recovered weight during one year of follow up, only 57% resumed regular menstrual cycles indicating the role of other factors besides energy availability [45].

Other Environmental Clues

As discussed above, the evidence of early puberty in children migrating for international adoption [10] and the possible involvement of endocrine disrupters in such a condition were suggested by the presence of a stable derivative of the estrogenic pesticide DDT in the serum of those children [46]. Furthermore, the stimulatory effects of DDT on GnRH secretion in vitro and in vivo were confirmed in a rodent model [reviewed in 41]. The endocrine disrupter effects on the reproductive system were known since vaginal adenocarcinoma were shown to occur in the female offspring of women treated with DES during pregnancy [47]. Fetal malnourishment as well as fetal exposure to endocrine disrupters such as DES and BPA were shown to possibly result in low birth weight, early puberty, ovulatory disorders, obesity in adulthood and metabolic syndrome [reviewed in 41]. The hypothesis was raised recently that EDC effects on adipose tissue and energy balance could be a toxicological factor in the obesity epidemic [48]. Thus, while some authors suggested that the obesity epidemic could account for the changes in pubertal timing in some countries, it can be hypothesized that endocrine disrupters are a common pathogenetic link of secular changes in adiposity and pubertal timing [41]. Thus, the global concept is that several factors including nutrition, stress and endocrine disrupters interplaying during fetal and early postnatal life could determine several disorders throughout life (fig. 3). It is likely that all those factors play some role in a condition such as internationally adopted children [49].

Neurodevelopmental Changes

Recent magnetic resonance imaging longitudinal studies of the Central Nervous System have highlighted important structural remodeling between childhood and adulthood with changing balance between limbic/subcortical and frontal lobe functions [50]. Though these observations cannot be correlated so far with neuroendocrine and behavioral changes in adolescence, they put emphasis on the need to further investigate the reciprocal interactions between suprahypothalamic nervous system and the neuroendocrine system in relation to pubertal and adolescent development.

Psychosocial Aspects of Physiological Variations in Pubertal Timing

On the one hand, psychosocial factors could influence pubertal timing in some conditions. For instance, among the subordinate female monkeys that are more vulnerable to social stressors than the dominant counterparts, puberty is delayed in individuals bearing a polymorphism (short variant) in the gene encoding serotonin reuptake transporter [51]. These findings nicely illustrate the interconnection between social factors and genetic susceptibility in influencing timing of maturation. In the male monkey, low social ranking is also associated with delayed puberty after early postnatal disruption of the pituitary gonadal axis [52].

On the other hand, pubertal timing could influence psychosocial factors. Besides the few patients with abnormally 'precocious' and 'delayed' puberty [see chapters by Sultan and Fenichel], attention has been paid during past decades to psychosocial maturation in the subjects starting puberty at the 'early' and 'late' edges of the physiological 4- to 5-year age window (fig. 1). Three theories have been proposed to account for the psychosocial implications of variations in pubertal timing [53]. According to the 'stage termination' or 'early timing' hypothesis, disturbed behavior and social maladjustment would be more likely to occur and possibly to persist when pubertal timing is early but not when it is late, physical immaturity being thus protective. Consistent with this theory, a longitudinal study in early Swedish girls reported increased behavioral problems that were partially persisting into adulthood [54]. Several studies further supported this hypothesis, including a recent report confirming increased psychopathology in young adult women who had experienced early but not late pubertal timing [55]. In a Swiss cohort of about 7,500 adolescents, Michaud et al. [56] reported increased dissatisfaction about self-image in early maturing girls and late boys. Early adolescents were more frequently involved in exploratory behaviors and sexually active. According to the 'deviance' or 'off-time' hypothesis, disturbed behavior and social maladjustment would be more likely to occur when pubertal timing lies out of the normal range, both in early and late conditions. In a recent study disordered eating behavior was correlated with pubertal timing self-assessed globally versus peers: 18 and 21% of the adolescent girls self rating her selves as early and late, respectively, showed elevated scores at the eating attitude test [57]. Graber et al. [55] found, however, that only boys were at increased risk of psychopathology after delayed puberty. A third 'accentuation' model was proposed by Caspi and Moffitt [53], pubertal events such as menarche being a stressful transition accentuating behavioural problems among girls who were predisposed to such problems earlier in childhood. In summary, it is recommended to evaluate perception of pubertal timing in the adolescent patients and integrate such information with the other relevant findings, e.g. networking with peers. It should be kept in mind that the relationship between pubertal timing and psychosocial issues in adolescence goes beyond simple reciprocal causality.

Conclusion

The variability in normal pubertal development is a still a moving reality that challenges the clinician through the continued requirement of updated local standards. It also challenges the scientist through the many new environmental factors influencing pubertal timing and their possible interaction with expression of genes that remain to be elucidated. Finally, emphasis has been put on the determination during fetal and early postnatal periods, of the pattern of sexual maturation and subsequent reproduction.

References

1 Tanner JM: Growth at Adolescence, ed 2. Oxford, Blackwell, 1962.

2 Schwanzel-Fukuda M, Pfaff DW: Origin of luteinizing hormone-releasing hormone neurons. Nature 1989;338:161–164.

3 Hardelin JP, Levilliers J, Young J, et al: Xp22.3 deletions in isolated familial Kallmann's syndrome. J Clin Endocrinol Metab 1993;76:827–831.

4 Grumbach MM, Styne DM: Puberty: ontogeny, neuroendocrinology, physiology, and disorders; in Wilson JD, Foster DW, Kronenberg HM, Larsen PR (eds): Williams' Textbook of Endocrinology, ed 9. Philadelphia, Saunders, 1998, pp 1509–1625.

5 Gluckman PD, Hanson MA, Beedle AS, Spencer HG: Predictive adaptive responses in perspective. Trends Endocrinol Metab 2008;19:109–110.

6 Barker DJ, Gluckman PD, Godfrey KM, et al: Fetal nutrition and cardiovascular disease in adult life. Lancet 1993;341:938–941.

7 Clavel-Chapelon F, E3N-EPIC Group: European Prospective Investigation into Cancer: evolution of age at menarche and at onset of regular cycling in a large cohort of French women. Hum Reprod 2002; 17:228–232.

8 Aksglaede L, Sorensen K, Petersen JH, Skakkebæk NE, Juul A: Recent decline in age at breast development: the COPENHAGEN Puberty Study. Pediatrics 2009;123:e932–e939.

9 Thodberg HH: Clinical review: An automated method for determination of bone age. J Clin Endocrinol Metab 2009;94:2239–2244.

10 Parent AS, Teilmann G, Juul A, et al: The timing of normal puberty and the age limits of sexual precocity: variations around the world, secular trends and changes after migration. Endocr Rev 2003;24:668–693

11 Herman-Giddens ME, Slora EJ, Wasserman RC, Bourdony CJ, Bhapkar MV, Koch GG, Hasemeier CM: Secondary sexual characteristics and menses in young girls seen in office practice: a study from the Pediatric Research in Office Settings network. Pediatrics 1997;99:505–512.

12 Sun SS, Schubert CM, Chumlea WC, Roche AF, Kulin HE, Lee PA, Himes JH, Ryan AS: National estimates of the timing of sexual maturation and racial differences among US children. Pediatrics 2002;110:911–919.

13 Wu T, Mendola P, Buck GM: Ethnic differences in the presence of secondary sex characteristics and menarche among US girls: the Third National Health and Nutrition Examination Survey, 1988–1994. Pediatrics 2002;110:752–757.

14 Ma HM, Du ML, Luo XP, Chen SK, Liu L, Chen RM, Zhu C, Xiong F, Li T, Wang W, Liu GL: Onset of breast and pubic hair development and menses in urban chinese girls. Pediatrics 2009;124: e269–e277.

15 Roelants M, Hauspie R, Hoppenbrouwers K: References for growth and pubertal development from birth to 21 years in Flanders, Belgium. Ann Hum Biol 2009;36:680–694.

16 Teilmann G, Pedersen CB, Skakkebaek NE, Jensen TK: Increased risk of precocious puberty in internationally adopted children in Denmark. Pediatrics 2006;118:e391–e399.

17 Ibanez L, Potau N, François I, et al: Precocious pubarche, hyperinsulinism, and ovarian hyperandrogenism in girls: relation to reduced fetal growth. J Clin Endocrinol Metab 1998;83:3558–3562.

18 Wildt L, Marshall G, Knobil E: Experimental induction of puberty in the infantile female rhesus monkey. Science 1980;207:1373.

19 Wildt L, Hausler A, Marshall G, et al: Frequency and amplitude of gonadotropin-releasing hormone stimulation and gonadotropin secretion in the rhesus monkey. Endocrinology 1981;109:376.

20 Mitsushima D, Hei DL, Terasawa E: Gamma-aminobutyric acid is an inhibitory neurotransmitter restricting the release of luteinizing hormone-releasing hormone before the onset of puberty. Proc Natl Acad Sci USA 1994;91:395–399.

21 Bourguignon JP, Jaeken J, Gérard A, et al: Amino acid neurotransmission and initiation of puberty: evidence from nonketotic hyperglycinemia in a female infant and gonadotropin-releasing hormone secretion by rat hypothalamic explants. J Clin Endocrinol Metab 1997;82:1899–1903.

22 Ojeda SR, Terasawa E: Neuroendocrine regulation of puberty; in Rubin RT, Pfaff DW (eds): Hormones, Brain and Behavior. New York, Elsevier Science, 2002, vol 4, pp 589–659.

23 El Majdoubi M, Sahu A, Ramaswamy S, Plant TM: Neuropeptide Y: A hypothalamic brake restraining the onset of puberty in primates. Proc Natl Acad Sci USA 2000;97:6179–6184.

24 de Roux N, Genin E, Carel JC, et al: Hypogonadotropic hypogonadism due to loss of function of the KiSS1-derived peptide receptor GPR54. Proc Natl Acad Sci USA 2003;100:10972–10976.

25 Seminara SB, Messager S, Chatzidaki EE, et al: The GPR54 gene as a regulator of puberty. N Eng J Med 2003;349:1614–1627.

26 Teles MG, Bianco SD, Brito VN, Trarbach EB, Kuohung W, Xu S, Seminara SB, Mendonca BB, Kaiser UB, Latronico AC: A GPR54-activating mutation in a patient with central precocious puberty. N Engl J Med 2008;358:709–715.
27 Clarkson J, Boon WC, Simpson ER, Herbison AE: Postnatal development of an estradiol-kisspeptin positive feedback mechanism implicated in puberty onset. Endocrinology 2009;150:3214–3220.
28 Ojeda SR, Roth C, Mungenast A, Heger S, Mastronardi C, Parent AS, Lomniczi A, Jung H: Neuroendocrine mechanisms controlling female puberty: new approaches, new concepts. Int J Androl 2006;29:256–263.
29 Parent AS, Lebrethon MC, Gérard A, Bourguignon JP: Factors accounting for perinatal occurrence of pulsatile gonadotropin-releasing hormone secretion in vitro. Biol Reprod 2005;72:143–149.
30 Matagne V, Rasier G, Lebrethon MC, Gérard A, Bourguignon JP: Estradiol stimulation of pulsatile GnRH secretion in vitro: correlation with perinatal exposure to sex steroids and induction of sexual precocity in vivo. Endocrinology 2004;145:2775–2783.
31 Kosut SS, Wood RI, Herbosa-Encarnacion C, Foster DL: Prenatal androgens time neuroendocrine puberty in the sheep: effect of testosterone dose. Endocrinology 1997;138:1072–1077.
32 Unsworth WP, Taylor JA, Robinson JE: Prenatal programming of reproductive neuroendocrine function: the effect of prenatal androgens on the development of estrogen positive feedback and ovarian cycles in the ewe. Biol Reprod 2005;72:619–627.
33 Gajdos ZKZ, Hirschhorn JN, Palmert MR: What controls the timing of puberty? An update on progress from genetic investigation. Curr Opin Endocrinol Diabetes Obes 2009;16:16–24.
34 Gorai I, Tanaka K, Inada M, Morinaga H, Uchiyama Y, Kikuchi R, Chaki O, Hirahara F: Estrogen-metabolizing gene polymorphisms, but not estrogen receptor-γ gene polymorphisms, are associated with the onset of menarche in healthy postmenopausal Japanese women. J Clin Endocrinol Metab 2003;88: 799–803.
35 Ojeda SR, Hill J, Hill DF, Costa ME, Tapia V, Cornea A, Ma YJ: The Oct-2 POU domain gene in the neuroendocrine brain: a transcriptional regulator of mammalian puberty. Endocrinology 1999;140:3774–3789.
36 Heger S, Mastronardi C, Dissen GA, Lomniczi A, Cabrera R, Roth CL, Jung H, Galimi F, Sippel W, Ojeda SR: Enhanced at puberty 1 (EAP1) is a new transcriptional regulator of the female neuroendocrine reproductive axis. J Clin Invest 2007;117:2145–2154.
37 Ong KK, Elks CE, Li S, et al: Genetic variation in LIN28B is associated with the timing of puberty. Nat Genet 2009;41:729–733.
38 Murray EK, Hien A, de Vries GJ, Forger NG: Epigenetic control of sexual differentiation of the bed nucleus of the stria terminalis Endocrinology 2009;150:4241–4247.
39 Lebrethon MC, Aganina A, Fournier M, Gérard A, Parent AS, Bourguignon JP: Effects of in vivo and in vitro administration of ghrelin, leptin and neuropeptide mediators on pulsatile gonadotrophin-releasing hormone secretion from male rat hypothalamus before and after puberty. J Neuroendocrinol 2007;19:181–188.
40 Ong KK, Emmett P, Northstone K, Golding J, Rogers I, Ness AR, Wells JC, Dunger DB: Infancy weight gain predicts childhood body fat and age at menarche in girls. J Clin Endocrinol Metab 2009;94:1527–1532.
41 Bourguignon JP, Rasier G, Lebrethon MC, Gérard A, Naveau E, Parent AS: Neuroendocrine disruption of pubertal timing and interactions between homeostasis of reproduction and energy balance. Mol Cell Endocrinol 2010;324:110–120.
42 Sloboda DM, Howie GJ, Pleasants A, Gluckman PD, Vickers MH: Pre- and postnatal nutritional histories influence reproductive maturation and ovarian function in the rat. PLoS ONE 2009;4:e6744.
43 Vickers MH, Gluckman PD, Coveny AH, Hofman PL, Cutfield WS, Gertler A, Breier BH, Harris M: Neonatal leptin treatment reverses developmental programming. Endocrinology 2005;146:4211–4216.
44 Williams NI, Helmreich DL, Parfitt DB, Caston-Balderrama A, Cameron JL: Evidence for a causal role of low energy availability in the induction of menstrual cycle disturbances during strenuous exercise training. J Clin Endocrinol Metab 2001;86: 5184–5193.
45 Van Elburg AA, Eijkemans MJC, Kas MJH, Themmen APM, de Jong FH, van Engeland H, Fauser BCJM: Predictors of recovery of ovarian function during weight gain in anorexia nervosa. Fert Steril 2007;87:902–908.
46 Krstevska-Konstantinova M, Charlier C, Craen M, et al: Sexual precocity after immigration from developing countries to Belgium: evidence of previous exposure to organochlorine pesticides. Hum Reprod 2001;16:1020–1026.
47 Herbst AL, Ulfelder H, Poskanzer DC: Adenocarcinoma of vagina: association of maternal stilbestrol therapy with tumor appearance in young women. N Engl J Med 1971;284:878–881.
48 Heindel JJ: Toxicological highlight: endocrine disruptors and the obesity epidemic. Toxicol Sci 2003; 76:247–249.

49 Dominé F, Parent AS, Rasier G, Lebrethon MC, Bourguignon JP: Assessment and mechanism of variations in pubertal timing in internationally adopted children: a developmental hypothesis. Eur J Endocrinol 2006;155:S17–S25.
50 Giedd JN: The teen brain: insights from neuroimaging. J Adolesc Health 2008;42:335–343.
51 Wilson ME, Kinkead B: Gene-environment interactions, not neonatal growth hormone deficiency, time puberty in female rhesus monkeys. Biol Reprod 2008;78:736–743.
52 Mann DR, Akinbami MA, Gould KG, Paul K, Wallen K: Sexual maturation in male rhesus monkeys: importance of neonatal testosterone exposure and social rank. J Endocr 1998;156:493–501.
53 Caspi A, Moffitt TE: Individual differences are accentuated during periods of social change: the sample case of girls at puberty. J Pers Soc Psychol 1991;61:157–168.
54 Stattin H, Magnusson D: Pubertal Maturation in Female Development. Hillsdale, Lawrence Erlbaum, 1990.
55 Graber JA, Seeley JR, Brooks-Gunn J, Lewinsohn PM: Is pubertal timing associated with psychopathology in young adulthood? J Am Acad Child Adolesc Psychiatry 2004;43:718–726.
56 Michaud PA, Suris JC, Deppen A: Gender specific psychosocial correlates of pubertal timing in a national sample of Swiss adolescents. Mol Cell Endocr 2006;254–255:172–178.
57 Berger U, Weitkamp K, Strauss B: Weight limits, estimations of future BMI, subjective pubertal timing and physical appearance comparisons among adolescent girls as precursors of disturbed eating behaviour in a community sample. Eur Eat Disorders Rev 2008;16:1–9.

Anders Juul
Department of Growth and Reproduction, Rigshospitalet Section 5064, University of Copenhagen
Blegdamsvej 9
DK–2100 Copenhagen (Denmark)
Tel. +45 3545 5085, Fax +45 3545 6054, E-Mail ajuul@rh.dk

Sultan C (ed): Pediatric and Adolescent Gynecology. Evidence-Based Clinical Practice. 2nd, revised and extended edition. Endocr Dev. Basel, Karger, 2012, vol 22, pp 24–39

Endocrine Evaluation of Reproductive Function in Girls during Infancy, Childhood and Adolescence

Anders Juul[a] · Casper P. Hagen[a] · Lise Aksglaede[a] · Kaspar Sørensen[a] · Annette Mouritsen[a] · Hanne Frederiksen[a] · Katharina M. Main[a] · Signe Sloth Mogensen[a] · Anette T. Pedersen[b]

Departments of [a]Growth and Reproduction and [b]Gynaecology, Rigshospitalet, University of Copenhagen, Copenhagen, Denmark

Abstract

Puberty is characterized by a series a hormonal events leading to the attainment of adult reproductive capacity. Clinical manifestations of the pubertal processes include breast development, pubic hair development, menarche and regular menstrual bleedings. Abnormal pubertal development includes a spectrum of disorders such as premature thelarche, premature adrenarche, central and peripheral precocious puberty, adolescent polycystic ovarian syndrome, functional ovarian hyperandrogenism, late-onset congenital adrenal hyperplasia, primary and secondary amenorrhea, and premature ovarian insufficiency. Diagnosis of these reproductive disorders includes biochemical as well as clinical evaluation. The biochemical evaluation of reproductive function includes measurement of basal reproductive hormone levels and dynamic pituitary or adrenal hormone testing. Correct interpretation of such test results requires detailed knowledge on the normal maturational changes in the hypothalamic-pituitary-ovarian and hypothalamic-pituitary-adrenal axes. Changes in basal reproductive hormone levels in infancy, childhood and adolescence as well as the GnRH and ACTH test procedures in girls and adolescents are described in this chapter.

Hypothalamic-Pituitary-Ovarian Axis

Ovarian Development

In the gonad of the XX fetus, the primordial germ cells are transformed at the 10th week of gestation into oogonia which enter first meiotic division. The oogonia stop further differentiation in the diplotene stage, during which they stay until ovulation. Oocytes are formed and peak in number during midgestation (6–7 million) with a subsequent decline [1]. At birth, 1–2 million oocytes are present in the ovaries of the

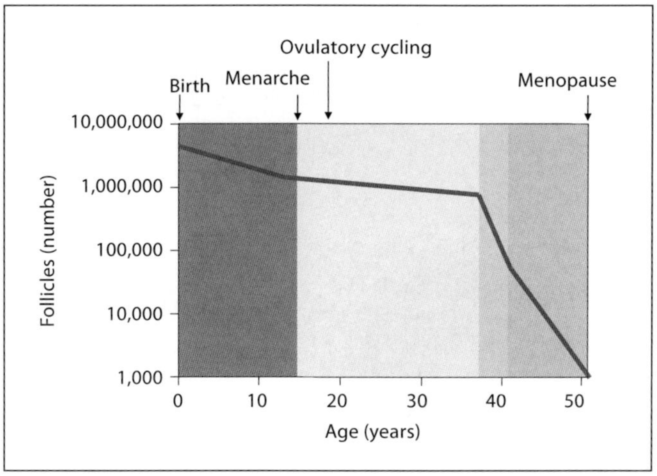

Fig. 1. Approximate number of ovarian follicles during pre- and postnatal life (line). Important reproductive milestones are indicated by arrows. Redrawn from Baker [1] and Wallace [2].

newborn girl. In postnatal life the number of ovarian germ cells decreases by 1–2% per year by programmed cell death (apoptosis). A minor part of the decreasing number of germ cells is caused by ovulation. From approximately 35–37 years of age, a much steeper rate of germ cell apoptosis occurs concurrent with markedly decreasing reproductive capacity until menopause (fig. 1).

Hormonal Regulation of Ovarian Function

In early pregnancy from around the 4th week of gestation placentally derived human chorionic gonadotropin (hCG) stimulates the undifferentiated gonads. In the presence of the *SRY* gene, the gonads develop into testes which secrete anti-Müllerian hormone (AMH). AMH causes regression of the Müllerian duct derivates in the male fetus. In the female gonads which do not produce AMH in early fetal life, the Müllerian structures develop into uterus, oviducts and proximal part of vagina. In the second trimester, the fetal pituitary gland takes over and regulates gonadal function. Hypothalamic gonadotropin-releasing hormone (GnRH) secretion stimulates the pituitary gonadotrophs to secrete follicle-stimulating hormone (FSH) and luteinizing hormone (LH) through activation of GnRH receptors. FSH and LH act via specific receptors on granulosa and theca cells of the ovary (fig. 2). The serum levels of fetal FSH and LH then decline until birth.

In postnatal life, the hypothalamic-pituitary-ovarian (HPO) axis is activated for the second time at approximately 3 months of age – the so-called minipuberty [3]. During early infancy, basal serum levels of FSH and LH reach those of adult cycling women. After the brief period of HPO activity the HPO axis is silenced during late infancy and childhood resulting in low circulating LH, but clearly detectable FSH levels [4] (fig. 3). With the onset of puberty, the HPO axis is again activated resulting in pulsatile secretion of gonadotropins. The diurnal rhythms of serum LH and

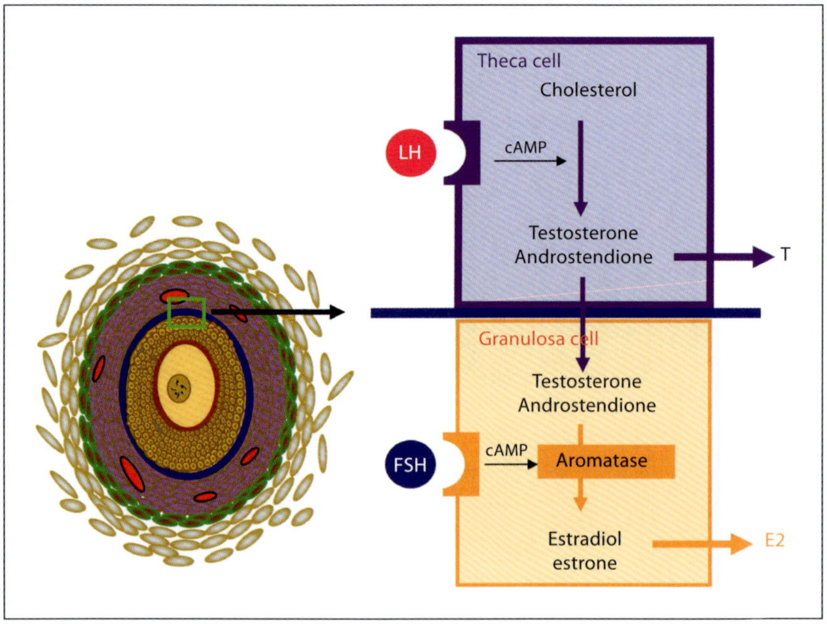

Fig. 2. Preantral ovarian follicle (left part of figure). The oocyte is surrounded by granulosa cells (yellow). The basal membrane (blue) marks the separation between the granulosa cells and the surrounding internal and external thecal cell layers (purple cells). Ovarian steroidogenesis is illustrated in the right part of the figure. Theca cells are stimulated by LH which stimulates steroidogenesis and production of testosterone. Testosterone passes the basal membrane to the granulosa cell where it is aromatized to estrogens, primarily estradiol. Aromatase actively is induced by FSH stimulation of the granulosa cell.

FSH already exist at 5–6 years of age, and serum levels increase before the onset of puberty [5–7]. This is reflected by elevations in urinary FSH and LH concentration before clinical signs of puberty are evident [8]. Altogether, these results suggest that preparation for the onset of female puberty begins already in 5- to 6-year-old girls.

Inhibin A and B

The pulsatile FSH and LH secretion stimulates ovarian steroidogenesis under feedback control from circulating estradiol. Granulosa cells also secrete a family of peptides (inhibin-activin-follistatin) in response to FSH stimulation. Two forms of inhibin (inhibin A and inhibin B) exist and consist of two heterodimers linked by disulfide bonds. Inhibin A consists of an α-subunit and a βA-subunit, whereas inhibin B consists of an α-subunit and a βB-subunit. Inhibins suppress pituitary FSH secretion. Serum inhibin B is low or undetectable in Tanner breast stage I. However, measurable levels of inhibin B in more than 60% of prepubertal girls indicate that some gonadotropin-responsive follicular activity is occurring at this early stage. Levels of

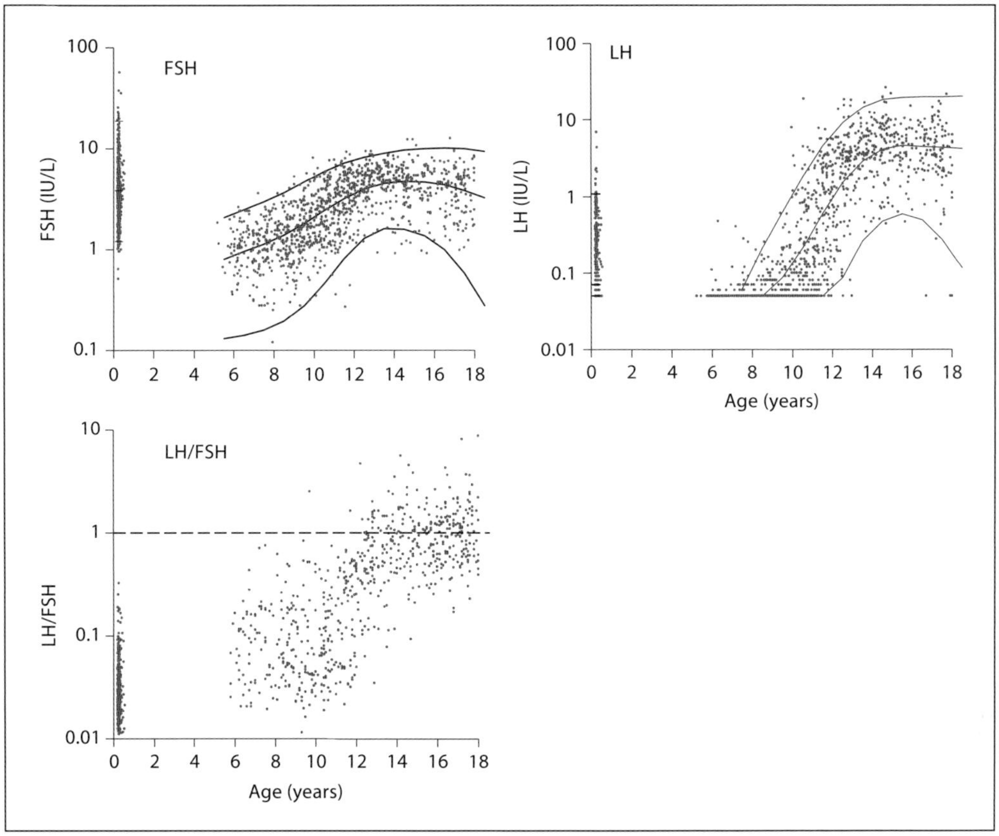

Fig. 3. Serum levels of FSH (upper left panel) and LH (upper right panel) according to chronological age in healthy females during infancy, childhood and adolescence. Lines represent geometric mean ±2 SD corresponding to the 95% prediction interval. LH/FSH ratios are shown according to age in the lower panel. The dashed line indicates LH/FSH ratio = 1. Data are combined from 3 different publications, and gonadotropin concentrations from the healthy subjects are measured using the same assays [3, 7, 10].

inhibin A increase progressively from Tanner stage I into adulthood. Inhibin A is only detectable in girls after menarche [9, 10], and is therefore a marker of ovulation. During the menstrual cycle, inhibin B levels are highest in the early and late follicular phases, decrease in the periovulatory phase, and are lower in the mid- and end-luteal phases. Serum inhibin A levels are lowest in the early follicular phase, increase significantly in the late follicular phase with maximal levels in the midluteal phase, with a subsequent decrease in the end-luteal phase [10].

Anti-Müllerian Hormone

AMH, also termed Müllerian inhibiting substance (MIS), is produced from gestational week 36 and onwards by granulosa cells of the antral follicles. AMH seems to reflect the follicle pool (ovarian aging) in adult women. The biological function of

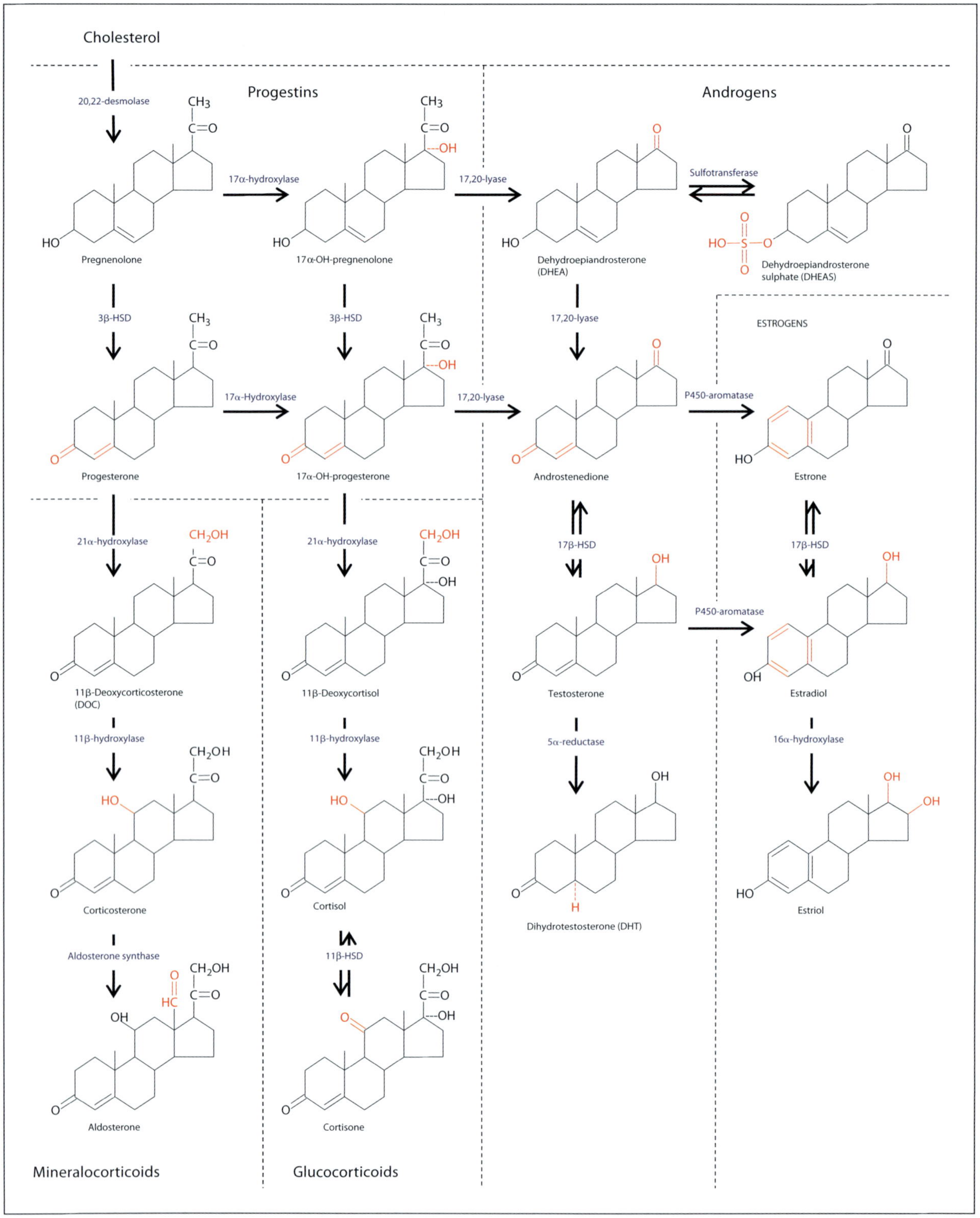
Cholesterol
Progestins
Androgens
20,22-desmolase
17α-hydroxylase
17,20-lyase
Sulfotransferase
Pregnenolone
17α-OH-pregnenolone
Dehydroepiandrosterone (DHEA)
Dehydroepiandrosterone sulphate (DHEAS)
3β-HSD
17,20-lyase
ESTROGENS
17α-Hydroxylase
P450-aromatase
Progesterone
17α-OH-progesterone
Androstenedione
Estrone
21α-hydroxylase
17β-HSD
11β-Deoxycorticosterone (DOC)
11β-Deoxycortisol
Testosterone
Estradiol
11β-hydroxylase
5α-reductase
16α-hydroxylase
Corticosterone
Cortisol
Dihydrotestosterone (DHT)
Estriol
Aldosterone synthase
11β-HSD
Aldosterone
Cortisone
Mineralocorticoids
Glucocorticoids

AMH in the ovary is largely unknown. Serum AMH levels are detectable in girls from 3 months of age with relatively constant levels until 35–40 years of age, followed by a decrease in AMH levels until menopause where AMH becomes undetectable. AMH shows only minor variation across the menstrual cycle [11] depending on the relative ovarian age rather than the chronologic age. Thus, the young ovary secretes higher mean AMH and inhibin B levels to the circulation, and a small rise in AMH during the follicular phase of the menstrual cycle is seen. This is in contrast to the aging ovary which is characterized by low mean AMH and inhibin B serum levels, shorter menstrual cycle lengths, and minimal variation in AMH levels during the cycle, suggesting diminished ovarian reserve. Thus, AMH is considered a promising marker of ovarian reserve [12]. It remains to be seen if pediatric AMH levels predict reproductive function in adult women.

Hypothalamic-Pituitary-Adrenal Axis

Adrenal Development

At approximately the 7th week of gestation, the fetal adrenal cortex is invaded by sympathetic neuronal structures, which differentiate into chromaffin cells which secrete catecholamines. The adrenal cortex consists of 3 zones (zona glomerulosa, zona reticularis and zona fasciculata). Their development depends on adrenocorticoptropic hormone (ACTH). The zona fasciculata and reticularis of the adrenal cortex produce cortisol and androgens. The zona glomerulosa of the adrenal medulla secretes primarily aldosterone which is stimulated by the renin-angiotensin system and potassium.

Hormonal Regulation of Adrenal Function

The hypothalamic corticotropin-releasing hormone stimulates pituitary ACTH secretion which is highly pulsatile. ACTH stimulates the adrenal cortex through its specific receptor (MC2R) to secrete glucocorticoids. The steroid biosynthesis pathway is illustrated in figure 4.

The ovary produces all 3 classes of sex steroids; estrogens, progestins, and androgens. The ovary is distinguished from the adrenal cortex by its lack of 21-hydroxylase and 11-hydroxylase reactions. Thus, glucocorticoids and mineralocorticoids are not produced in the normal ovary.

Fig. 4. Steroidogenic pathways in the adrenal and ovary. Cholesterol is taken up by ACTH-dependent mechanisms, and converted into progestins. Progestins are converted into 4 classes of steroids; mineral- and glucocorticoids (exclusively in the adrenal gland), and androgens and estrogens (adrenal and ovary). Cortisol, testosterone and estradiol are end products which are further converted in non-steroidogenic tissues to cortisone (inactive), DHT (potent) and estriol (inactive), respectively. Enzymes are written in blue, and structural changes in the steroids compared to the former steroid metabolite are marked in red.

Steroidogenesis is characterized by a series of enzymatic reactions mediated by steroidogenic enzymes which are members of the cytochrome P450 group of oxidases. All steroids are of similar structure with relatively small chemical differences resulting in major changes in biochemical activity. Conversion of cholesterol to pregnenolone involves hydroxylation at the carbon 20 and 22 positions. The acute regulation of this conversion is controlled by the steroidogenic acute regulatory protein (StAR) which is mediated by ACTH. Following the formation of pregnenolone further conversion can take 2 pathways; the Δ5-pathway via 17-hydroxy-pregnenolone and DHEA, and the Δ4-pathway via progesterone and 17-hydroxy-progesterone.

Steroids are named according to the number of carbon atoms to designate the basic name; pregnane resulting in progestins and corticoids, androstane resulting in androgens, or estrane resulting in estrogens. Glucocorticoids have a C21-structure, and are also referred to as 17-hydroxycorticosteroids. The most important glucocorticoid is cortisol (also known as compound F or hydrocortisone). The interconversion of cortisol and cortisone is catalyzed by 11β-hydroxysteroid dehydrogenase 2, which is present in many peripheral non-steroidogenic tissues including the kidney. Androgens have a C19- structure and are produced in the zona fasciculata and reticularis of the adrenal gland as well as in the gonads. Androgens promote growth and have androgenic effects. Estrogens have a C18-structure, and are converted by aromatase activity from androgens. Estrogen production occurs in the adrenal cortex and gonads, but aromatization of androgens also occurs in peripheral tissues.

DHEAS is the predominant marker of adrenarche in serum which represents an altered pattern of adrenocortical response to ACTH. This is characterized by disproportionately increasing Δ5-steroid intermediates (17OH-pregnenolone and DHEA) compared to Δ4-steroid metabolites (17OH-progesterone and androstenedione). This results from decreasing expression of 3β-HSD in the zona reticularis from 6 to 8 years of age throughout life, which promotes DHEA and DHEAS production. CYP21 expression does not seem to change in the zona reticularis with increasing age, suggesting that adrenarche does not rely on alterations in CYP21 expression. Altogether, the initiation and regulation of adrenarche is poorly understood.

Reproductive Disorders in Girls and Adolescents which Require Biochemical Evaluation

Precocious puberty is defined as clinical signs of puberty before the age of 8 years in girls.

Central Precocious Puberty

Central precocious puberty is caused by activation of the hypothalamic-pituitary-ovarian (HPO) axis, termed central or gonadotropin-dependent precocious puberty (CPP). Central precocious puberty is idiopathic (ICPP) in the majority of cases, but may be secondary to a brain abnormality like hamartomas, gliomas and hydrocephalus (organic CPP) in 15–20% of cases.

Peripheral Precocious Puberty

Alternatively, precocious puberty is caused by an abnormal steroid production in peripheral steroidogenic organs which is not the result of sustained activation of the HPO-axis. This condition is termed peripheral or gonadotropin-independent precocious puberty.

Isolated forms of abnormal precocious puberty like premature thelarche or premature adrenarche are also not caused by central activation of the HPO axis.

Isolated premature thelarche is considered a benign, self-limiting condition, characterized by premature breast development, and no other clinical signs of sexual maturation. There are two types of premature thelarche; one type (classical) manifesting itself in the first year of life, following which it tends to resolve by 2 years of age. Another type of premature thelarche manifests itself after 2 years of age and tends to be more persistent. Commonly, breast development fluctuates over a period of time, and can disappear and reappear within months. Premature thelarche is characterized by overnight gonadotropin secretion, but circulating estradiol concentrations are commonly undetectable by conventional immunoassays. A GnRH test will demonstrate a prepubertal LH rise, and a predominant FSH response. The ovaries are small on ultrasound but may contain large follicular cysts which vary in size in synchrony with the fluctuating breast development. Typically, no acceleration of linear growth is seen, and bone age is not advanced. However, this form of premature thelarche may progress into a true central precocious puberty in some cases.

The distinction between central precocious puberty and premature thelarche may not always be straightforward as intermediate slowly progressing forms (thelarche variant forms) exist.

Isolated premature adrenarche is characterized by isolated pubic or axillary hair development before 8 years of age in girls, and may be associated with other cutaneous manifestations of androgen excess (like microcomedonal acne, greasy hair and body odor). Also, behavioral changes are seen and bone age may be slightly advanced. Suspicion of adrenal pathology increases, the more bone age is advanced.

Androgen-producing adrenal tumors are characterized by a rapidly progressing form of puberty, and serum testosterone are usually high (>5–6 nmol/l). Adrenal tumors are nevertheless extremely rare in children, and may be combined with symptoms of Cushing.

Congenital adrenal hyperplasia (CAH) is most commonly due to 21-hydroxylase deficiency (CYP21 mutation), but also other enzyme deficiencies resulting in CAH exist. CAH is typically diagnosed in the neonatal period due to national screening programs, or during the first weeks of life due to clinical symptoms like failure to thrive, salt wasting (hyponatremic crisis) or ambiguous genitalia. However, milder forms of CAH (late-onset CAH) exist, which may present in childhood with varying degrees of virilization including pubic hair development. Late-onset CAH (CYP21 mutation) is diagnosed by an ACTH test during which 17-OH-progesterone is significantly elevated. Thus, isolated premature adrenarche is an exclusion diagnosis which is relatively common, especially in overweight children and children born small for gestational age. It appears that children born from mothers with PCOS may be at increased risk of premature adrenarche.

Polycystic ovary syndrome (PCOS) is a heterogeneous syndrome of unexplained chronic hyperandrogenism and oligo-anovulation, with a polycystic ovary on sonography being one of the alternative diagnostic criteria [13, 14]. Half of the patients lack one or several of the classical criteria (menstrual irregularity, hirsutism, obesity, and polycystic ovaries).

Functional ovarian hyperandrogenism (FOH) is usually the source of androgen excess in adolescent girls and is characterized by 17-OH-progesterone hyperresponsiveness to GnRH stimulation or to hCG testing, and subnormal suppressibility of serum testosterone by dexamethasone. However, FOH is often accompanied by functional adrenal hyperresponsiveness, which is characterized by 17-OH-progesterone or DHEA hyperresponsiveness to ACTH [15]. These test are primarily used for research purposes.

Absent puberty or primary amenorrhea may result from hypogonadotropic hypogonadism (HH) due to mutations in selected genes (*KAL1, FGFR1, GPR54, PROK2, TAC3, TAC3R*) which account for only 20–30% of cases with HH. Familial delayed puberty may be suspected based on family history once a 45,X karyotype, hyperprolactinemia or anorexia/ortorexia are excluded. Idiopathic HH will result in low FSH and LH levels, and GnRH testing is of limited value in such conditions.

Evaluation of Basal Serum Hormone Levels

FSH and LH are glycoproteins which are not single proteins, but consist of a number of heterogeneous forms of varying biological activity. Thus, 20–30 different LH and FSH isoforms are present in the circulation. FSH, LH and hCG are dimers which are composed of 2 glycosylated polypeptide subunits, the α- and β-subunits, that are tightly noncovalently bound. FSH, LH, and hCG share a common α-subunit (92 amino acids), whereas the β-subunits differ in amino acid and carbohydrate content. Sensitive and accurate gonadotropin assays are critical for diagnosis and monitoring of pubertal disorders. Random LH and FSH levels follow a distinct developmental pattern. In prepubertal girls, FSH levels are low, whereas LH levels are usually undetectable by currently available sensitive immunoassays [10]. With the onset of puberty, gonadotropin levels rise gradually in puberty (fig. 3) until the adult cyclic pattern is obtained (fig. 5).

LH/FSH Ratio

In prepubertal children FSH levels are higher than those of LH (LH/FSH ratio <1), but half of healthy adolescent children has LH/FSH ratio >1 (fig. 3). This is due to the

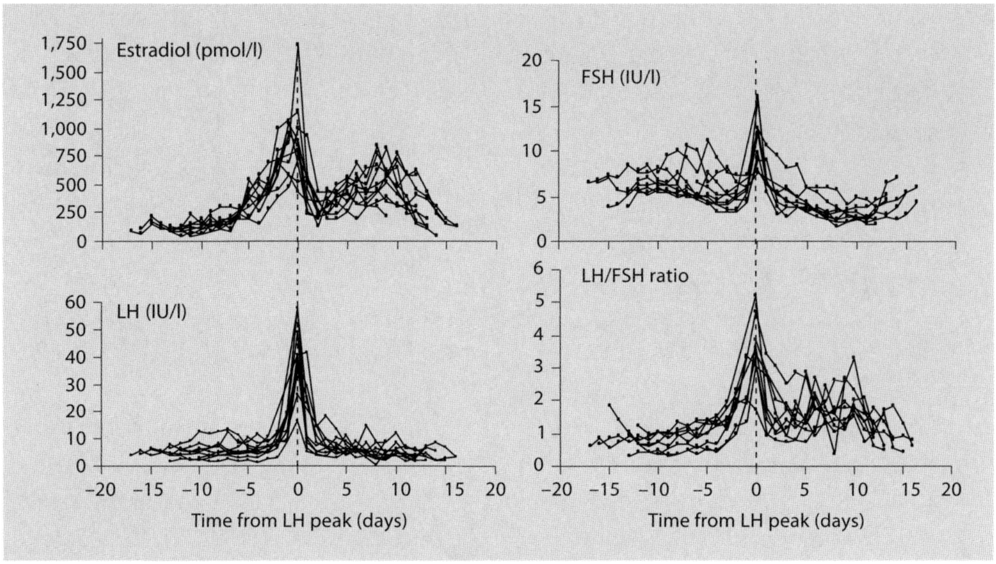

Fig. 5. Serum levels of estradiol, LH, FSH and LH/FSH ratio during the menstrual cycles in healthy regularly menstruating young women. Values from individual women are illustrated according to days from ovulation (LH peak). Data derived from Juul et al. [9].

fact that the LH/FSH ratio is elevated at ovulation and in the luteal phase of a normal menstrual cycle (fig. 5). Thus, a random LH/FSH >1 in an adolescent girl is not pathological *per se*, whereas an increased follicular phase LH/FSH ratio is indicative of PCOS in cases of oligomenorrhea/hyperandrogenism. The LH/FSH ratio should not be used as part of the diagnostic criteria for PCOS [13, 14].

Estrogens

Estrogens, primarily 17β-estradiol and estrone, are produced in the ovarian granulosa cell following aromatization of their precursors Δ4-Androstenedione and testosterone. Estrogens act through two types of estrogen receptors (ER-α and ER-β). Estrogen production is elevated during minipuberty and with the onset of puberty, whereas levels are typically below the detection limit of commonly used immunoassays in prepubertal children (fig. 6).

Our knowledge of the biological significance of low prepubertal sex steroid levels is hampered by the fact that most available analytical methods are not sensitive enough to assess the low levels of estrogenic and androgenic hormones and metabolites in serum of prepubertal children. Available data on sex steroid levels in prepubertal children differ substantially depending on the assay used and remain controversial. Immunoassays are the most commonly used methods for analysis of estradiol levels. However, for clinical and research applications most immunoassays have insufficient sensitivity resulting in substantial inaccuracy and high intra- as

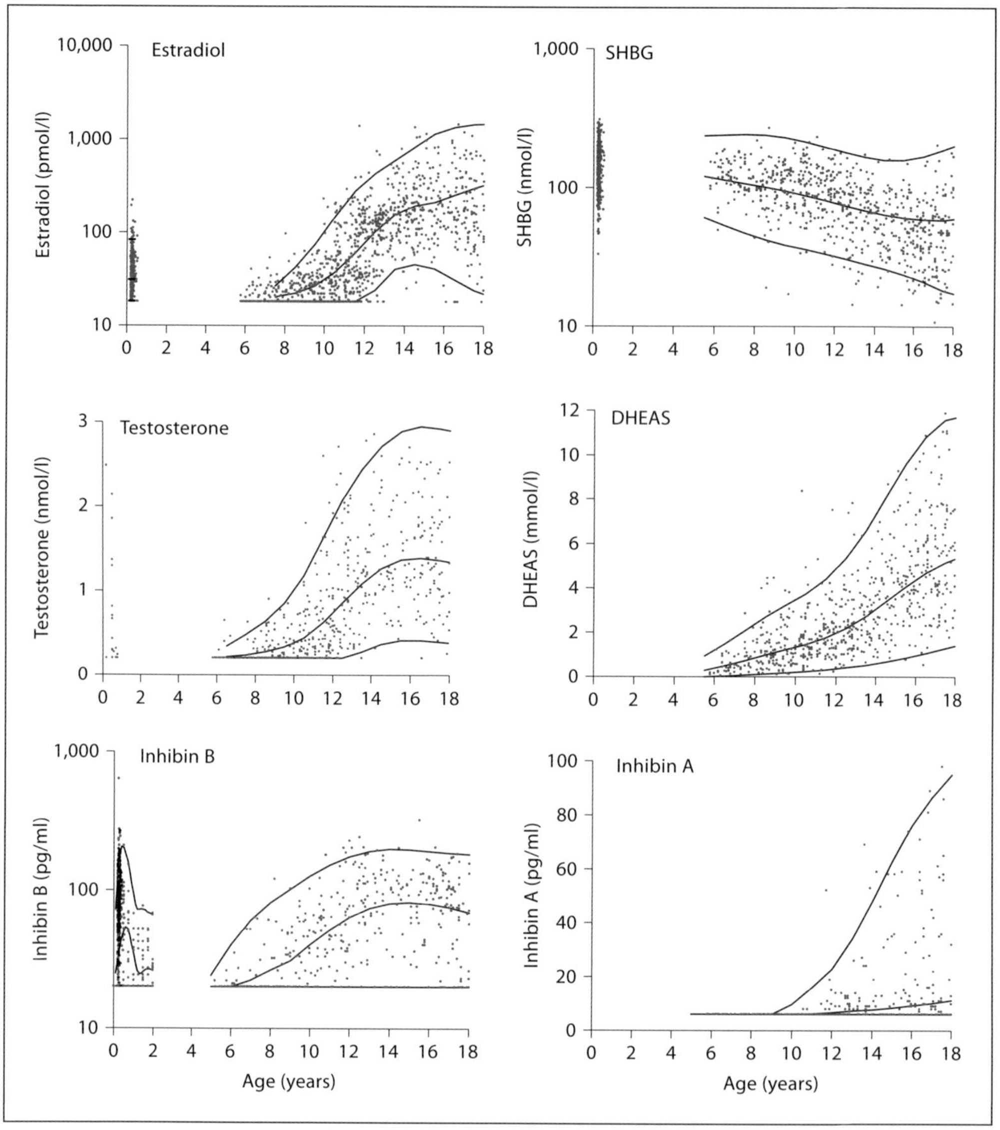

Fig. 6. Serum levels of estradiol, SHBG, testosterone, DHEAS, inhibin B and inhibin A according to chronological age in 2,406 healthy girls. Lines represent geometric means ±2 SD corresponding to the 95% prediction interval. Data for DHEAS are not available for infant girls. Please note the logarithmic scale for estradiol SHBG, testosterone and inhibin B. [data derived from refs. 3, 7, 10, 19].

well as interassay variations in the low concentration range. The sensitivity of the most sensitive immunoassays is in the order of 10–18 pmol/l, whereas ultrasensitive recombinant cell bioassays (RCBA) or gas chromatography-tandem mass spectrometry (GC-MS/MS) methodologies have lower detection limits (0.7–1.8 pmol/l) [16–18]. This may be of clinical relevance for instance in girls with premature thelarche in whom estradiol is usually below the detection limit of commercially available immunoassays, but clearly elevated compared to prepubertal children using a RCBA [16].

Sex Hormone-Binding Globulin
Estradiol is bound to sex hormone-binding globulin (SHBG), thus a minor part of circulating estradiol is in its free biologically active form. SHBG is regulated by estrogens, androgens, thyroid hormones, insulin and liver function. SHBG seems to reflect the degree of physiological insulin resistance seen in mid-puberty [19, 20].

Androgens
DHEAS levels are low during childhood but start to increase before other hormonal changes of puberty take place, a process termed adrenarche. DHEAS levels are high in patients with adrenal cortical tumors, whereas lesser elevations are seen in patients with congenital adrenal hyperplasia, and moderate elevations are seen in children with precocious adrenarche.

17-OH-Progesterone
17-OH-progesterone is produced by the adrenal as well as the ovary. In classical CAH due to 21-hydroxylase deficiency 17-OH-progesterone is clearly elevated, whereas it is only marginally elevated in late-onset CAH.

Urinary Excretion of Steroids
The polycyclic carbon ring of steroids is not degraded during metabolism, but is transformed by a series of reductions and hydroxylations. Active steroids are glucuronidated or sulfated and thereby water-soluble, and can be excreted into urine. Generally, glucuronidation reduces the activity of a steroid, but glucuronidated steroids can be deconjugated in peripheral tissues, restoring their biological activity locally. Cortisol is excreted as tetrahydrocortisol (THE) and tetrahydrocortisone (THF) is conjugated with glucuronic acid.

Determination of steroid excretion rates in a 24-hour urine sample is a non-invasive way of estimating the combined output of adrenal and gonadal steroid production. A urinary sample of 5–20 ml is required for urinary steroid profiling by GC-MS/MS methodology. Samples can be sent to the laboratory at room temperature, and should be processed within 3 days. A 24-hour collection allows determination of excretion rates (relevant for diagnosis of Cushing or adrenal insufficiency), whereas a spot urine is sufficient for diagnosis of enzymatic defects in the steroidogenic pathway or tumors.

CAH due to 21-hydroxylase deficiency is characterized by elevated urinary levels of 17-hydroxypregnanolone, pregnanediol, and pregnanetriol, whereas CAH due to 11-hydroxylase deficiency is characterized by elevated urinary tetrahydro-11-deoxycortisol. CAH due to 3β-HSD deficiency show increased urinary levels of

DHEA, 16-hydroxy-DHEA, pregnanetriol and 17-hydroxypregnanetriol. Children with adrenocortical tumors will typically have markedly elevated urinary levels of DHEA. Thus, urinary steroid profiling is useful in a wide variety of clinical conditions. Urinary cortisol metabolites are increased in Cushing's disease and low or undetectable in adrenal insufficiency.

Adrenocorticotropic Hormone
ACTH can be determined in a single blood sample, but is extremely unstable in blood. Thus, care should be taken at blood sampling and the following sample handling procedure should be followed: heparin or EDTA plasma tubes should be placed immediately on ice, centrifuged and the plasma frozen within 15 min. ACTH is elevated in cases of adrenal insufficiency (or pituitary Cushing), but results are typically difficult to interpret.

GnRH Testing

Measurement of basal LH and FSH levels is sufficient for some reproductive disorders, but a GnRH test is necessary for diagnosis of CPP. Luteinizing hormone-releasing hormone (LHRH; 100 μg Relefact®) is injected intravenously, and blood samples are drawn before and 30 min after the injection of a bolus. Blood samples are analyzed for LH and FSH. The test is easy to perform, and can be performed in an outpatient setting at any time during the day. The upper normal range of stimulated LH levels in prepubertal children depends on the LH assay, and may vary from 3.3 to 5–6 IU/l. A peak LH level >5 IU/l [21, 22] and/or stimulated LH/FSH ratio >0.66 IU/l [23] has been suggested as cut off limits for a pubertal response during GnRH testing in accordance with the recent consensus guidelines [24] (fig. 7). Furthermore, girls presenting with breast development and a basal LH level above 0.3 IU/l are assumed to have CPP [22].

ACTH Testing

A short standard ACTH test using tetracosactrin (the synthetic 1–24 subunit of ACTH) is the most commonly used test. A blood sample is drawn and tetracosactrin (Synacthen®) is injected intravenously as a bolus dose of 250 or 36 μg/kg body weight in infants. Blood samples are drawn 30 and 60 min after injection. Firstly, the blood samples are used for cortisol measurements to rule out adrenal insufficiency. Secondly, steroidogenic metabolites (21-OH-progesterone, 11-OH-progesterone or DHEA) may be analyzed during the short ACTH test to evaluate possible CYP21, CYP11 or 3βHSD defects.

A Synacthen test is easy to perform, and can be performed at any time of the day, does not require fasting or bed rest, and Synacthen can also be administered

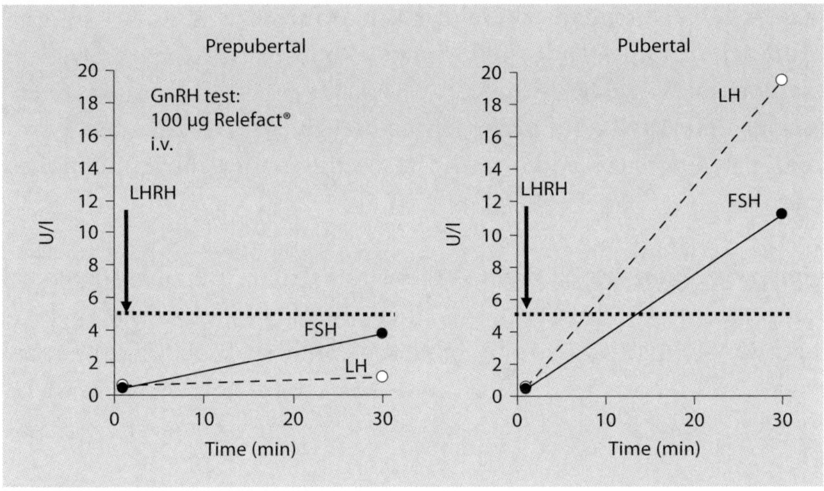

Fig. 7. Serum LH and FSH at baseline and 30 min following a GnRH intravenous injection (100 µg LHRH, Relefact). The left panel illustrates a typical prepubertal response to a GnRH agonist challenge with FSH predominance (stimulated LH/FSH ratio <1) and maximal LH level below 5 IU/l. The right panel illustrates a typical pubertal GnRH test with a stimulated LH level above 5 IU/l and a LH/FSH ratio >1.

intramuscularly. A normal cortisol response during an ACTH test is a rise to >500 nmol/l (or a rise of >250 nmol/l). In neonates, the cortisol responses are higher. Ongoing or recent treatment with glucocorticoids may interfere with cortisol measurements by immunoassays, and chromatographic separation is needed in such cases. Furthermore, use of oral contraceptives may result in erroneously high cortisol levels due to the induction of corticosteroid binding globulin, and should be stopped for 4 weeks before ACTH testing is valid.

Conclusions

In girls with *premature breast development* initial biochemical evaluation may include:

1 basal FSH, LH, E2, SHBG, inhibin A and inhibin B,
2 GnRH test (FSH, LH),
3 AMH (can be used if granulosa cell tumor is suspected).

In girls with *premature pubic hair* initial biochemical evaluation may include:

1 basal testosterone, DHEAS, Δ4-androstenedione, 17-OHP,
2 Synacthen test (cortisol, 17-OHP),
3 GnRH test (FSH, LH, 17-OHP).

In girls with *hirsutism* initial biochemical evaluation may include:
1 basal testosterone, DHEAS, Δ4-androstenedione, 17-OHP,
2 Synacthen test (cortisol, 17-OHP),
3 fasting glucose, insulin, HbA1C (or preferably an oral glucose tolerance test).

Urinary steroid profiling may additionally be useful in the above-mentioned conditions.

In girls with *primary amenorrhea* or premature ovarian failure initial biochemical evaluation may include:
1 Basal FSH, LH, E2, SHBG, testosterone, inhibin A, inhibin B, AMH, prolactin, karyotype.

References

1 Baker TH: A quantitative and cytological study of germ cells in human ovaries. Proc R Soc Lond 1963; 158:417.
2 Wallace WH, Kelsey TW: Human ovarian reserve from conception to the menopause. PLoS One 2010; 5:e8772.
3 Chellakooty M, Schmidt IM, Haavisto AM, Boisen KA, Damgaard IN, Mau C, Petersen JH, Juul A, Skakkebæk NE, Main KM: Inhibin A, Inhibin B, Follicle-stimulating hormone, luteinizing hormone, estradiol, and sex hormone binding globulin levels in 473 healthy infant girls. J Clin Endocrinol Metab 2003;88:3515–3520.
4 Andersson AM, Toppari J, Haavisto AM, Petersen JH, Simell T, Simell O, Skakkebaek NE: Longitudinal reproductive hormone profiles in infants: peak of inhibin B levels in infant boys exceeds levels in adult men. J Clin Endocrinol Metab 1998;83:675–681.
5 Goji K, Tanikaze S: Comparison between spontaneous gonadotropin concentration profiles and gonadotropin response to low-dose gonadotropin-releasing hormone in prepubertal and early pubertal boys and patients with hypogonadotropic hypogonadism: assessment by using ultrasensitive, time-resolved immunofluorometric assay. Pediatr Res 1992;31:535–539.
6 Mitamura R, Yano K, Suzuki N, Ito Y, Makita Y, Okuno A: Diurnal rhythms of luteinizing hormone, follicle-stimulating hormone, testosterone, and estradiol secretion before the onset of female puberty in short children. J Clin Endocrinol Metab 2000;85:1074–1080.
7 Aksglaede L, Sorensen K, Petersen JH, Skakkebæk NE, Juul A: Recent decline in age at breast development: the COPENHAGEN Puberty Study. Pediatrics 2009;123:e932–e939.
8 Demir A, Voutilainen R, Juul A, Dunkel L, Alfthan H, Skakkebæk NE, Stenman U-H: Increase in first morning voided urinary luteinizing hormone levels precedes the physical onset of puberty. J Clin Endocrinol Metab 1996;81:2963–2967.
9 Juul A, Scheike T, Pedersen AT, Main K, Pedersen LM, Skakkebæk NE: The impact of endogenous sex steroids on serum growth hormone, insulin-like growth factor (IGF)-I, IGF binding proteins (IGFBP-1 and -3) levels and urinary GH excretion during menstrual cycle in normal women. Human Reprod 1997;12:101–106.
10 Sehested A, Juul A, Andersson AM, Petersen JH, Müller J, Skakkebæk NE: Serum inhibin A and inhibin B in healthy prepubertal, pubertal and adolescent girls and adults women: relation to age, stage of puberty, menstrual cycle, FSH, LH and estradiol levels. J Clin Endocrinol Metab 2000;85:1634–1640.
11 Sowers M, McConnell D, Gast K, Zheng H, Nan B, McCarthy JD, Randolph JF: Anti-Müllerian hormone and inhibin B variability during normal menstrual cycles. Fertil Steril 2010;94:1482–1486.
12 Hagen CP, Aksglaede L, Sørensen K, Main KM, Boas M, Cleemann L, Holm K, Gravholt CH, Andersson AM, Pedersen AT, Petersen JH, Linneberg A, Kjaergaard S, Juul A: Serum levels of anti-Müllerian hormone as a marker of ovarian function in 926 healthy females from birth to adulthood and in 172 Turner syndrome patients. J Clin Endocrinol Metab 2010;95:5003–5010.

13 Azziz R, Carmina E, Dewailly D, Diamanti-Kandarakis E, Escobar-Morreale HF, Futterweit W, Janssen OE, Legro RS, Norman RJ, Taylor AE, Witchel SF, Androgen Excess Society: Positions statement: criteria for defining polycystic ovary syndrome as a predominantly hyperandrogenic syndrome: an Androgen Excess Society guideline. J Clin Endocrinol Metab 2006;91:4237–4245.

14 Rotterdam ESHRE/ASRM-Sponsored PCOS Consensus Workshop Group: Revised 2003 consensus on diagnostic criteria and long-term health risks related to polycystic ovary syndrome. Fertil Steril 2004;81:19–25.

15 Rosenfield RL: Identifying children at risk for polycystic ovary syndrome. J Clin Endocrinol Metab 2007;92:878–896.

16 Klein KO, Mericq V, Brown-Dawson JM, Larmore KA, Cabezas P, Cortines A: Estrogen levels in girls with premature thelarche compared with normal prepubertal girls as determined by an ultrasensitive recombinant cell bioassay. Pediatrics 1999;134:190–192.

17 Paris F, Servant N, Terouanne B, Balaguer P, Nicolas JC, Sultan C: A new recombinant cell bioassay for ultrasensitive determination of serum estrogenic activity in children. J Clin Endocrinol Metab 2002; 87:791–797.

18 Courant F, Aksglaede L, Antignac JP, Monteau F, Sørensen K, Andersson AM, Skakkebæk NE, Juul A, Le Bizec B: Assessment of circulating sex steroid levels in prepubertal and pubertal boys and girls by a novel ultrasensitive gas chromatography-tandem mass spectrometry method. J Clin Endocrinol Metab 2010;95:82–92.

19 Sørensen K, Andersson AM, Skakkebaek NE, Juul A: Serum sex hormone binding globulin in healthy children and in girls with precocious puberty before and during GnRH agonist treatment. J Clin Endocrinol Metab 2007;92:3189–3196.

20 Sørensen K, Aachmann-Andersen NJ, Petersen JH, Hilsted L, Helge JW, Juul A: Sex hormone-binding globulin levels predict insulin sensitivity, disposition index and cardiovascular risk during puberty. Diabetes Care 2009;32:909–914.

21 Neely EK, Hintz RL, Wilson DM, Lee PA, Gautier T, Argente J, Stene M: Normal ranges for immunochemiluminometric gonadotropin assays. J Pediatr 1995;127:40–46.

22 Neely EK, Wilson DM, Lee PA, Stene M, Hintz RL: Spontaneous serum gonadotropin concentrations in the evaluation of precocious puberty. J Pediatr 1995;127:47–52.

23 Oerter KE, Uriarte MM, Rose SR, Barnes KM, Cutler GB Jr: Gonadotropin secretory dynamics during puberty in normal girls and boys. J Clin Endocrinol Metab 1990;71:1251–1258.

24 Carel JC, Eugster EA, Rogol A, et al: Consensus statement on the use of gonadotropin-releasing hormone analogs in children. Pediatrics 2009;123: e752–e762.

Anders Juul
Department of Growth and Reproduction, Rigshospitalet Section 5064, University of Copenhagen
Blegdamsvej 9
DK–2100 Copenhagen (Denmark)
Tel. +45 3545 5085, Fax +45 3545 6054, E-Mail ajuul@rh.dk

Sultan C (ed): Pediatric and Adolescent Gynecology. Evidence-Based Clinical Practice. 2nd, revised and extended edition. Endocr Dev. Basel, Karger, 2012, vol 22, pp 40–55

Diagnostic Methods in Pediatric and Adolescent Gynecology

Dvora Bauman

Pediatric and Adolescent Gynecology, Bikur Holim Hospital, Jerusalem, Israel

Abstract

The evolving role of imaging techniques and endoscopic tools used in gynecologic practice has become essential over the last several years. Pelvic organs of the young girl are deeply hidden in the abdomen and the vagina is narrow and atrophic. The presence of an intact hymen provides an additional obstacle to vaginal examination. Therefore, bimanual pelvic (vaginal/rectal) examination has a limited advantage in this population. It could cause unnecessary discomfort and hamper further 'patient-doctor' dialog. Imaging techniques are constantly improving in sensitivity, thus providing more accurate diagnoses. Ultrasonography which is a safe and available modality provides real-time images of multiple planes and therefore is ideal for pelvic evaluation. It should be an integral part of child and young adolescent examination. Additional modalities such as CT and MRI should be reserved for cases which are ultrasonography doubtful and be applied as a subsequent evaluation. Vaginoscopy and laparoscopy, although invasive, are used for final diagnosis and provision of treatment as 'see and treat' procedures. These main modalities used in the diagnosis of gynecologic disorders in the young are described in this chapter.

Ultrasonography

Ultrasonography (US) is the modality of choice for imaging the pediatric female pelvis. It remains the most useful modality used in pediatric and adolescent gynecology and often the only one necessary prior to therapeutic intervention.

The principle of ultrasound involves the use of high-frequency sound waves to detect the interface of two tissues with different densities. Energy is reflected based on the density of the tissue and converted into two- or three-dimensional images.

Three approaches utilizing different ultrasonic probes, might be applied for imaging of the female pelvis. The transabdominal sector probe is most widely used in pediatric gynecology and suffices for most indications. Transvaginal probe used only in sexually active adolescents and the perineal approach may be useful in young children with lower genital tract pathologies.

The high-frequency transducers applied to scan the pelvic organs, varying in wavelength, are based upon the age of the patient and the distance of the pelvic viscera from the scanned area. Neonates are classically examined with 9- to 7.5-MHz transducers, children's pelvis best visualized with 5- or 7.5-MHz transducers and teenagers with the 5- to 3.5-MHz transducers.

Abdominal sonographic imaging requires an adequately distended urinary bladder which allows transmissions of sound into deeper structures of the pelvis and displaced gas-filled bowel loops out of the pelvis allowing easier identification of the uterus and ovaries. This can be achieved by hydration either by drinking, the common use, or by intravenous supply of fluids in patients with impending surgical intervention. In very young infants who cannot hold a distended bladder, a 100 ml fluid package could be placed on the infants lower abdomen with the US probe scanning through this 'artificial' bladder [1].

Doppler US and color Doppler imaging are based on sound waves that encounter a moving object; the reflected frequency is changed and can be detected. This shift in frequency is proportional to the velocity of the moving object and can be used to evaluate blood flow. It allows rapid identification of normal vessels and abnormal vascular structure, thus making the diagnosis more accurate [2].

Normal Ultrasonographic Anatomy of Genital Organs in Children and Adolescents

The Uterus

Uterine anatomy changes during childhood. The neonatal uterus is enlarged under the influence of maternal and placental hormones. The cervix is more prominent than the fundus (fundus-to-cervix ratio = 1/2), the uterine length is approximately 3.5 cm, and the maximum thickness is approximately 1.4 cm, with echogenic endometrial lining. Some fluid can also be seen within the endometrial cavity in about 25%.

In the prepubertal child, during the remarkable decline in sex steroids levels between the ages of 6–12 months up to puberty, the size of the uterus and ovaries decrease progressively. The uterus develops a tubular configuration (anteroposterior cervix equal to anteroposterior fundus) or sometimes a spade shape (anteroposterior cervix larger than anteroposterior fundus). The length is approximately 2.5 cm and the thickness does not exceed 10 mm. The endometrium is normally not apparent; however, high-frequency transducers can demonstrate the central lining in some cases (fig. 1).

At puberty when the hormones achieve the adult levels, the uterus gets the adult pear configuration (fundus larger than cervix) (fundus-to-cervix ratio = 2/1 to 3/1) and is 5–8 cm long, 3 cm wide, and 1.5 cm thick. The endometrial lining is seen and varies with the phases of the menstrual cycle. Difference in bladder distension can modify the uterine shape [3].

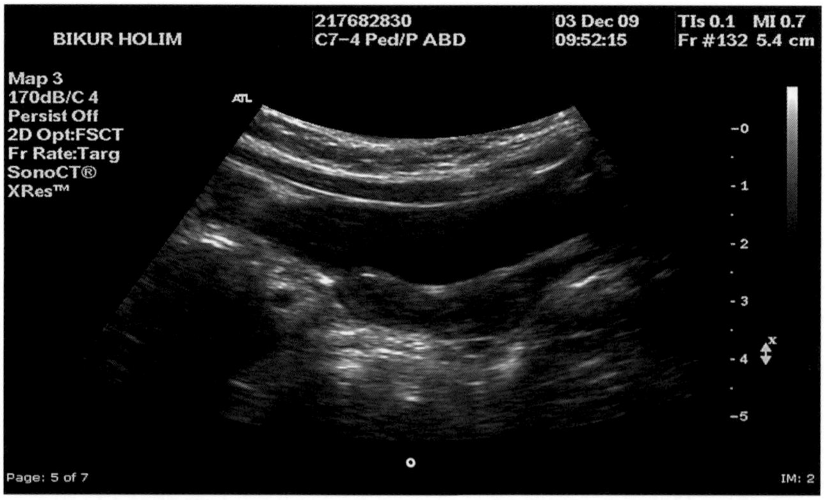

Fig. 1. Infantile uterus.

The Ovaries

Ovarian size is usually described by assessment of the ovarian volume: V = 1/2 length • width • depth (simplified formula for a prolate ellipse). In infants, measurements are slightly greater than 1 cm^3 for the first year of life and 0.67 cm^3 for the second year. The mean ovarian volume in girls less than 6 years of age is less than or equal to 1 cm^3 (fig. 2).

The increase in ovarian volume begins after 6 years of age at the time of increasing hypothalamic activity. In prepubertal girls (6–10 years old), ovarian volumes range from 1.2 to 2.3 cm^3, with the upper limit for normal size up to 4–5 cm^3. In premenarchal girls (11–12 years old), it ranges from 2 to 4 cm^3. After menarche, the ovarian volume reaches the normal adult size –8 cm^3 (range, 2.5–20 cm^3) [4].

The ovary contains follicles at all ages, usually <9 mm in size in the prepubertal period. Those follicles are routinely imaged (in 84% of cases from birth to 24 months of age and in 35.5% of cases between 2 and 9 years of age) [5] (fig. 3).

The normal size of the ovaries and the uterus during childhood and adolescence is listed in table 1.

Ultrasonography appears as a useful tool in the follow-up of puberty process.

Pubertal development is characterized by increased gonadotropic activity and heightened estrogen levels. Estrogen stimulation is indicated by thickness and volume of the uterus, swelling of the fundus and the presence of an echogenic endometrium. The appearance of the ovaries is less useful because of the overlapping measurements and because of the normal visibility of follicles at all ages.

Doppler of the uterine artery is a useful complementary parameter to follow puberty. The narrow systolic flow waves found in prepubertal girls is progressively

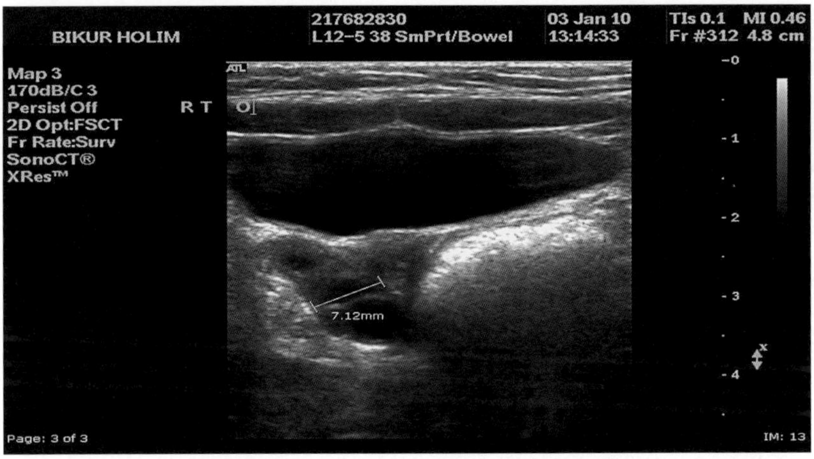

Fig. 2. Prepubertal ovaries. Note the presence of small follicles.

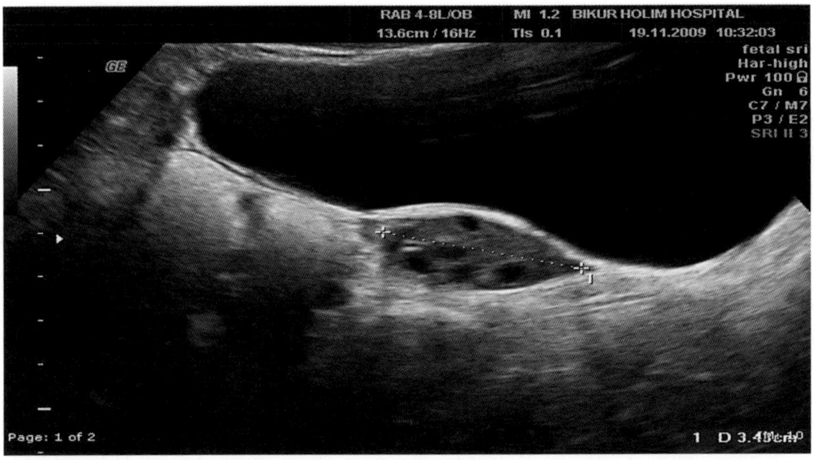

Fig. 3. Normal appearance of ovary at the beginning of puberty (microcystic). Note the small multiple follicles.

Table 1. Normal volume of the ovaries and uterus

Age	Ovarian volume ml	Uterine volume ml	Uterine shape	Endometrial stripe
Neonate	1–3.6	2.6–4	spade shape	echogenic
3 months to 1 year	1–2.7	0.8-1-.3	tubular shape	hypoechoic
1–2 years	<1–1.6	0.8–1.3	tubular shape	hypoechoic
2–8 years	1–4.3	0.8–1.6	tubular shape	hypoechoic
8–16 years	2–18.3	0.8–25	pear shape after puberty	cyclical changes after puberty

Adapted with permission from Stranzinger and Strouse [4].

replaced by a systolic-diastolic flow wave. This modification of the Doppler pattern will appear earlier than the changes in size and morphology of the internal genital organs [2].

Ultrasonographic Imaging of Pathologic Conditions

Precocious Puberty

The erroneous pubertal development occurring before the age of 8 years old is defined as precocious puberty.

US can demonstrate adult size ovaries with increase in follicle size and number. The uterus changes from tubular shape to pear shape with increased echogenicity and thickness of the endometrium. Prominent endometrium suggests that pubertal concentrations of estrogen have been attained and can be used for monitoring of effective inhibitory treatment. Endometrium of 6–8 mm thickness implies imminent menarche.

These changes are expected in true precocious puberty but not in premature isolated telarche or adrenarche.

Doppler study of uterine artery is helpful in the follow-up of girls with precocious puberty, the technique will also help to monitor the effect of medical treatment [6].

Ambiguous Genitalia

Most cases of ambiguous genitalia consist of female pseudohermaphroditism due to congenital adrenal hyperplasia. The role of sonography in sex assignment is to document the presence of uterus and ovaries. The clinical signs of ambiguous genitalia together with the US findings of a uterus and enlarged adrenals are almost pathognomonic of congenital adrenal hyperplasia. Absence of the ovaries (the very small uterus could be missed) should rise the suspicion of XY genotype.

Foreign Body

Vaginal bleeding and blood-stained, foul-smelling discharge are considered to be the main clinical manifestations of vaginal foreign bodies. Although not infrequent in occurrence, the insertion of the object is often forgotten by the child. Toilet tissue in the form of amorphous material is the most common type of vaginal foreign body found and it is usually radiolucent and can occasionally be demonstrated as a slight indentation of the posterior bladder wall [7].

Sonographic vaginogram performed by retrograde injection of water into the vagina while viewing the vaginal lumen transabdominally can improve the detection of a foreign body [8].

Turner Syndrome

Patients with XO karyotype have a prepubertal uterus (could be even undetectable) and nonvisualized or streaky ovaries. In girls with Turner's mosaic karyotype (40–

50%), varying ovarian activity has been demonstrated. In those patients ultrasound antral follicular count (AFC) may be used for predicting future fertility, contributing to decision whether perform early ovarian cryopreservation [9].

US might be useful in the monitoring of hormone replacement treatment for achieving sexual characteristics and estrogen treatment should be followed by adding cyclic progesterone just after pubertal concentrations of estrogen have been attained, as demonstrated by thickening of the endometrium.

Obstructive Uterovaginal Anomalies

Teenagers with obstructive uterovaginal anomalies present with amenorrhea and cyclic abdominal pain. Imperforated hymen, most frequent anomaly, sonographically characterized by a fluid-filled mass posterior to the bladder representing the dilated vagina (hematocolpus) and possibly a fluid-filled uterus (hematometrocolpos).

Sonographically, the fluid-filled vagina appears as an oval thin-walled structure with absent or low level internal echoes or may contain a urine mucus level.

US is very valuable in differentiating the frequent case of hemato(metro)colpos due to imperforate hymen or transverse vaginal septum from the rare case of hematometra due to cervical dysgenesis or other Müllerian system anomalies. The diagnosis of those in the pediatric age is possible if there is high grade of suspicion. In girls with Mayer-Rokitansky-Kunster-Hauser syndrome, functioning endometrial tissue may present in 6–10% as unilateral hematometra and cause cyclic abdominal pain. Renal anomalies such as renal agenesis and pelvic kidney occur in 30–50% of the cases [10].

Three-Dimensional Sonography

Three-dimensional ultrasound has improved the ability to characterize congenital uterine anomalies, but may still be limited in patients where the uterine horns are incompletely visualized secondary to patient body habitus or bowel gas. The visualization of the external uterine contour is important in the distinction between bicornuate and septate uteri since a uterine septum can be removed with hysteroscopic resection. The distinction criteria are summarized in table 2, based on the external contour of the uterus and the depth of fundal midline indentation.

Pelvic Pain

US is the initial imaging modality in children or adolescents with acute or subacute pelvic pain.

Adnexal Torsion

Torsion of the ovarian pedicle is the fifth most common gynecologic emergency, occasionally resulting in late diagnosis and treatment due to inconsistency of its clinical presentation. The most common ultrasound finding in ovarian torsion is an enlarged ovary, more than double in size compared to the normal ovary. The involved ovary may have multiple enlarged follicles at the periphery measuring

Table 2. Criteria for fundal contour in the distinction between bicornuate and septate uteri

Bicornuate uterus	Septate uterus	Author, year
>10 mm indentation	≤10 mm	Fedele, 1989
Flat or concave	convex	Carrington, 1990
≥10 mm indentation	flat or convex	Letterie, 1995
Not specified	flat or convex	Fielding, 1996
Fundal midpoint <5 mm over the interostial line, or below it	over the interostial line	Homer, 2000

Adapted with permission from Levine [10].

8–12 mm in diameter, these cysts seem related to transudation of fluid into the follicles as a result of vascular congestion (found in 74% of twisted ovaries). The ovarian parenchyma shows a spectrum of findings ranging from edema to necrosis [11].

Absence of flow at color Doppler US is not a reliable diagnostic criteria because Doppler waveforms are not obtained in about 30% of normal ovaries in young girls. Indeed, arterial flow (peripheral or even central) can be seen in surgically proved twisted ovaries, reflecting the dual blood supply from the uterine and ovarian vessels. The whirlpool sign, visible as a clockwise or counterclockwise wrapping of the hypoechoic vessels around the central axis, was demonstrated in all cases with approved torsion [12].

Pelvic Inflamatory Disease

Clinical presentation may have vague symptoms and signs. Ultrasonographic imaging supplies additional clues to the diagnosis.

In the early stage, an 'ill-defined uterus' can be seen due to indistinct demarcation between the uterus and ovaries. When pyosalpinx is presented, a tubular structure containing internal echoes can be observed. In the late stage of the disease, the tubo-ovarian abscess presents initially as a solid mass and may appear later, when necrosis and liquefaction occurs, as a uni- or multilocular cystic mass with irregular, thickened walls. Color Doppler imaging can show hypervascularization of the inflamed ovary [13].

Chronic Pelvic Pain

Abnormalities causing chronic pelvic pain as endometriotic implants, adhesions and others are hardly seen on US. Pelvic congestion syndrome occasionally involved in the pathogenesis of chronic pelvic pain can be demonstrated as positive Doppler flow in enlarged multiple tortuous hypoechoic vessels that are consistent with pelvic varices [14].

Ovarian Masses

Ovarian Cysts

Functional ovarian cysts are the most common cystic pelvic mass. Sonographically detected cysts are present in 84% of ovaries identified during the first 2 years of life and in 68% of ovaries identified in children aged 2 through 12 years.

The size of normal ovarian follicles in children is usually 9 mm in diameter. However, cysts up to 2 cm are still defined as follicles. Larger cysts (more than 2 cm) may be pathologic, particularly if persistent. Follow-up ultrasound of ovarian cysts is recommended to ensure resolution.

Other cystic masses which can be seen in the pelvis include hematocolpos, ovarian neoplasms, mesenteric cysts, meconium pseudocysts, duplication cysts, urachal remnants, Meckel diverticulum, ureteroceles, dilated ureters, hydronephrosis, vascular and lymphatic malformations, abscess, hematoma and endometrioma.

Hemorrhagic Ovarian Cyst

Ultrasonography imaging of a corpus luteum cyst shows a complex adnexal mass with increased through transmission, thus reflecting its cystic nature. Free fluid can often be observed. Hemorrhagic cysts are avascular at color Doppler sonography. A changing sonographic appearance over time caused by clot lysis is an important diagnostic feature [3].

Ovarian Neoplasms

Benign tumors and functional cysts are much more common than any malignant ovarian tumor in the young patient (2/3 benign, 1/3 malignant) and sonography can suggest a histological diagnosis in up to 50% of the cases (fig. 4).

Benign mature teratoma (Dermoid cyst), the most frequent neoplasm, is commonly discovered by chance. It has a typical appearance of hypoechoic mass with an echoic/solid nodule associated with distal acoustic shadowing representing either calcification or mixture of sebum, air and teeth (fig. 5).

Knowing the high sensitivity of US diagnosis (97.4%) as well as the low malignant potential (0.17%), those tumors could be followed up conservatively [15].

Malignant pelvic neoplasms of gynecologic origin are rare in children and include sex cord stromal tumors (granulosa cell, theca cell, fibroblast, Leydig and Sertoli cells) and germ cell tumors (dysgerminoma, malignant teratoma, endodermal sinus tumor, embryonal carcinoma, choriocarcinoma).

Indicators of malignancy at US are mostly the presence of peritoneal implants, ascites, lymphadenopathy, or hepatic metastases; the characteristics of the mass are less indicative.

Vaginal rhabdomyosarcoma (botryoid) appears as a large heterogeneous or hypoechoic mass posterior to the bladder; the mass effect may cause distortion of the bladder base [4].

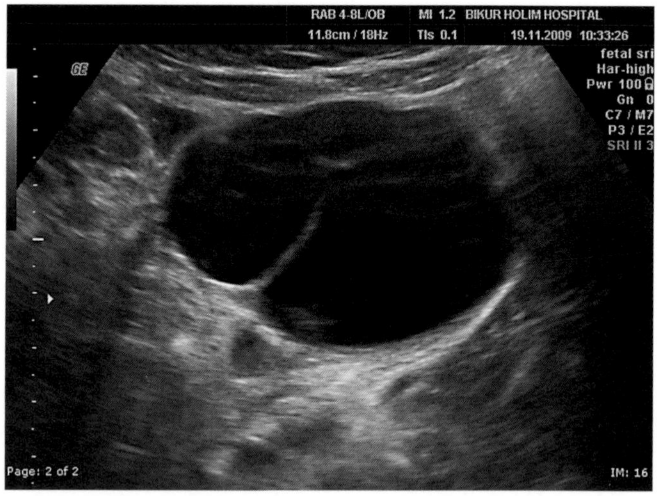

Fig. 4. Ovarian serous cystadenoma in a 9-year-old girl.

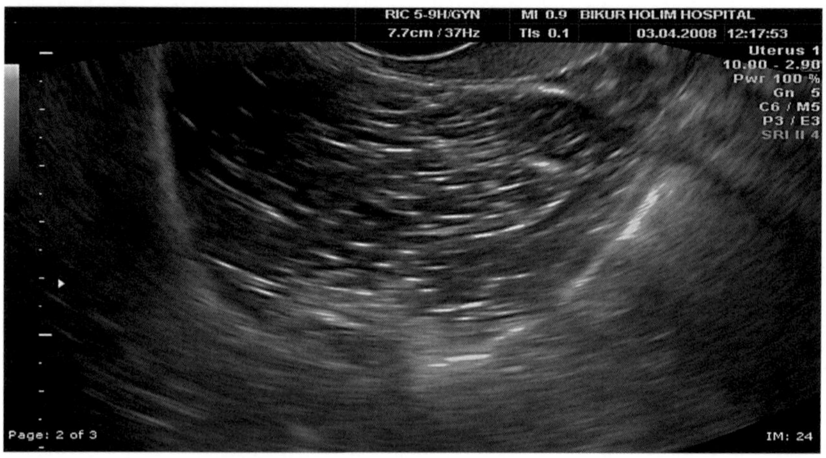

Fig. 5. Mature cystic teratoma (dermoid cyst). Note the typical 'snow storm' appearance.

Polycystic Ovaries

There is growing acceptance that polycystic ovaries, as appearing on US, are important markers of polycystic ovary syndrome (PCOS).

Ovaries are enlarged 1.5–3 times larger and more echogenic than normal with stromal hypertrophy. Multiple small immature cortical cysts are seen at the periphery of the ovary (fig. 6). The current ultrasound guidelines supported by the ESHRE/ASRM consensus characterize the polycystic ovary as containing 12 or more follicles measuring 2–9 mm and/or an increased ovarian volume of >10 cm^3. The cutoff value for an increased ovarian volume was derived from cumulative reports of a larger

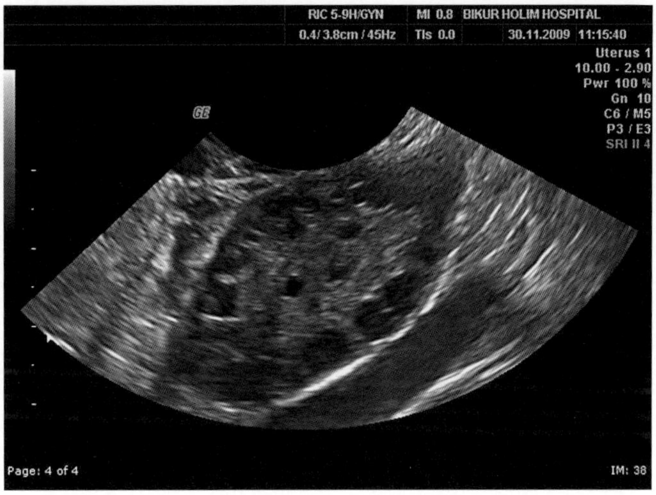

Fig. 6. Polycystic ovary in a 16-year-old patient.

mean volume for polycystic ovaries compared to a mean volume of <10 cm^3 for normal ovaries. A subjective assessment of stromal echogenicity and follicle distribution pattern is no longer included [16].

Computed Tomography and Magnetic Resonance Imaging

These techniques, although less available and not easy performed as sonography, may still be advantageous when the sonographic findings are incomplete or inconclusive. In these cases, CT and MRI are helpful in clarifying abnormalities.

The choice between CT and MRI should take into account the need to sedate (especially for MRI), accessibility to the technique (especially for MRI), and irradiation (CT).

Conscious sedation is usually required for CT and MRI of young children. MRI often requires a relatively longer examination period and is extremely sensitive to motion artifact, so most patients younger than 7 years of age require sedation.

Computed Tomography

The principles of CT involve variable attenuation (absorption) of an X-ray beam as it passes through tissue based on the tissue's density, providing the computer with information to generate cross-sectional images. The technological advantage of CT is that CT can distinguish a difference in tissue attenuation of 0.1%, unlike conventional radiographs that record differences in attenuation of about 10%, preventing detailed characterization of various soft-tissue densities.

For ovarian masses, CT allows delineation of the lesion and surpasses US and MRI in the ability to detect the presence of subtle areas of calcium or fat within

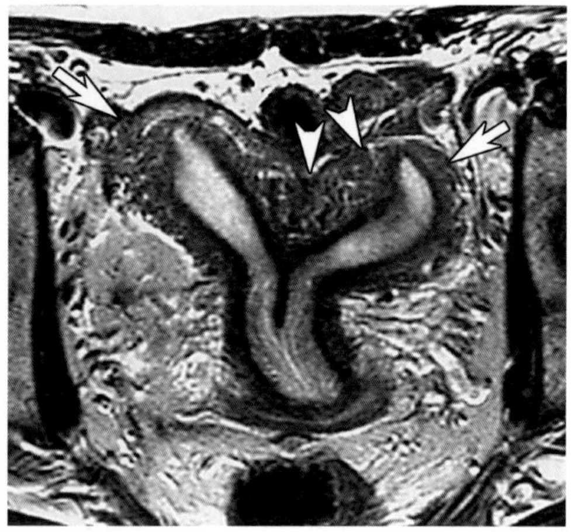

Fig. 7. Bicornuate uterus. Note the concave fundal contour as demonstrated by MRI.

the pelvic mass, which can sometimes be fine and not visible using other imaging techniques.

It can be a useful adjunct to sonography for confirmation of the diagnosis in cases of teratoma (dermoid cyst) because of its ability to characterize the fat and calcification present in most teratomas.

CT remains the most useful imaging modality for tumor staging before operative treatment and for further follow-up [3].

Magnetic Resonance Imaging

MRI is based on the fact that a nucleus with an odd number of protons or neutrons has inherent spin, allowing it to behave as a magnet. MRI takes advantage of the ability to induce and monitor the resonance of the magnetic moment of nuclei in magnetic fields. The interplay of the relaxation times (T1 and T2) and the concentration of hydrogen ions in tissue determine the intensity of signals that are converted to images. Each tissue has a characteristic T1 and T2 relaxation time as well as hydrogen ion concentration, whereby specific characteristics can be detected.

MRI provides precise demonstration of anatomic features in multiple planes in cases of complex anomalies like urogenital sinus or persistent cloaca when US findings are nonspecific (although with the increasing availability of three-dimensional sonography, this is a less important consideration) (fig. 7).

It is particularly useful in evaluating masses of musculoskeletal and those arising in the presacral space [14].

MRI is also helpful in evaluating complex adnexal masses such as endometriomas and cystic teratomas in circumstances where the sonographic diagnosis is unclear. In a study on the impact of MRI on adnexal mass treatment in 49 patients scheduled for surgery, 73% either did not have surgery or had a less-invasive procedure after MR evaluation [17].

It can be more useful than CT in determining the site of the original tumor, local tissue invasion, tumor staging and response to therapy, as well as showing local invasion, inguinal adenopathy and distant metastases.

Endometriosis is a particularly difficult diagnosis in virgin patients. Endometrial implants are scattered throughout the pelvis and abdomen. These are typically not visualized sonographically but can be seen as regions of high signal intensity on T_1-weighted gadolinium-enhanced fat-suppressed images. Since very small lesions can be missed by MRI, laparoscopy remains the gold standard for diagnosis.

The diagnosis of simple hydrosalpinx is typically made by sonography. However, in the case of a complex cystic adnexal mass, it may not be possible to establish the tubular nature of the process by sonography and MRI can be helpful in demonstrating incomplete septations and a separate normal ovary.

In cases of ovarian torsion with nonspecific clinical and sonographic appearance, to suggest an immediate surgical approach, MRI can be helpful. Findings on MRI include enlarged ovary with multiple peripherally displaced follicles. The ovarian stroma is of low signal intensity on T_1-weighted images and of high signal intensity on T_2-weighted images due to the edema. Lack of enhancement after administration of gadolinium is diagnostic.

Vaginoscopy

Inspection of the vagina may be necessary in childhood whenever abnormal bleeding or persistent vulvovaginitis occurs. The narrow hymenal orifice is a significant obstacle to the physician. Traditionally, use of a pediatric speculum can cause unnecessary discomfort and a further psychosexual negative impact.

The vaginoscope is used to minimize invasive evaluation of the vagina without hymen injury. Nowadays, endoscopes are available measuring 3–5 mm in their outer diameter, in accord with the diameter of a hymen orifice. Due to cold light sources supplied by optical fibers, as well as an integrated system magnifying the picture, contemporary vaginoscopes provide fair visualization of the vaginal wall and vaginal part of the uterine cervix (fig. 8). Continuous flow vaginoscopy is performed by irrigating fluid with normal saline (NaCl 0.9%) or glycine 1.5% solution for distension of the vagina and clearing the view. The lubricated hysteroscopy is gently inserted through the vaginal orifice with one hand while the other hand softly compresses the vulvar tissue around the hysteroscope in order to prevent fluid leakage. The diagnostic procedure requires less than 2 min and the child can be discharged after 2 h [18]. Additional equipment, such as forceps used to remove foreign objects, facilitate simultaneous therapeutic management, eliminating the cause of complaints.

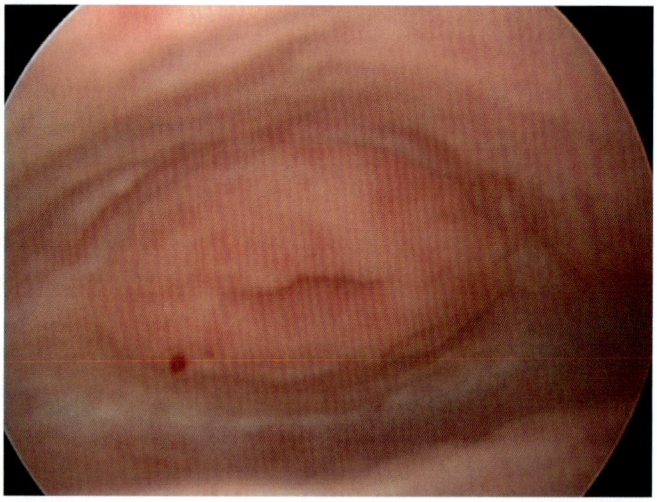

Fig. 8. Vaginal walls and ectocervix as seen by vaginoscopy in a 5-year-old girl.

The necessity of sedation, or even general anesthesia, should always be considered individually based on the age of the patient and taking into account the possibility of psychological injury. For younger children, vaginoscopy under general anesthesia might be the preferred method; however, it can be used as an office-based procedure without anesthesia in virginal teenage girls.

The yield of the procedure was shown to be as high as 36% of the cases with abnormal findings at the time of vaginoscopy performed for abnormal bleeding, prolonged vaginal discharge and suspected anomalies [19].

Abnormal appearance of genitalia or suspected vaginal malformation should be explored by vaginoscopy. The diagnosis transverse vaginal septum is based upon direct visualization. This procedure facilitates precise evaluation of type and localization of the septum. The diagnosis of a complete septum obstructing menstrual blood flow is an indication of early resection of the septum. In case of a partial septum, it is possible to postpone the procedure until the initiation of sexual activity, as the septum has to be removed only when the disorder causes dyspareunia. In case of uterine malformations such as bicornuate or septate, it is recommended to postpone the surgery until fertility desire [20].

The safety, easy implementation and high efficiency of vaginoscopy place it as a useful procedure in the evaluation of vaginal disorders.

Laparoscopy

Laparoscopy, although invasive, still remains the 'gold-standard' diagnostic tool for many pelvic organ disorders, and is often used for final diagnosis and provision of treatment as a 'see and treat' procedure.

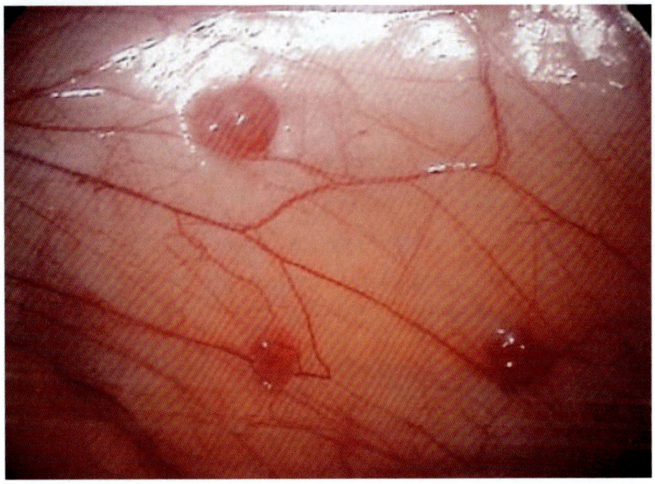

Fig. 9. Endometriosis in an adolescent girl. Note the clear vesicular lesions.

Endometriosis

Even though suspicion of endometriosis is based upon clinical presentation adjunct to physical signs and imaging findings, laparoscopy still remains the most reliable diagnostic modality.

The final diagnosis of endometriosis is histological confirmation through surgical biopsy. Once the abdomen is entered, a careful systematic evaluation of the pelvic and abdominal cavities should be done. A stepwise approach begins with exploring the anterior cul the sac followed by the ovarian fossae and the posterior cul de sac. The uterosacral ligaments should be carefully inspected for fibrosis tethering and asymmetry. Once the pelvis is evaluated, attention is then turned to the abdominal cavity [21].

Evaluation of the peritoneal surfaces is performed by filling the pelvic cavity with saline solution (NaCl 0.9%) and bringing the immersed laparoscope close to the surface, looking for any irregularities such as small clear papules and red lesions (typical in adolescents) [22] (fig. 9).

Diagnosis of endometriosis should not be delayed as it postpones symptomatic relief and may also endanger the patient's future fertility and allow the disease to progress.

Pelvic Inflammatory Disease

Laparoscopy plays a role in the diagnosis and treatment of this devastating condition. The early diagnosis of pelvic inflammatory disease is key to reducing the sequelae of this infection. In situations where clinical diagnosis is difficult, laparoscopy can be helpful [21].

Adnexal Mass

Laparoscopic diagnosis of adnexal masses has been found to be reliable, with a sensitivity of 100% for diagnosis of malignancy. The majority of benign ovarian neoplasms could be managed by means of laparoscopy as well as chosen cases of malignant tumors.

Ovarian Torsion

Sonography is not reliable in the diagnosis or exclusion of ovarian torsion. Thus, a strategy of earlier and liberal use of diagnostic laparoscopy, particularly with characteristic clinical presentation and a pelvic mass of approximately 5 cm, may improve ovarian salvage. Because pathology is predominantly benign, the edematous detorsed ovary is safe to salvage [23].

Müllerian Malformations

The prompt diagnosis and treatment of obstructed uterovaginal or uterine duplication malformations is crucial. Those patients may develop endometriosis from retrograde menstruation as a result of delayed diagnosis and jeopardize their future fertility performance.

Another malfunction diagnosed and treated by means of endoscopic techniques is an asymmetric bicornuate uterus with an obstructed uterine horn. In case of the obstruction and clinical symptoms connected to menstrual blood retention, it is recommended to surgically remove the obstructed horn [24].

The variety of imaging modalities used to demonstrate genital organs of the child and adolescent can bring the physician to the appropriate diagnosis and treatment.

References

1 Garel L, Dubois J, Grignon A, et al: US of the pediatric female pelvis: a clinical perspective. Radiographics 2001;21:1393–1407.

2 Ziereisen F, Heinrichs C, Dufour D, et al: The role of Doppler evaluation of the uterine artery in girls around puberty. Pediatr Radiol 2001;31:712–719.

3 Ziereisen F, Gussard G, Damry N, et al: Sonographic imaging of the pediatric female pelvis. Eur Radiol 2005;15:1296–1309.

4 Stranzinger E, Strouse PJ: Ultrasound of the pediatric female pelvis. Semin Ultrasound CT MR 2008;29:98–113.

5 Qublan HS, Abdel-Hadi J: Simple ovarian cysts: frequency and outcome in girls aged 2–9 years. Clin Exp Obstet Gynecol 2000;27:51–53.

6 Battaglia C, Mancini F, Regnani G, et al: Pelvic ultrasound and color Doppler findings in different isosexual precocities. Ultrasound Obstet Gynecol 2003;22:277–283.

7 Caspi B, Zalel Y, Katz Z: The role of sonography in the detection of vaginal foreign bodies in young girls: the bladder indentation sign. Pediatr Radiol 1995;25(suppl 1):S60–S61.

8 Stricker T, Navratil F, Sennhauser FH: Vaginal foreign bodies. J Paediatr Child Health 2004;40:205–207.

9 Giuseppe L, Attilio G, Edoardo DN, et al: Ovarian function after cancer treatment in young women affected by Hodgkin disease (HD). Hematology 2007;12:141–147.

10 Levine D: Solving the problem pelvic ultrasound with magnetic resonance imaging. Ultrasound Q 2006;22:159–168.

11 Shadinger LL, Andreotti RF, Kurian RL: Preoperative sonographic and clinical characteristics as predictors of ovarian torsion. J Ultrasound Med 2008;27:7–13.

12 Vijayaraghavan SB: Sonographic whirlpool sign in ovarian torsion. J Ultrasound Med 2004;23:1643–1649; quiz 1650–1651.
13 Siegel MJ: Pediatric gynecologic sonography. Radiology 1991;179:593–600.
14 States LJ, Bellah RD: Imaging of the pediatric female pelvis. Semin Roentgenol 1996;31:312–329.
15 Caspi B, Appelman Z, Rabinerson D: The growth pattern of ovarian dermoid cysts: a prospective study in premenopausal and postmenopausal women. Fertil Steril 1997;68:501–505.
16 Jonard S, Robert Y, Cortet-Rudelli C: Ultrasound examination of polycystic ovaries: is it worth counting the follicles? Hum Reprod 2003;18:598–603.
17 Schwartz LB, Panageas E, Lange R, et al: Female pelvis: impact of MR imaging on treatment decisions and net cost analysis. Radiology 1994;192:55–60.
18 Golan A: Continuous flow vaginoscopy in children. J Low Genit Tract Dis 2001;5:85–86.
19 Smorgick N, Padua A, Lotan G, et al: Diagnosis and treatment of pediatric vaginal and genital tract abnormalities by small diameter hysteroscope. J Pediatr Surg 2009;44:1506–1508.
20 Zimmer M, Pomorski M, Wiatrowski A, et al: Application of endoscopy in pediatric and adolescent gynecology. Neuroendocrinol Lett 2008;29: 1–5.
21 Broach AN, Mansuria SM, Sanfilippo JS: Pediatric and adolescent gynecologic laparoscopy. Clin Obstet Gynecol 2009;52:380–389.
22 Templeman C: Adolescent endometriosis. Obstet Gynecol Clin North Am 2009;36:177–185.
23 Oltmann SC, Fischer A, Barber R, et al: Cannot exclude torsion – a 15-year review. J Pediatr Surg 2009;44:1212–1216.
24 Breech LL, Laufer MR: Müllerian anomalies. Obstet Gynecol Clin North Am 2009;36:47–68.

Dvora Bauman, MD
Pediatric and Adolescent Gynecology, Bikur Holim Hospital
IL–97756 Jerusalem (Israel)
E-Mail bauman_d@netvision.net.il

Sultan C (ed): Pediatric and Adolescent Gynecology. Evidence-Based Clinical Practice. 2nd, revised and extended edition. Endocr Dev. Basel, Karger, 2012, vol 22, pp 56–71

Disorders of Sex Development: Neonatal Diagnosis and Management

Françoise Paris[a,b] · Laura Gaspari[a,b] · Pascal Philibert[b] · Laurent Maïmoun[b] · Nicolas Kalfa[a,c] · Charles Sultan[a,b]

[a]Unité d'Endocrinologie-Gynécologie Pédiatriques, Département de Pédiatrie, Hôpital A. de Villeneuve, [b]Service d'Hormonologie (Développement et Reproduction), Hôpital Lapeyronie, et [c]Service de Chirurgie Pédiatrique, Hôpital Lapeyronie, CHU Montpellier et Université Montpellier 1, Montpellier, France

Abstract

The disorders of sex development (DSD) refer to the insufficient virilization of the external genitalia of a 46,XY fetus or the excessive virilization of those of the 46,XX fetus. Some of these disorders are associated with karyotype abnormalities. DSD arise from abnormal gonadal determination or sex differentiation, as in the case of the abnormal testosterone synthesis or androgen insensitivity of 46,XY DSD. The impact of environmental endocrine disrupting chemicals during fetal life requires further investigation. The basic investigations should include SRY gene sequencing and measurement of 17-hydroxyprogesterone, anti-Mullerian hormone, and testosterone. Choosing the sex of rearing is difficult and the decision must be made by an experienced multidisciplinary team.

Malformations of the external genitalia, formerly referred to as ambiguous genitalia, are today categorized as disorders of sex differentiation (DSD) [1]. They are secondary to the undervirilization of the 46,XY fetus or the excessive masculinization of the 46,XX fetus. These malformations are usually discovered in the neonatal period during the systematic examination of the newborn's external genital organs. However, they can also be detected during prenatal ultrasonography. These situations are extremely distressful for the families and optimal management is therefore imperative so that the sex of rearing can be determined as quickly as possible. DSD management is thus the response to a medical emergency. It requires a multidisciplinary team that should include a pediatric endocrinologist, pediatric urological surgeon, geneticist, and psychologist. The clinical, biological and genetic investigations, along with imaging studies and surgical and psychological management, should suggest the better choice of sex orientation or at least the less onerous one.

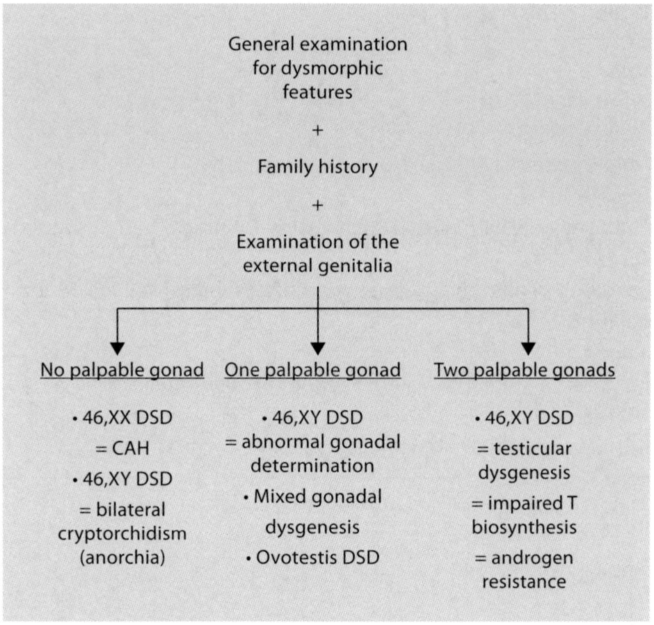

Fig. 1. Clinical orientation for DSD.

Diagnosis of the Disorders of Sex Differentiation

Clinical Diagnosis

A scrupulous clinical examination will permit the diagnosis of a disorder of sex differentiation (DSD) (fig. 1) and will also determine whether it has occurred in a context of malformation. The genital bud, genital ridges (scrotum in boys and labia majora in girls) and urogenital sinus (closed in boys and open in girls) should be very carefully examined. It is important to determine whether the family has had other cases of DSD or neonatal salt-wasting.

In some cases, the external genitalia are 'ambiguous' and are associated with:

- a genital bud that is midway between a penis and a clitoris
- genital ridges that are incompletely fused (forked scrotum)
- the urethral opening on the underside of the penis (hypospadias) or a single perineal orifice at the base of the genital bud, between the genital ridges
- gonads that are impalpable or palpable in the inguinal position.

In other cases the malformation is less clear cut and attention should be focused on:

- bilateral cryptorchidism
- posterior hypospadias
- cryptorchidism associated with hypospadias
- micropenis (<2.5 cm)
- clitoral hypertrophy

Table 1. The Prader scores

Stage 0
Normal female external genitalia
Stage 1
Female external genitalia with clitoromegaly
Stage 2
Clitoromegaly with partial labial fusion forming a funnel-shaped urogenital sinus
Stage 3
Increased phallic enlargement; complete labioscrotal fusion forming a urogenital sinus with a single opening
Stage 4
Complete scrotal fusion with urogenital opening at the base or on the shaft of the phallus
Stage 5
Normal male external genitalia

- a nonvisible vaginal orifice with posterior fusion of the genital ridges in a newborn with female phenotype
- palpation of a uni- or bilateral mass in the inguinal position or in the labia majora.

The degree of the DSD should be evaluated according to the Prader classification (stages I–V) (table 1).

Genetic Investigations

The presence of the SRY gene should be determined with PCR and the results should be ready within 24 h. This will determine whether the case is an undervirilization of a 46,XY fetus or the excessive virilization of a 46,XX fetus. It is essential to determine the karyotype, as this will enable the diagnosis of chromosomal abnormalities like 45X/46,XY mosaicism. However, this type of diagnosis will take from a couple of days to several weeks.

Hormonal Investigations

The hormone work-up should be performed between 6 and 36 h after birth. The following measurements are crucial: 17-hydroxyprogesterone (17-OHP), testosterone (T) and anti-Mullerian hormone (AMH). If possible, follicle-stimulating hormone (FSH), luteinizing hormone (LH), and delta4androstenedione (Δ4A) measurements should be associated.

High 17-OHP suggests congenital adrenal hyperplasia (CAH), which is usually due to a deficiency in 21-hydroxylase that results in a 46,XX DSD.

The values of T and AMH are crucial for evaluating DSD with the 46,XY karyotype. The T, FSH and LH levels should be reevaluated during the minipuberty

Table 2. Comparison between the old and new DSD classification (ESPE Consensus, 2006)

Previous classification *Sexual ambiguities*	New classification *Disorders of sexual development*
MPH (male pseudohermaphrodisms)	46,XY DSD
FPH (female pseudohermaphrodisms)	46,XX DSD
True hermaphroditism	Ovotestis, DSD
46,XX male	46,XX testicular DSD
45,XO, 46,XX Klinefelter syndrome 47,XXY	DSD with chromosomic abnormalities

(days 15–90), which is the period of activation of the hypothalamic-pituitary-gonadal axis. During other periods, T and its precursors should be evaluated after the hCG stimulation test. Most often the long test is used (1,500 IU 1d/2 × 7). All these investigations should be able to differentiate 46,XY DSD secondary to insufficient androgen production (gonadal dysgenesis or defective androgen synthesis) from those secondary to androgen resistance associated with normal T production.

Imaging

Fetal ultrasonography sometimes reveals a uterus. Genitography can show evidence of Mullerian derivatives. Urogenital endoscopy under general anesthesia can be used to specify the implantation height of the Mullerian cavity when it is present.

Causes of DSD in Newborns

According to the 2006 consensus statement of the ESPE [1] (table 2), we differentiate between 46,XX DSD, 46,XY DSD, DSD with ovotestis, and DSD associated with chromosome abnormalities.

46,XX DSD

46,XX DSD is due to the masculinization of the 46,XX fetus because of excessive exposure to androgens during intrauterine life, whether of endogenous or exogenous origin. It may also be due to abnormal ovarian determination.

Fetal Hyperandrogenism

In the great majority of cases (75%), the 46,XX fetus has been overexposed to fetal androgens in the context of congenital adrenal hyperplasia (CAH). The excessive adrenal androgens produced upstream of an enzymatic block are peripherally converted to T and dihydrotestosterone (DHT) and cause fetal virilization (fig. 2).

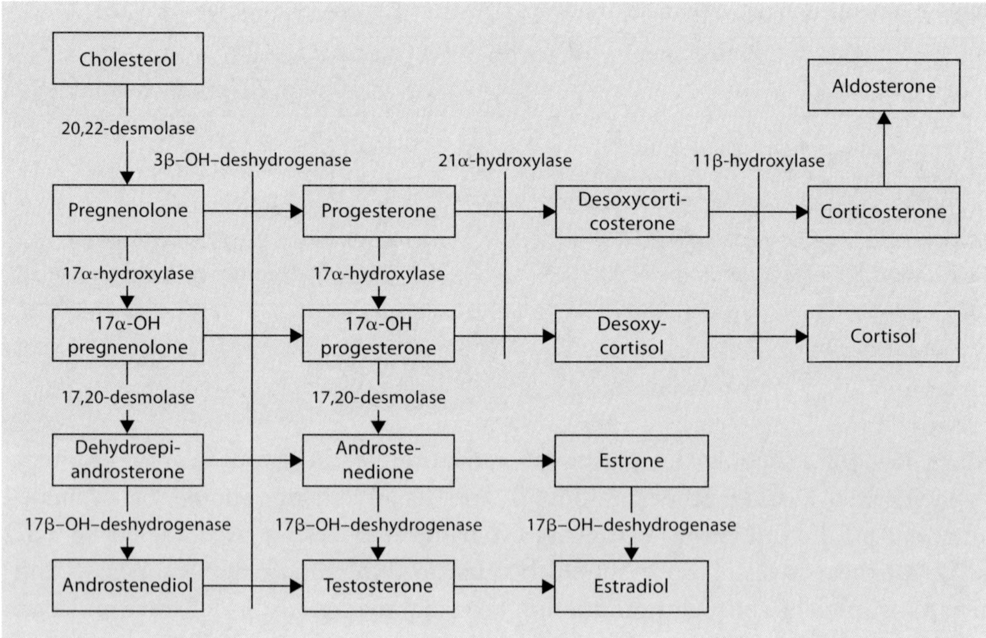

Fig. 2. Steroidogenesis.

21-OH deficiency is the most frequent (90%-95%) of the enzymatic blocks, accounting for 1/14,000 births. Systematic screening with blotting paper is performed on the third day of life. A salt-wasting condition with hyponatremia may be associated with the virilization because of aldosterone and glucocorticoid defects downstream of the enzymatic block. The elevated plasma 17-OHP is generally >50 ng/ml. Treatment with glucocorticoids and mineralocorticoids should be undertaken as soon as possible. Molecular study of the CYP21A2 gene will confirm the diagnosis, since this disorder is transmitted recessively [2]. The sex of rearing of these newborns is almost always female; however, given the excessive androgen exposure during fetal life and the evidence of disturbed gender identification in adulthood, some authors have questioned systematic female orientation in the case of highly virilized CAH [3].

Other forms of CAH can be encountered, though these are rarer. The 11-beta-hydroxylase block is seen in 5% of the cases. No salt-wasting occurs. The diagnosis is based on simultaneously elevated S-component and desoxycorticosterone, and a ratio of Δ4/17-OHP >1 is highly suggestive. Study of the CYP11B1 gene will confirm the diagnosis, since transmission is autosomal recessive [4]. Careful substitutive therapy with glucocorticoids should be undertaken. The 3-beta-hydroxysteroid dehydrogenase block is rare (1%). It associates salt-wasting and moderate virilization. During hormonal investigations, high 17-OH pregnenolone is evident and moderately elevated 17-OHP is also frequently noted, probably due to the effect of the hepatic 3-beta-hydroxysteroid dehydrogenase. An HSD3B2 gene abnormality will confirm the diagnosis, since transmission is recessive [5]. Substitutive therapy with gluco- and mineralocorticoids should be prescribed.

More rarely, the virilization of the 46,XX fetus may be caused by a lipoid adrenal hyperplasia secondary to a mutation of the StAR gene, which codes for the steroidogenic acute regulatory protein (StAR). Transmission is autosomal recessive. The StAR protein is involved in the cholesterol transport in mitochondria, which is the first step in adrenal and gonadal steroidogenesis. Lipoid adrenal hyperplasia is thus characterized by a major deficit in adrenal and gonadal steroidogenesis, evidenced by severe adrenal insufficiency and a female phenotype in both 46,XX and 46,XY fetuses. However, less severe forms – characterized by adrenal insufficiency but less pronounced undervirilization – have recently been reported [6].

The P450-oxidoreductase (POR) deficit is a possible etiology of 46,XY DSD, as well as 46,XX DSD [7]. These forms are dealt with more extensively in the chapter on 46,XY DSD.

Exogenous Hyperandrogenism

This type of fetal hyperandrogenism may be secondary to placental aromatase gene mutation, which is recessively transmitted. This abnormality is rare and is characterized by maternal virilization in the third trimester of pregnancy with spontaneous regression after delivery [8]. Another cause of exogenous androgens is one of the rare ovarian tumors, such as luteoma of pregnancy or maternal adrenal tumors [9].

Abnormalities in Gonadal Determination

Abnormalities in gonadal determination lead to 46,XX testicular DSD, and affected individuals were formerly termed XX males. These patients may present genital abnormalities during the neonatal period or a normal male phenotype. In the latter case, the diagnosis is made in adult life, frequently because of infertility. Since about 10% of patients are SRY negative, other genes are probably involved in testis determination. It has been hypothesized that these abnormalities are secondary to either an underexpression of ovary-determining genes or an overexpression of testis-determining genes [10], and both hypotheses have been reinforced by evidence [11]. Moreover, Camerino et al. [11] reported an RSPO1 gene mutation in the family of a 46,XX patient with male phenotype associated with palmoplantar hyperkeratosis.

Regarding the potential role of the testis-determining genes, the overexpression of the Sox9 gene – which has its major role during testicular development – was reported in a 46,XX man [12,13].

46,XY DSD

46,XY DSD refers to the case of 46,XY newborns with undermasculinization. One or both gonads are usually palpated at birth. The hormonal levels of T, AMH, FSH and

LH, as well as the presence of Mullerian derivatives at pelvic ultrasonography, will differentiate gonadal dysgenesis (associated with insufficient gonadal secretion of T and AMH) from T production defects or T insensitivity.

Gonadal Dysgenesis

Gonadal dysgenesis is a defect in testis determination characterized by a variable alteration in Leydig and Sertoli cell function. This disorder may be secondary to mutations in any of the several genes taking part in the differentiation process of the primitive gonad to a testis.

SRY Gene Abnormalities

SRY gene abnormalities express with a clinical picture of 46,XY sex reversal with female phenotype. If gonads are not palpated at birth, it is probable that the diagnosis will be made in the pubertal period in the context of primitive amenorrhea associated with pubertal delay. However, some patients may present partial pubertal development, often caused by an association with a secreting gonadoblastoma [14]. This picture of 46,XY sex reversal is associated with a SRY gene mutation in 20% of the cases.

Abnormalities in Other Sex Determination Genes

About 80% of the cases of gonadal dysgenesis are not caused by a SRY gene abnormality. They may be secondary to abnormalities in the other genes that take part in testis determination, however, and they are autosomal or X-linked.

Some cases of gonadal dysgenesis have been linked to SF1 gene mutation. This gene is involved in the development of male gonads and the adrenal glands [15]. The phenotype is variable, from severe expression [16] with isolated clitoral hypertrophy to moderate expression with hypospadias or isolated micropenis [17]. Adrenal insufficiency may be associated but is not systematically observed [18].

In some patients, the gonadal dysgenesis is associated with renal dysfunction. In these cases, the diagnosis of Drash syndrome – defined as Wilms' tumor associated with renal insufficiency – or Frasier syndrome – which is proteinuria secondary to focal glomerular sclerosis – may be made. Both syndromes are due to WT1 gene abnormalities that are nevertheless quite specific for each syndrome. In particular, heterozygous mutations in the open reading frame have been associated with Drash syndrome [19], while intron mutations leading to splicing abnormalities have been found in Frasier patients [20].

Sox9 gene abnormalities have been reported. Sox9 is a key gene in early male sex determination [15]. Several mutations have been identified in patients with severe skeletal malformations like campomelic dysplasia, associated in some cases with sex reversal and gonadal dysgenesis [21–23].

Homozygous or composite heterozygous mutations of the desert hedgehog (DHH) gene, which is involved in testis differentiation and perineal development, have been identified. The virilization defect is frequently severe, the phenotype is often female, and a neuropathy may be associated.

A linkage study recently identified an MAP3K1 mutation in two families with several cases of 46,XY DSD, thus indicating another player in male sex determination [24].

In addition, duplications in the short arm of the X chromosome [dosage-sensitive sex-reversal (DSS) locus, DAX1 gene] have been reported in several cases of gonadal dysgenesis. A DSS locus duplication was found in 46,XY DSD patients with female phenotype (46,XY complete dysgenesis). Both the DAX1 (DSS-AHC critical region on X chromosome, gene 1) and NR0B1 (nuclear receptor 0B1) genes have been identified in this locus. The NR0B1 gene belongs to the nuclear receptor family and, through its linkage with other transcription factors such as SF1, it has an 'anti-testis' effect during the process of male sex determination, proportional to the gene dosage. Thus, the overexpression of the DAX gene, as in the case of duplication in a 46,XY patient, may contrast with normal testis differentiation, leading to gonadal dysgenesis [25].

Last, a CBX2 gene mutation was recently identified in a newborn with complete female phenotype but a 46,XY karyotype, which had been determined in the prenatal period because of concerns about maternal age. This testis differentiation abnormality nevertheless differed from the previously presented cases of gonadal dysgenesis in that ovaries with primordial follicles were detected [26]. A mutation in the CBX2 gene, which is known for activating SF1 transcription, was identified in this patient. The CBX2 gene thus seems to actively repress ovarian development in 46,XY gonads.

Defects in Testosterone Production

Defects in T production are rare and are characterized by variable degrees of external genital undervirilization. Conversely, no Mullerian derivatives are present because AMH is normally secreted by the Sertoli cells. These defects are due to an enzymatic defect in T biosynthesis or they may be secondary to an LH receptor gene abnormality.

Defect in 3-Beta-Hydroxysteroid Dehydrogenase

This defect is associated with a variable but insufficient virilization of the 46,XY fetus, ranging from a female phenotype to minor forms of DSD, such as isolated micropenis or salt-wasting conditions. The biological and genetic investigations are the same as for 46,XX DSD.

Defect of 17-Alpha-Hydroxylase

The phenotype in cases of a 17-alpha-hydroxylase defect may also be extremely variable. In some individuals, the diagnosis is made only in the pubertal period because of pubertal delay or stagnation associated with gynecomastia. A desoxycorticosterone excess causes hypertension during puberty. The plasma levels of pregnenolone, progesterone and corticosterone are elevated, which contrasts with the low values of T and D4 that are unresponsive to stimulation. The genetic abnormality concerns the CYP17 gene with recessive transmission.

Defect of 17-Beta-Hydroxysteroid Reductase

This is a rare testicular block that causes a deficit in testicular T production. The phenotype is more frequently female at birth. The diagnosis is based on a striking elevation in plasma D4 contrasting with a low T level. The mutation involves the 17β-HSD type 3 gene, which is expressed only in testis, and its transmission is recessive. Virilization occurs at puberty associated with gynecomastia.

P450-Oxydoreductase (POR) Deficit

A POR deficit may cause 46,XY DSD as well as 46,XX DSD [7]. The cytochrome P450 oxidoreductase protein enables the electron transport from NADPH to P450 cytochromes localized in microsomes. Several cytochromes take part in cholesterol biosynthesis, while three are involved in steroid biosynthesis: P450C17 (17a-hydroxylase/17,20 lyase), P450C21 (21-hydroxylase), and P450CYP19 (aromatase). Transmission of POR gene mutations is autosomal recessive, and the study of several of these mutations has provided greater insight into DSD in association with combined deficits in 21-OH and 17-OH in cases where molecular analysis of CYP21 and CYP17 was normal. In addition to DSD, several patients present craniofacial malformations, suggestive of Antley-Bixler syndrome. The great variability in the phenotype and endocrine findings makes this diagnosis very difficult. This may be due in part to the varying degrees of the enzymatic defects and to the differences in the ability of each mutation to alter enzyme function [27].

Leydig Cell Agenesis or Hypoplasia

This is a rare form of 46,XY DSD, first identified in a patient with female phenotype associated with the 46,XY karyotype. She presented primary amenorrhea and no breast development at puberty, associated with low T at baseline and after hCG stimulation testing. The discrepancy between increased LH and normal FSH levels is generally evocative. This condition is determined by a homozygous or double heterozygous inactivating mutation of the LH receptor gene. Since the identification of these genetic abnormalities, the phenotypic expression has expanded to include conditions that range from ambiguous genitalia to partial forms such as hypospadias or isolated micropenis [28].

Androgen-Resistance Disorders

The androgen-resistance disorders are characterized by normal/high T and AMH production, in contrast to undermasculinization. These disorders are classified as 46,XY DSD, which was previously termed male pseudohermaphroditism with normal or high T.

Androgen Insensitivity

Androgen insensitivity (AI) represents more than 50% of 46,XY DSD in our experience and is caused by a T receptor abnormality. Clinically, a gonad is palpable in the inguinal region in the majority of cases. AI is due to a recessive X-linked mutation that alters the androgen receptor (AR) gene and leads to variable degrees of undervirilization.

Regardless of the initial condition, testes are present and functional, despite cryptorchidism. They secrete T and AMH, and there are thus no Mullerian derivatives, such as uterus, Fallopian tubes or the upper part of the vagina [29]. The AI conditions are classically distinguished by two forms: complete androgen insensitivity (CAI), which is typically monomorphic, and partial androgen insensitivity (PAI), which is conversely far more heterogeneous, with phenotypes varying from Prader scores of I–V (table 1).

CAI leads to the most severe phenotype of a normal female newborn. The diagnosis is often made only in the pubertal period, when primary amenorrhea associated with normal breast development and sparse axillary and pubic hair suggests this diagnosis. This adolescent also presents no acne, which is a further sign of no androgen action on target tissues.

Conversely, PAI is a quite variable condition, with phenotypes expressing all degrees of lost AR function. The range is extremely wide, with the most severe forms characterized by female external genitalia with moderate clitoral hypertrophy to the least severe forms like isolated micropenis [30] or male sterility with no external genital malformation, which is the so-called minimal androgen insensitivity syndrome (MAIS). Between these two extreme conditions, there are all degrees of undervirilization, most frequently with one or both gonads palpable. It is important to note that almost all patients develop gynecomastia in the pubertal period.

The endocrine investigations performed in neonatal PAI patients show normal or high plasma T and AMH, along with a high LH level. Conversely, in CAI patients, the T and LH levels are not always increased. In addition, the LH and T peak level observed around the 6th week of life in normal boys may be absent. The absence of Mullerian derivatives during echography or genitography is an important diagnostic element. An AR gene mutation will confirm this diagnosis. Choosing the sex of rearing at birth is relatively straightforward for CAI patients, who are always raised as females. Conversely, the choice of gender orientation for PAI patients is more difficult and needs to take into account the technical difficulties of virilizing these patients during the pubertal period. It is also important to note the absence of correlation between genotype and phenotype for several AR gene mutations, which may, moreover, express with variable phenotypes within the same family. Since most mutations are transmitted, it is important to screen all women to faciltate prenatal diagnosis.

5αR Deficiency

In the case of 5αR deficiency, T is not converted to dihydrotestosterone (DHT), which is responsible for external genital virilization. The phenotype is usually female, but it may assume all degrees of undervirilization. Clitoral hypertrophy and the association of hypospadias and micropenis were the most frequently reported findings in a recent study enrolling a large cohort of patients with a 5αR defect [31]. If the diagnosis was not made in the neonatal period, it is usually made at puberty because of amenorrhea, absence of breast development, striking virilization associated with hirsutism, clitoral hypertrophy, significant muscle development, and a masculinization in behavior. The virilization is due to the presence of an isoenzyme expressed after puberty. The hormonal investigations usually reveal an increased T/DHT ratio >10. However, 5αR defects have also been identified in patients with a normal T/DHT ratio. The diagnosis of a 5αR deficit should always be considered for a 46,XY DSD patient with increased T and AMH plasma values, regardless of the T/DHT ratio. The molecular abnormality concerns the gene coding for 5αR2. This enzyme is expressed in genital skin and prostate during fetal life and transmission is autosomal recessive; conversely, the 5αR1 enzyme expressed at puberty remains functional in skin. There is high genotype/phenotype variability, as in androgen insensitivity. In severe forms, the gender orientation is often female; conversely, this choice is more difficult in less severe cases. Sex behavior, male identity, pubertal virilization, and preserved fertility in some men with the 5αR mutation [32] provide arguments for male orientation [1].

MALD1 Gene Mutations

CXorf6 or MAMLD1 is a new gene, discovered during a study on myotubular myopathy (MTM1 gene). This muscle disease is associated with genital malformations, since the MAMLD1 gene, which is near MTM1, is deleted. MAMLD1 is temporarily expressed in fetal gonad and may thus take part in fetal steroidogenesis. Mutations in this gene are associated with severe forms of hypospadias in a context of DSD [33]; however, this mutation has been also identified in patients with isolated hypospadias and elevated plasma T [34].

46,XY DSD and the Environment

In some cases of 46,XY DSD with elevated plasma T, no genetic abnormality is identified, leading to the diagnosis of 'idiopathic' 46,XY DSD. In these cases, it is important to investigate the parental domestic and occupational exposure to environmental endocrine disrupting chemicals (EDCs) in order to identify possible fetal contamination.

Over the past 30 years, several studies have reported the undervirilization of wild animals, as well as an increasing trend in the prevalence of external genital malformations in male newborns. This trend includes isolated hypospadias [35, 36], cryptorchidism [37], and the association of two or more external genital malformations [38]. Several EDCs are known to present anti-androgenic and/or estrogenic activity, which has led to the suspicion that these chemicals may interfere with male sex differentiation during fetal life [39]. Moreover, many epidemiological studies have reinforced the EDC hypothesis by evidencing an elevated prevalence of these malformations in especially polluted areas [40, 41], and others have demonstrated an augmented concentration of EDCs in the mothers' milk of 46,XY DSD newborns [42]. In addition, animal studies have demonstrated the potentiating effect of an EDC mixture

[43]. It is thus probable that the environment plays an important role in this increasing trend of external genital malformations [38–44]. We found increased estrogenic bioactivity in three 46,XY patients who were apparently exposed to EDCs during fetal life [45]. However, a geographic variation in the prevalence of these external genital malformations has also been noted, with a sharp north/south gradient in Europe, which has raised the suspicion of a genetic susceptibility to EDCs [38]. In addition to DSD, the incidence of testis cancer has increased parallel to the decline in male fertility. Based on all this evidence, Skakkebaek et al. [46] hypothesized in 2001 that the increasing trend in external genital malformations in males, the decline in spermatogenesis, and the rise in testis cancer have a common origin: fetal exposure to EDCs, or the so-called testicular dysgenesis syndrome.

True Hermaphroditism

True hermaphroditism is now called ovotesticular DSD, following the ESPE consensus statement of 2006 [1]. This denomination has the advantage of referring directly to the pathology, which is characterized by the coexistence of testicular and ovarian tissue. The clinical phenotype depends on the predominant tissue and may thus express any degree of DSD. It has also been reported that several virilized patients were diagnosed only in the pubertal period because of gynecomastia and growth stagnation [47]. Diagnosis is based on the histological examination of a gonadal biopsy sample, which generally shows the presence of an ovotestis or ovarian tissue on one side and testicular tissue in the contralateral side. The ovarian tissue is normal; conversely, the testicular tissue is normal in the neonatal period but becomes dysgenetic with age [48]. The karyotype is 46,XX in the majority of these patients, as the SRY gene is found in only 30% of cases, and the 46,XY karyotype is more rarely seen. In much rarer cases, 46,XX/46,XY mosaicism is observed. Female orientation is frequently recommended because of the presence of uterus in 75% of patients and the differentiated ovarian tissue. In addition to DSD management, surgery can preserve the gonadal tissue according to the choice of gender orientation [48].

DSD Caused by Chromosomal Abnormalities

Mixed gonadal dysgenesis is among the chromosomal abnormalities that cause DSD; the karyotype is 45,X0/46,XY. This genetic condition leads to DSD of variable degrees, frequently with an asymmetry characterized by one palpable gonad in the inguinal or scrotal region and the other gonad, generally a streak, in the abdominal region. The presence of Mullerian derivatives, usually on one side only, is confirmed by genitography. The choice of gender orientation may be male or female, depending on the virilization of the external and internal genitalia and the presence of Mullerian derivatives. When female gender is chosen, a gonadectomy is generally performed to eliminate the high risk of gonadoblastoma. When male gender is chosen, the gonads are surgically lowered and fixed in the scrotum to facilitate screening for gonadoblastoma.

In this classification, we find also the Klinefelter syndromes, whose karyotype is 47,XXY. The phenotype is more usually male and the diagnosis is generally made at adolescence because of pubertal delay or stagnation associated to gynecomastia and low testis volume. Much more rarely, this syndrome is associated with a mild defect of virilization such as micropenis or cryptorchidism [49].

Elements for Gender Declaration

The choice of gender orientation should always involve a multidisciplinary team and the decision must be made very carefully. Although the orientation of highly virilized 46,XX DSD is today under discussion, the choice of gender orientation for 46,XY DSD remains an extremely difficult step. The presence of testicular tissue is not an essential factor; conversely, the surgical possibilities and the potential for virilization under treatment at puberty are key factors for orientation:

- in testicular dysgenesis: female orientation is standard if vaginoplasty can easily be performed;
- in testicular T synthesis abnormality: female orientation is advised, since the possibility of performing a masculinizing genitoplasty is low;
- in androgen resistance: female orientation is indisputable in newborns with complete androgen resistance; conversely, in partial forms the female orientation should be considered because of the risk of insufficient virilization at puberty;
- in 5α-reductase deficiency: theoretically, the orientation should be toward male gender since pubertal virilization will enable subnormal penile development, normal pubic hair, and male identity;
- in the rare ovotestis DSD: female orientation is most often adopted.

Conclusions

In conclusion, scrupulous clinical examination and hormonal, imaging, genetic and molecular investigations all lead to the confirmation of DSD diagnosis in newborns (fig. 3).

The families should be informed in a calm and balanced manner of the treatment options and their respective difficulties.

The choice of gender orientation should not be made by one physician, but instead a multidisciplinary team should be involved in all diagnostic investigations, the gender choice, and treatment.

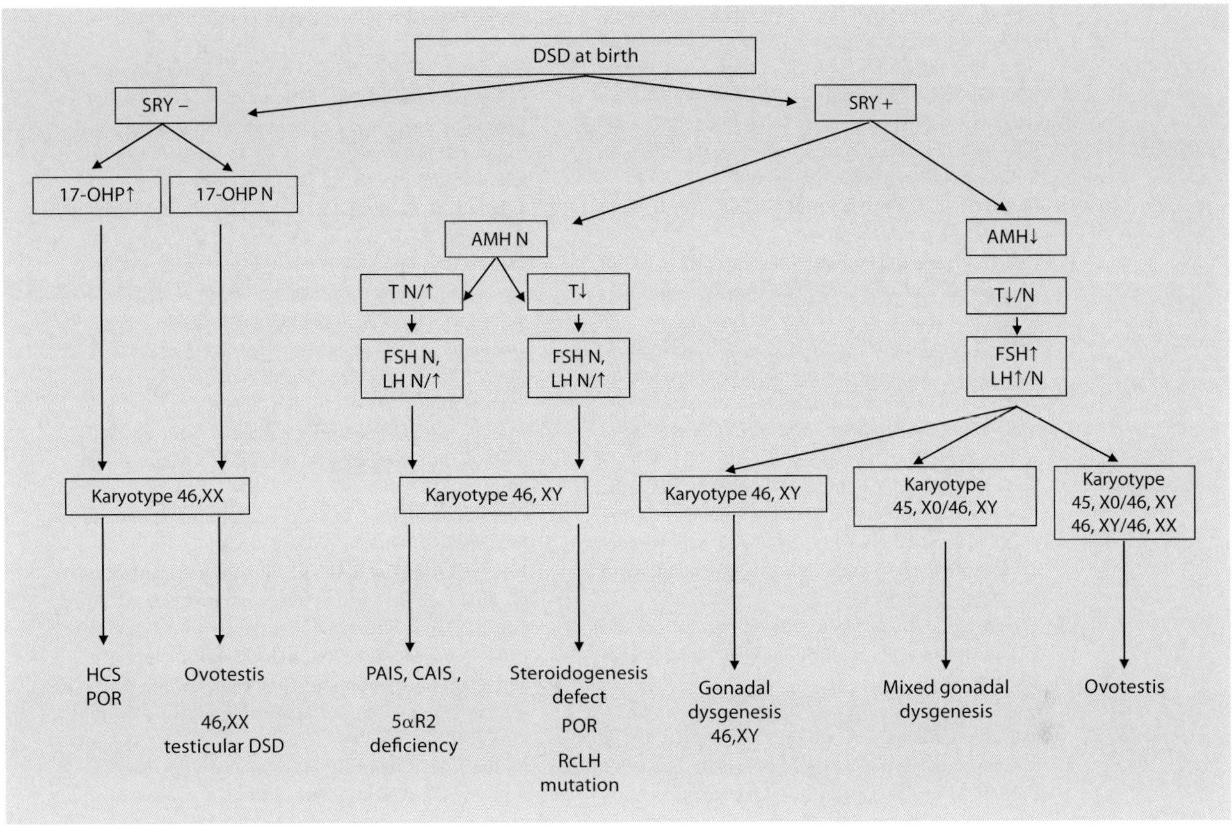

Fig. 3. Management of DSD.

References

1 Hughes IA, Houk C, Ahmed SF, Lee PA: Consensus statement on management of intersex disorders. Arch Dis Child 2006;91:554–563.

2 Balsamo A, Baldazzi L, Menabo S, Cicognani A: Impact of molecular genetics on congenital adrenal hyperplasia management. Sex Dev 2010;4:233–248.

3 Houk CP, Lee PA: Approach to assigning gender in 46,XX congenital adrenal hyperplasia with male external genitalia: replacing dogmatism with pragmatism. J Clin Endocrinol Metab 2010;95:4501–4508.

4 Nimkarn S, New MI: Steroid 11beta-hydroxylase deficiency congenital adrenal hyperplasia. Trends Endocrinol Metab 2008;19:96–99.

5 Krone N, Arlt W: Genetics of congenital adrenal hyperplasia. Best Pract Res Clin Endocrinol Metab 2009;23:181–192.

6 Sahakitrungruang T, Soccio RE, Lang-Muritano M, Walker JM, Achermann JC, Miller WL: Clinical, genetic, and functional characterization of four patients carrying partial loss-of-function mutations in the steroidogenic acute regulatory protein (StAR). J Clin Endocrinol Metab 2010;95:3352–3359.

7 Scott RR, Miller WL: Genetic and clinical features of p450 oxydoreductase deficiency. Horm Res 2008; 69:266–275.

8 Lin L, Ercan O, Raza J, Burren CP, Creighton SM, Auchus RJ, Dattani MT, Achermann JC: Variable phenotypes associated with aromatase (CYP19) insufficiency in humans. J Clin Endocrinol Metab 2007;92:982–990.

9 Spitzer RF, Wherrett D, Chitayat D, Colgan T, Dodge JE, Salle JL, Allen L: Maternal luteoma of pregnancy presenting with virilization of the female infant. J Obstet Gynaecol Can 2007;29:835–840.
10 Hughes IA: Disorders of sex development: a new definition and classification. Best Pract Res Clin Endocrinol Metab 2008:22:119–134.
11 Parma P, Radi O: Forgetting RSPO1. Fertil Steril 2010;94:e39, author reply e40.
12 Cox JJ, Willatt L, Homfray T, Woods CG: A SOX9 duplication and familial 46,XX developmental testicular disorder. N Engl J Med 2011;364:91–93.
13 Refai O, Friedman A, Terry L, Jewett T, Pearlman A, Perle MA, Ostrer H: De novo 12;17 translocation upstream of SOX9 resulting in 46,XX testicular disorder of sex development. Am J Med Genet A 2010; 152A:422–426.
14 Paris F, Philibert P, Lumbroso S, Baldet P, Charvet JP, Galifer RB, Sultan C: Primary amenorrhea in a 46,XY adolescent girl with partial gonadal dysgenesis: identification of a new SRY gene mutation. Fertil Steril 2007;88;1437, e21–e25.
15 Sekido R, Lovell-Badge R: Sex determination and SRY: down to a wink and a nudge? Trends Genet 2009;25:19–29.
16 Lin L, Philibert P, Ferraz-de-Souza B, Kelberman D, Homfray T, Albanese A, Molini V, Sebire NJ, Einaudi S, Conway GS, Hughes IA, Jameson JL, Sultan C, Dattani MT, Achermann JC: Heterozygous missense mutations in steroidogenic factor 1 (SF1/Ad4BP, NR5A1) are associated with 46,XY disorders of sex development with normal adrenal function. J Clin Endocrinol Metab 2007;92:991–999.
17 Paris F, De Ferran K, Bhangoo A, Ten S, Lahlou N, Audran F, Servant N, Poulat F, Philibert P, Sultan C: Isolated 'idiopathic' micropenis: hidden genetic defects? Int J Androl 2011, doi: 10.1111/j.1365-2605.2010.01135.x. [2011].
18 Philibert P, Paris F, Audran F, Kalfa N, Polak M, Thibaud E, Pinto G, Houang M, Zenaty D, Leger J, Mas JC, Pienkowski C, Einaudi S, Damiani D, Ten S, Sinha S, Poulat F, Sultan C: Phenotypic variation of SF1 gene mutations. Adv Exp Med Biol 2011;707: 67–72.
19 Chiang PW, Aliaga S, Travers S, Spector E, Tsai AC: Case report: WT1 exon 6 truncation mutation and ambiguous genitalia in a patient with Denys-Drash syndrome. Curr Opin Pediatr 2008;20:103–106.
20 Bache M, Dheu C, Doray B, Fothergill H, Soskin S, Paris F, Sultan C, Fischbach M: Frasier syndrome, a potential cause of end-stage renal failure in childhood. Pediatr Nephrol 2010;25:549–552.
21 Gentilin B, Forzano F, Bedeschi MF, Rizzuti T, Faravelli F, Izzi C, Lituania M, Rodriguez-Perez C, Bondioni MP, Savoldi G, Grosso E, Botta G, Viora E, Baffico AM, Lalatta F: Phenotype of five cases of prenatally diagnosed campomelic dysplasia harboring novel mutations of the SOX9 gene. Ultrasound Obstet Gynecol 2010;36:315–323.
22 Lecointre C, Pichon O, Hamel A, Heloury Y, Michel-Calemard L, Morel Y, David A, Le Caignec C: Familial acampomelic form of campomelic dysplasia caused by a 960 kb deletion upstream of SOX9. Am J Med Genet A 2009;149A:1183–1189.
23 Okamoto T, Nakamura E, Nagaya K, Hayashi T, Mukai T, Fujieda K: Patient reports: two novel frameshift mutations in the SOX9 gene in two patients with campomelic dysplasia who showed long-term survival. J Pediatr Endocrinol Metab 2011; 23:1189–1193.
24 Pearlman A, Loke J, Le Caignec C, White S, Chin L, Friedman A, Warr N, Willan J, Brauer D, Farmer C, Brooks E, Oddoux C, Riley B, Shajahan S, Camerino G, Homfray T, Crosby AH, Couper J, David A, Greenfield A, Sinclair A, Ostrer H: Mutations in MAP3K1 cause 46,XY disorders of sex development and implicate a common signal transduction pathway in human testis determination. Am J Hum Genet 2010;87:898–904.
25 Barbaro M, Oscarson M, Schoumans J, Staaf J, Ivarsson SA, Wedell A: Isolated 46,XY gonadal dysgenesis in two sisters caused by a Xp21.2 interstitial duplication containing the DAX1 gene. J Clin Endocrinol Metab 2007;92:3305–3313.
26 Biason-Lauber A, Konrad D, Meyer M, DeBeaufort C, Schoenle EJ: Ovaries and female phenotype in a girl with 46,XY karyotype and mutations in the CBX2 gene. Am J Hum Genet 2009;84:658–663.
27 Miller WL, Agrawal V, Sandee D, Tee MK, Huang N, Choi JH, Morrissey K, Giacomini KM: Consequences of POR mutations and polymorphisms. Mol Cell Endocrinol 2011;336:174–179.
28 Mendonca BB, Domenice S, Arnhold IJ, Costa EM: 46,XY disorders of sex development (DSD). Clin Endocrinol (Oxf) 2009;70:173–187.
29 Werner R, Grotsch H, Hiort O: 46,XY disorders of sex development–the undermasculinised male with disorders of androgen action. Best Pract Res Clin Endocrinol Metab 2010;24:263–277.
30 Bhangoo A, Paris F, Philibert P, Audran F, Ten S, Sultan C: Isolated micropenis reveals partial androgen insensitivity syndrome confirmed by molecular analysis. Asian J Androl 2010;12:561–566.

31 Maimoun L, Philibert P, Cammas B, et al: Phenotypical, biological, and molecular heterogeneity of 5{alpha}-reductase deficiency: an extensive international experience of 55 patients. J Clin Endocrinol Metab 2011;96:296–307.
32 Matsubara K, Iwamoto H, Yoshida A, Ogata T: Semen analysis and successful paternity by intracytoplasmic sperm injection in a man with steroid 5alpha-reductase-2 deficiency. Fertil Steril 2010;94: 2770, e7–e10.
33 Fukami M, Wada Y, Miyabayashi K, Nishino I, Hasegawa T, Nordenskjold A, Camerino G, Kretz C, Buj-Bello A, Laporte J, Yamada G, Morohashi K, Ogata T: CXorf6 is a causative gene for hypospadias. Nat Genet 2006;38:1369–1371.
34 Kalfa N, Liu B, Klein O, Audran F, Wang MH, Mei C, Sultan C, Baskin LS: Mutations of CXorf6 are associated with a range of severities of hypospadias. Eur J Endocrinol 2008;159:453–458.
35 Boisen KA, Chellakooty M, Schmidt IM, Kai CM, Damgaard IN, Suomi AM, Toppari J, Skakkebaek NE, Main KM: Hypospadias in a cohort of 1072 Danish newborn boys: prevalence and relationship to placental weight, anthropometrical measurements at birth, and reproductive hormone levels at three months of age. J Clin Endocrinol Metab 2005;90:4041–4046.
36 Lund L, Engebjerg MC, Pedersen L, Ehrenstein V, Norgaard M, Sorensen HT: Prevalence of hypospadias in Danish boys: a longitudinal study, 1977–2005. Eur Urol 2009;55:1022–1026.
37 Cortes D, Kjellberg EM, Breddam M, Thorup J: The true incidence of cryptorchidism in Denmark. J Urol 2008;179:314–318.
38 Main KM, Skakkebaek NE, Virtanen HE, Toppari J: Genital anomalies in boys and the environment. Best Pract Res Clin Endocrinol Metab 2010;24: 279–289.
39 Stoker TE, Cooper RL, Lambright CS, Wilson VS, Furr J, Gray LE: In vivo and in vitro anti-androgenic effects of DE-71, a commercial polybrominated diphenyl ether (PBDE) mixture. Toxicol Appl Pharmacol 2005;207:78–88.
40 Fernandez MF, Olmos B, Granada A, López-Espinosam MJ, Molina-Molina JM, Fernandez JM, Cruz M, Olea-Serrano F, Olea N: Human exposure to endocrine-disrupting chemicals and prenatal risk factors for cryptorchidism and hypospadias: a nested case-control study. Environ Health Perspect 2007;115:8–14.
41 Gaspari L, Paris F, Jandel C, Kalfa N, Orsini M, Daurès JP, Sultan C: Prenatal environmental risk factors for genital malformations in a population of 1442 French male newborns: a nested case-control study. Hum Reprod 2011;26:3155-3162.
42 Brucker-Davis F, Ducot B, Wagner-Mahler K, Tommasi C, Ferrari P, Pacini P, Boda-Buccino M, Bongain A, Azuar P, Fenichel P: Environmental pollutants in maternal milk and cryptorchidism. Gynecol Obstet Fertil 2008;36:840–847.
43 Christiansen S, Scholze M, Axelstad M, Boberg J, Kortenkamp A, Hass U: Combined exposure to anti-androgens causes markedly increased frequencies of hypospadias in the rat. Int J Androl 2008;31: 241–248.
44 Kalfa N, Philibert P, Baskin LS, Sultan C: Hypospadias: interactions between environment and genetics. Mol Cell Endocrinol 2011;335:89–95.
45 Paris F, Jeandel C, Servant N, Sultan C: Increased serum estrogenic bioactivity in three male newborns with ambiguous genitalia: a potential consequence of prenatal exposure to environmental endocrine disruptors. Environ Res 2006;100:39–43.
46 Skakkebaek NE, Rajpert-De Meyts E, Main KM: Testicular dysgenesis syndrome: an increasingly common developmental disorder with environmental aspects. Hum Reprod 2001;16:972–978.
47 Alonso G, Pasqualini T, Busaniche J, Ruiz E, Chemes H: True hermaphroditism in a phenotypic male without ambiguous genitalia: an unusual presentation at puberty. Horm Res 2007;68:261–264.
48 Verkauskas G, Jaubert F, Lortat-Jacob S, Malan V, Thibaud E, Nihoul-Fekete C: The long-term follow-up of 33 cases of true hermaphroditism: a 40-year experience with conservative gonadal surgery. J Urol 2007;177:726–731, discussion 731.
49 Mazen I, El-Ruby M, El-Bassyouni HT: Variable associations of Klinefelter syndrome in children. J Pediatr Endocrinol Metab 2010;23:985–989.

Prof. Charles Sultan, MD, PhD
Unité d'Endocrinologie-Gynécologie Pédiatriques
Département de Pédiatrie
Hôpital A. de Villeneuve
FR–34295 Montpellier cedex 5 (France)
Tel. +33 467 33 86 96, E-Mail c-sultan@chu-montpellier.fr

Sultan C (ed): Pediatric and Adolescent Gynecology. Evidence-Based Clinical Practice. 2nd, revised and extended edition. Endocr Dev. Basel, Karger, 2012, vol 22, pp 72–83

Vulvovaginitis and Other Common Vulvar Disorders in Children

Ellen S. Rome

Section of Adolescent Medicine, Cleveland Clinic, Cleveland Clinic Lerner College of Medicine at Case, Cleveland, Ohio, USA

Abstract

Vulvovaginitis, labial adhesions, and other vulvar disorders occur commonly in children and can provoke high anxiety in both the parent and child. Performed correctly, the pediatric gynecologic examination can diagnose and treat, educate and reassure both parent and child. This examination requires patience, sensitivity, direct communication with the child as well as with the parent, and an open manner that inspires trust in both parties to manage a potentially anxiety-provoking situation. This chapter will review common vulvar disorders, including vulvovaginitis, lichen sclerosis et atrophicus, bubble bath vaginitis, labial adhesions, urethral prolapse, and other common problems. A discussion of childhood sexual abuse is beyond the scope of this chapter, with appropriate references available elsewhere. Practical pearls will be offered to make this exam easy for the primary care clinician and/or subspecialist.

Approach to the Vaginal Exam

Many pediatricians and family practitioners are quite comfortable with palpation of testes during examination of boys from infancy onward. The girls, once out of diapers, may not be looked at again until a first pelvic examination – which the American College of Obstetricians and Gynecologists has now delayed until age 21 years. A key point for physician education is that all girls, from infancy onward, require routine inspection of the external genitalia. Making this a normal, expected part of yearly physicals provides an opportunity to inspect for labial adhesions and other common problems, educate on hygiene and proper terminology, and make sure little girls learn from an early age that 'private parts are private'. This latter aspect can also help parents initiate conversations about 'stranger danger', have a vocabulary and an opportunity to talk about sensitive topics with their child. Moreover, when a gynecologic examination is required due to vaginitis or other symptomatology, the pediatrician has already made the vaginal examination a routine occurrence, minimizing the stress that naturally accompanies vaginal or vulvar problems. The clinician can help the parents learn to answer children's questions simply and directly, with correct anatomical terms, in a developmentally appropriate fashion.

Obtaining a History

The physical examination is shaped by what history is obtained, with vaginal bleeding prompting a separate set of questions than pruritis. Signs of precocious puberty, vaginal discharge in a young child, a pungent smell, or allegations of abuse all prompt a more thorough evaluation. The child should be asked directly if she has any worries or concerns about her body or her health. If the child looks to the parent for guidance, the clinician can redirect questions to the parent or care provider, yet still try to draw the child in with a pertinent question in a nonthreatening way ('Does it itch anywhere? Where?') The child and then parent can be asked about where and when the symptom has occurred; is it in her vagina or bottom ('where she poops', or other culturally appropriate translation), is there any discharge or dysuria (again, with use of vocabulary understandable to the child and parent), use of bubble bath or lotions/powders/ perfumed body washes, funny or distinct odors, bleeding, and duration and timing of the symptom. Lines of questioning by specific disease processes can be found in table 1. In the context of vaginal bleeding or when sexual abuse is a concern, directly ask the child if anyone has ever touched her private parts, with an open-ended next question such as, simply, 'Tell me about it'. This style of nonjudgmental questions creates less opportunity for suggestibility. Questions should be asked nonjudgmentally without stern looks or tone. Good eye contact should be maintained with the child to help ensure that she feels safe to answer, has the chance to ask questions, and can see herself as an important member of the team. Particularly in cases of potential abuse, the child's words should be documented verbatim in quotations.

'The Rules' of the Gynecologic Exam

The gynecologic examination in a prepubertal child provides a real-time opportunity to practice the Hippocratic Oath, 'Above all, do no harm'. Ideally, children have been taught that 'private parts are private' – but that it is okay for a doctor to look at them, especially if Mommy is there. This visit provides an opportunity to educate that it is okay for a physician to do an examination, but that it is not okay for other adults or children to see or touch her private parts. The astute clinician also has the chance to do an informal role play: 'You know that it is okay for a doctor to look at your private parts, with a mommy here. But it's not okay for another adult or teen or child to look at or touch your private parts – that's why we call them private! If someone tried to do

Table 1. Useful questions relevant for specific diagnoses

Suspected problem	Specific questions
Vaginitis	Timing of onset of symptoms Type of discharge Recent infection (Streptococcal, staph, pinworms) Recent or past use of antibiotics Skin conditions (eczema, psoriasis) Methods used for perineal hygiene Use of bubble baths, perfumed soaks/lotions Frequent masturbation noted Sexual abuse questions ('Has anyone ever tried to touch your private parts?')
Abuse	Behavioral changes: timing, onset Somatic symptoms: abdominal pain, headaches Enuresis, especially new Who takes care of the child?
Vaginal bleeding	Growth history Timing of changes noted (pubic hair, breast development) Use of skin creams (may contain estrogen) Family members' use of contraceptives Pattern of bleeding Vaginal discharge History of foreign bodies found in any orifice

that, what would you do?' Parents may not have had the opportunity or trusted their own skill set to initiate this conversation, so the clinician may be role modeling for them, as well. In our clinic, we often hold this conversation in terms of sharing The Rules, with the first one being that 'private parts are private, and it is okay to touch your own private parts in private, but not another person's when you are a child. If they are a stranger, we call that Stranger Danger. But if they are someone you know, it still doesn't make it right, and it is worth talking to your parents and your doctor about that.' The second rule is 'that you don't let poop get near your girl parts. That is why we wipe from front to back (demonstrating), so that the poop stays away from where you tinkle.' Culturally appropriate words can be substituted, but also with reference or translation into the proper anatomical terms. Use of a mirror can be used to help teach a child simple anatomy and the proper way to wipe after elimination. The clinician should use reassuring words when describing findings, e.g. 'everything is in the right place' or 'your vagina looks normal.' The child must feel in total control over the examination; in situations of high anxiety, it sometimes takes more than one visit to complete the examination. In emergent cases, such as traumatic vaginal bleeding, the exam may need to be performed under anesthesia. Use of 'tricks' such as hiding behind drapes, use of headphones, or ceiling murals are not recommended as this

Table 2. Helpful hints on hygiene (adapted from Jonathan Trager, MD)

The Do's
Do wipe from front to back
Do use sitz baths when itchy or irritated
Do pat – don't rub – the vulva dry with a clean towel
Do wear loose fitting clothes
Do take off underwear at bedtime
Do use unscented, nonirritating cleansers
Do use baby shampoo instead of bubble bath to avoid vaginal irritation
Do urinate with knees wide apart to prevent urine pooling in the vagina
The Dont's
Don't use bubble bath
Don't douche
Don't scrub the vulva – treat it gently!
Don't use perfumed soaps or powders
Don't stay in a wet bathing suit for a long time
Don't wear tight-fitting clothing
Don't sleep in restrictive garments or footy pajamas if vaginal problems occur

strategy further allows dissociation if sexual abuse has occurred; rather, the clinician should strive to partner with the child to raise the child's comfort level and make the examination 'safe'. A calm manner, with time to educate and reassure, can do more to promote health in parent and child than use of exam 'tricks.' Useful 'Do's' and 'Don'ts' for the parent and child can be found in table 2.

The Prepubertal Genital Examination

Examination of the child with any vulvar concern should include measuring height, weight, and body mass index, a visual inspection from head to toe, including head, neck, heart, lungs, abdomen, Tanner staging, breasts (inspection with palpation for masses or discharge), and skin for rashes/lesions. Use of gentle traction can help better visualize the external genitalia; in the anxious child, she can be an active participant in the exam by helping with the traction under the clinician's guidance. Hymenal anatomy should be documented; figure 1 outlines various hymenal configurations. The inguinal area should be examined for hernias or masses.

Positioning of the child for the examination should have a goal of demystifying the examination while keeping the patient comfortable. Most children will easily lie supine on the exam table with a parent close by (fig. 2, 3). With the anxious child, the clinician can help her have a sense of control by asking if she prefers to be on the table

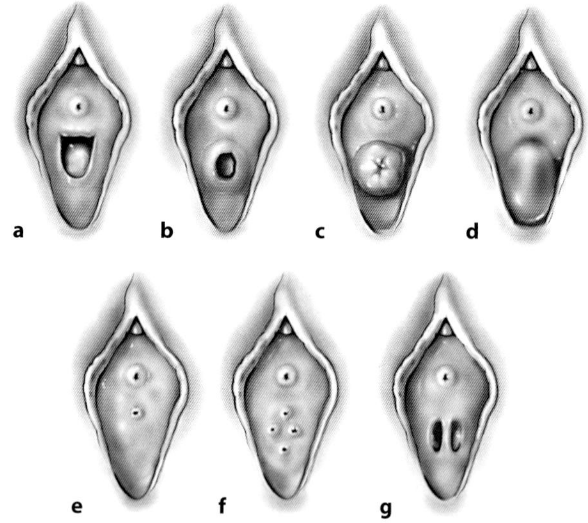

Fig. 1. Variations on hymenal anatomy.

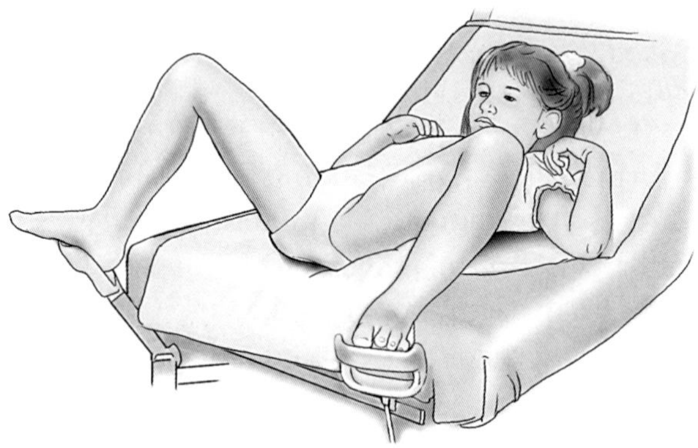

Fig. 2. Child in lithotomy position.

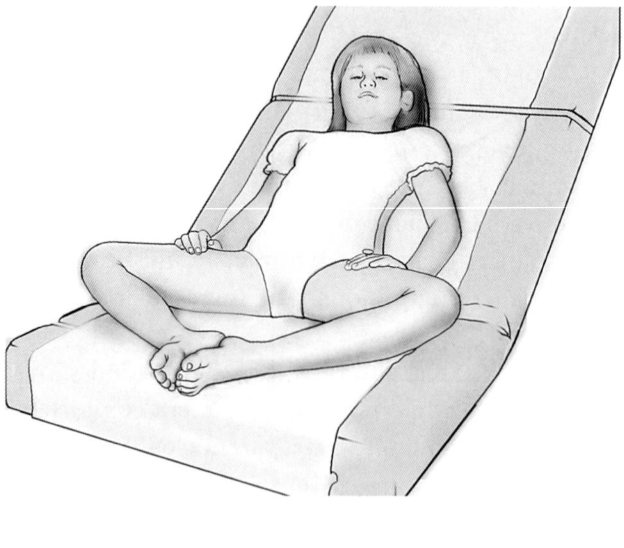

Fig. 3. Frog-leg position on exam table.

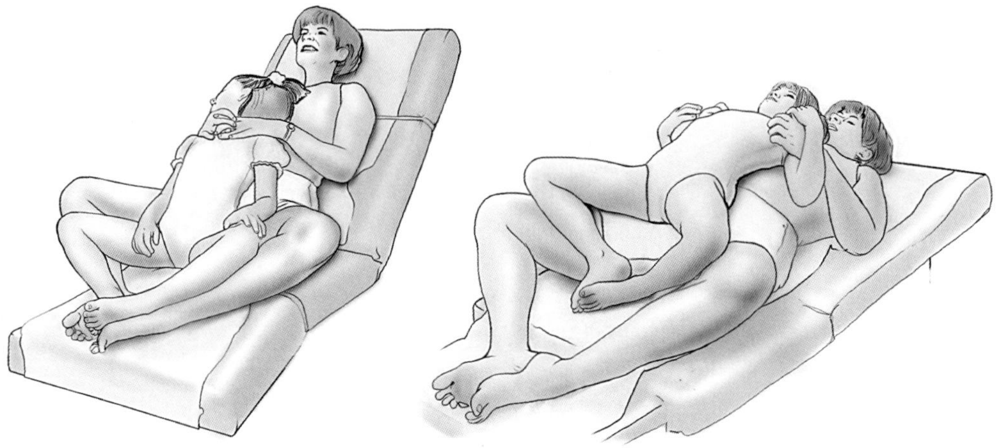

Fig. 4. Child on parent's lap.

herself or on her mommy's lap for the exam. For the latter, the parent can be placed in a semireclining position on the exam table with the parent's feet in the stirrups and the child's legs straddling the parents' thighs (fig. 4). Even fathers can be taught to assume this position, with the child on their lap – a good learning experience all around! In cases of extreme anxiety in either parent or child, this position can be tried with the patient in clothes prior to performing the actual exam. Use of a hand-held mirror allows the clinician to educate the patient (and parent) on normal anatomy while engaging the child in the process. The child can also have a sense of control by being asked to assist in holding her labia apart. The clinician sets the tone – if he or she presents as relaxed and confident, both patient and parent tend to respond positively [1]. An abrupt or hurried approach will exacerbate anxiety and can result in a child's refusal to continue; patience and a calm, confident tone remain essential for the safe examination of the child.

The external genitalia should be examined with use of gentle traction for better visualization, noting hymenal anatomy (fig. 5) and documenting all findings. The vagina can easily be visualized in a frog-leg position. If this position provokes anxiety or concerns about a foreign body exist, the child can be placed in the knee-chest position (fig. 6); the child can be asked to flip over onto her stomach, placing her bottom in the air and her head on her hands, 'just as she might have slept when she was a baby'. An otoscope can be used to illuminate the area, and the child herself or her parent can be recruited to gently spread the buttocks. Two-thirds of the vagina and even the cervix may be visualized using this technique. Foreign bodies can be more easily viewed from this position, with bits of toilet paper or other objects easily removed via flushing. A butterfly catheter of any size with the needle removed can be attached to a tuberculin syringe with 1 ml of saline, and then placed inside a 12-inch red rubber bladder catheter to irrigate the genitalia [2]. This catheter within a catheter can be

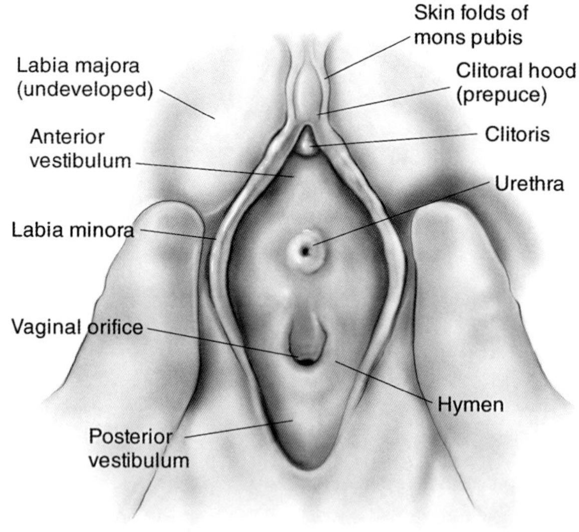

Fig. 5. External genitalia.

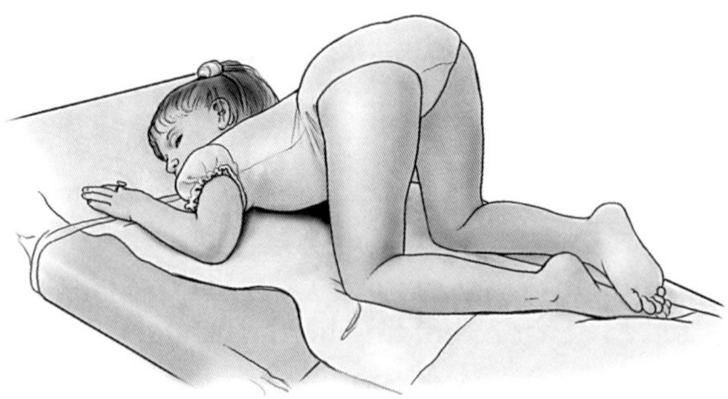

Fig. 6. Knee-chest position.

squirted onto the patient's arm or leg, teaching her how it works, and telling her that it may feel 'cold and wet' (fig. 7).

Causes of Vulvovaginitis in the Child

Poor hygiene, lack of estrogenization, lack of protective hair and labial fat pads, and proximity of vagina to the anus contribute to the frequency of vulvovaginitis in the prepubertal child. Spandex and tight jeans, nylon tights and underwear, wet bathing suits worn poolside or at the beach, and sweat may cause nonspecific vulvar itching or overgrowth of candida, which flourishes in moist areas such as the vagina or folds of the groin. Also common is 'bubble bath vaginitis', or a chemical irritation caused by perfumed soaps, bath soaps/oils or gels. Pinworms (*Enterobius vermicularis*)

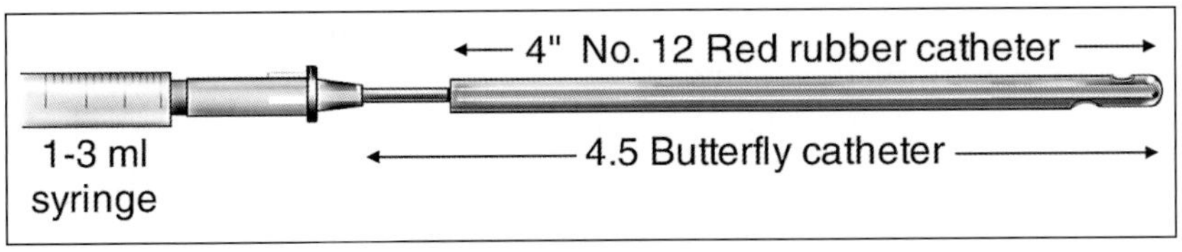

Fig. 7. A catheter in a catheter for irrigation.

remain another common cause of itchy bottoms, with the thin, white worms often seen around the anus at night where they surface to lay their eggs. These ova are easily visualized by pressing scotch tape onto the perianal skin for several seconds, then sticking that tape briefly against a slide. Pinworms are easily treatable with 100 mg of mebendazole, repeated in 2 weeks [1].

In several studies, nonspecific vaginitis was found in 25–75% of cases of vulvovaginitis seeking care in referral centers [3–6]. *Bacteroides, Peptostreptococcus* and *Candida* have been detected more commonly in girls with vaginal discharge and/or with vulvovaginitis than in asymptomatic girls [6]. In a study of 80 prepubertal girls aged 2 to 12 years with vulvovaginitis, pathogenic bacteria were isolated from vaginal swab in 36% of cases, with group A beta hemolytic streptococcus detected in 59% of this group [7]. Pathogenic bacteria (including *Staphylococcus aureus, Streptococcus pneumoniae, Streptococcus pyogenes, Haemophilus influenzae, Moraxella catarrhalis, Neisseria meningitides, Shigella* and *Yersinia entercolitica*) correlated with the presence of leukocytes in vaginal secretions with a sensitivity of 83% and a specificity of 59% [1,7]. Less vaginitis caused by *H. influenzae* may be found in the past decade due to the unplanned yet positive effect of universal vaccination against that organism. *Escherichia coli* vaginal colonization is relatively common in girls beyond the toddler years; it was detected in 36% of girls presenting with vaginitis versus 23% of asymptomatic girls [8]. Another study found that 90% of girls less than 3 years of age had *E. coli* vaginal colonization, as compared to 15% of asymptomatic girls ages 3–10 years [9]. This finding may correlate with improved hygiene with age. In one case report, a prepubertal girl at age 7 and two thirds years was diagnosed with a prolonged course of vulvovaginitis caused by antibiotic-resistant *Shigella flexneri* [10]. Although uncommon in the prepubertal child, bloody discharge should warrant culture using a nasopharyngeal Calgiswab moistened with nonbacteriostatic saline [10, 11]. As noted above, most vulvovaginitis in the prepubertal child is noninfectious; infection correlates with more severe inflammation and vaginal discharge [12]. Also, positive culture may represent colonization rather than true infection. When predominantly one organism grows via culture, clinicians should consider infection.

Treatment of prepubertal vulvovaginitis may often simply consists of removal of the offending agent (e.g. the foreign body, perfumed lotion, or bubble bath) combined with sitz baths. Environmental irritants may include ammonia, bleach or other solutions left in the tub with overzealous cleaning and should be discontinued or better diluted prior to use of the bath. Sexual abuse should be considered when specific patterns of injuries occur or with suspicious histories.

When vaginal bleeding occurs, anxiety can run higher, and the clinician should maintain a sensitive and careful approach. Newborn vaginal bleeding can occur from withdrawal of maternal estrogen. Foreign bodies remain a common cause of bleeding in the toddler and older child. The differential diagnosis for vaginal bleeding includes vulvovaginitis, lichen sclerosis, precocious puberty, urethral prolapse, hemangiomas, and more rarely tumors. A careful history should include timing and duration of the bleeding, any history of trauma, rectal bleeding, dysuria and hematuria, symptoms of vaginitis, pubertal development, and opportunities for potential abuse. Thelarche and adrenarche in a child under 7–8 years of age, especially with accelerated linear growth, may indicate precocious puberty. Thrombocytopenia can be associated with vaginal bleeding, along with evidence of bleeding elsewhere, such as petechiae, easy bruising, or epistaxis [3].

Specific Genital Findings in Prepubertal Children

Lichen sclerosis et atrophicus

Associated with hypoestrogenism, lichen sclerosis occurs in both prepubertal children and postmenopausal women. Symptoms in girls include itching, soreness, dysuria, vaginal or perineal bleeding, and more rarely, constipation. On exam, classically, the clinician will see what looks like an hourglass or figure 8 demarcation of hypopigmented skin from above the clitoris to the anus with scattered telangiectasia, with or without perineal fissuring. Treatment consists of midpotency to stronger topical corticosteroids, with the goal of providing relief with the lowest steroid formulation possible. Mid-potency steroids include hydrocortisone valerate 0.2% (Westcort); high potency steroids include fluocinonide 0.05% (Lidex). Rarely, a patient will need a super-potent steroid, such as clobetasol proprionate 0.05% (Temovate) or halobetasol proprionate 0.05% ointment (Ultravate). Creams will sting more than ointments when applied to a sensitive area. Emollients such as diaper rash ointments, Vaseline or Aquaphor can also help. The steroid cream can be applied sparingly twice a day for 2 weeks, then once a day for 2–4 weeks, then every other day for 2 weeks. Chronic use of steroids can lead to atrophy, telangiectasias, striae, hypopigmentation, and superinfection (fungal or viral), so the clinician must educate both parent(s) and child with close follow-up.

Atopic Dermatitis

Some children may be overly sensitive to specific diaper brands, wipes or creams. These children present with a brightly erythematous perineum without the satellite lesions common with *Candida* that extinguishes when a nonsensitive brand or cream is used. Usually, a simple brand change will suffice, but in extreme cases, the parent can be advised to wipe with water on a soft washcloth and avoid use of commercially available wipes. Atopic dermatitis tends to spare the diaper area, aiding in diagnosis. For instance, chemicals found in new factory-produced clothes that have not been washed before wearing can cause a contact dermatitis everywhere but in the diaper area. In contrast, nondiluted bleach-cleaned changing tables will create an erythematous area solely in the diaper area where skin-to-table contact has occurred. Superinfection with *Staphylococcus aureus* or Streptococcal species may occur in those children with atopic dermatitis who scratch; fortunately, *S. aureus* infections rarely involve the vagina [13]. As with lichen sclerosis, use of emollients, hypoallergenic soaps, and lightly used 1% hydrocortisone cream may help relieve symptoms.

Other Systemic Diseases

Infectious mononucleosis and other systemic illnesses may present with vulvar findings. Desquamation and the finding of vulvar ulcers may mimic herpes simplex virus [13, 14]; the former can be an early or late sign of Kawasaki syndrome. Vulvar or perianal desquamation can also be seen with Stephens-Johnson syndrome. Crohn's disease can cause perianal ulcerations and more rarely fistulae to the vagina. Behcet's disease, an autoimmune disorder characterized by the clinical triad of oral and genital ulceration plus iridocyclitis, may initially present with vulvovaginitis. These children may first present with oral apthous ulcers, with genital ulcers showing up later. Ocular symptoms tend to emerge in the teenage years [13, 15, 16]. In Behcet's and other ulcerative diseases, the parent may fear that the painful ulcers and vulvar excoriations represent a sexually transmitted disease such as herpes. Acrodermatitis enteropathica, associated with zinc deficiency, presents with lateral cracking of the lips/mouth, and can cause an eroded bilateral vulvar rash with a well-demarcated edge [17, 18].

Psoriasis

Children are more likely than adults to have psoriasis in the vulvar area, presenting with an itchy, well-demarcated, nonscaly, brightly erythematous, symmetrical plaque involving the vulva, perineum, and/or gluteal folds. Children with psoriasis may also have pitting of the nails, posterior auricular erythema, or scaling rash found elsewhere. As with lichen sclerosis, the clinician should start with low to midpotency topical corticosteroids, increasing in strength only as necessary. Some children require maintenance therapy with lower dose topical steroids. Any concurrent infection should be treated.

Genital Tumors

Although rare, genital tumors should be considered in any child presenting with (1) chronic genital ulceration, (2) nontraumatic swelling of the external genitalia, (3) protrusion of a mass from the vagina, (4) foul-smelling bloody discharge and no evidence of foreign body, and (5) virilization or precocious puberty. Botyroid sarcoma, or embryonal carcinoma of the vagina, has a peak incidence in 2-year-olds, with 90% of cases in children under 5 years of age. In children over age 10 years, this tumor tends to affect the upper vagina or cervix, whereas in younger children, it is found in the lower vagina [13]. Originating from undifferentiated mesenchyme in the lamina propria, this tumor spreads rapidly below the vaginal epithelium, infiltrating the vaginal wall. It looks like a cluster of grapes, bulging outward with polypoid growths containing edematous stroma and dilated blood vessels. Treatment consists of chemotherapy, conservative surgery, and sometimes radiation therapy. The survival rate is 80–90% in girls with localized pelvic rhabdomyosarcoma [3, 19, 20].

Malignant vulvar melanomas can be found rarely in young girls. Langerhans' cell histocytosis may involve the genital area. Other rare findings include congenital perineal lipomas and prolapsed ectopic ureterocoeles. Condyloma accuminata can be congenitally acquired or via sexual abuse.

Labial Adhesions

Labial adhesions can occur commonly in babies and children with most appearing as an incidental finding on exam, more worrisome to the parent rather than the child. Occasionally, a secondary dermatitis is caused by pooling urine or vaginal secretions in those children with adhesions extending from above the urethra past the vagina. Children with labial adhesions may also get urinary tract infections.

Labial adhesions are easily treatable with topical estrogen cream (Premarin vaginal cream; Ayerst, New York, N.Y., USA) applied directly to the area by finger or Q-tip in tiny amounts daily. The skin of this area can act like a sticky adhesive, causing adhesions to recur easily. Parents should be instructed on restarting premarin if adhesions recur, and especially on how to apply topical estrogen in insufficient amounts to promote systemic estrogen effects.

Conclusions

Vulvovaginitis can be found frequently in girls, causing angst to the parent and bothersome symptoms to the child. In performing the pediatric gynecologic examination, the astute clinician has the opportunity to diagnose and treat pathology, prevent future symptomatology, educate on hygiene, and allay fears in the process. Engaging the child and parent in the discussion can teach 'the rules' of the gynecologic exam, role model frank discussions on how to avoid 'stranger danger' or sexual abuse, answer questions on normal functions and aspects of sexuality. Using proper positioning and simple office tools such as a catheter within a catheter as shown in figure 7, foreign bodies can be flushed out painlessly and simply. Systemic diseases such as Behcet's disease, Kawasaki syndrome, and infectious mononucleosis may present with ulceration or desquamation of the perineal area. Lichen sclerosis can affect the bottoms of the old and young, with a picture worth a thousand words in recognizing and then treating. Labial adhesions provide another simple means of problem detection, reassurance, education and treatment. Other common problems such as bubble bath vaginitis or contact dermatitis require removal of the causative agent, and when in doubt, sitz baths help. With patience, care and sensitivity, the pediatric gynecologic examination can be performed by pediatricians, primary care clinicians, and subspecialists, emphasizing what is normal, with a focus on prevention as well as treatment.

References

1 Emans SJ, Laufer MR, Goldstein DP: Pediatric and Adolescent Gynecology, ed 5. Philadelphia, Lippincott Williams & Wilkins, 2005.
2 Pokorny, SF, Stormer LVN: Atraumatic removal of secretions from the prepubertal vagina. Am J Obstet Gynecol 1987;157:950–956.
3 Emans SJ, Goldstein DP: The gynecologic examination of the prepubertal child with vulvovaginitis: use of the knee-chest position. Pediatrics 1980; 65:758.
4 Heller RH, Joseph JH, David HJ: Vulvovaginitis in the premenarchal child. J Pediatr 1969;74:370.
5 Pippo S, Lenko H, Vuento R: Vulvar symptoms in paediatric and adolescent patients. Acta Paediatr 2000;9:431.
6 Stricker T, Navratil F, Sennhauser FH: Vulvovaginitis in prepubertal girls. Arch Dis Child 2003;88:324–326.
7 Emans SJ, Woods ER, Allred EN, Grace E: Hymenal findings in adolescent women: impact of tampon use and consensual sexual activity. J Pediatr 1994; 125:153.
8 Alexander ER: Misidentification of sexually transmitted organisms in children: medicolegal implications. Pediatr Infect Dis J 1988;7:1.
9 Whittington WL, Rice RJ, Biddle JW, et al: Incorrect identification of *Neisseria gonorrhoeae* from infants and children. Pediatr Infect Dis J 1988;7:3.
10 Centers for Disease Control and Prevention: Screening tests to detect *Chlamydia trachomatis* and *Neisseria gonorrhoeae* infections 2002. MMWR 2002;51(RR-15):1.
11 Centers for Disease Control and Prevention: Sexually transmitted diseases treatment guidelines. MMWR 2006;55 (RR-11):1–94.
12 Paradise JE, Compos JM, Friedman HM, et al: Vulvovaginitis in premenarchal girls: clinical features and diagnostic evaluation. Pediatrics 1982;70: 193.
13 Mroueh J, Muram D: Common problems in pediatric gynecology: new developments. Curr Opin Obset Gynecol 1999;11:463–446.
14 Sisson BA, Glick L: Genital ulceration as a presenting manifestation of infectious mononucleosis. J Pediatr Adolesc Gynecol 1998;11:185–187.
15 Uziel Y, Brik R, Padeh S, et al: Juvenile Behcet's disease in Israel. The Pediatric Rheumatology Study Group of Israel. Clin Exp Rheumatol 1998;16:502–505.
16 Elem B, Onur C, Ozen S: Clinical features of pediatric Behcet's disease. J Pediatr Ophthalmol Strabismus 1998;35:159–161.
17 Fischer GO: Vulvar disease in pre-pubertal girls. Australasian J Dermatol 2001;42:225–236.
18 Stapleton KM, O'Loughlin E, Relic JP: Transient zinc deficiency in a breast-fed premature infant. Australasian J Dermatol 1995;36:157–159.
19 Copeland LJ, Gershenson DM, Saul PB, et al: Sarcoma botyroides of the female genital tract. Obstet Gynecol 1985;66;262.
20 Arndt CA, Donaldson SS, Anderson JR, et al. What constitutes optimal therapy for patients with rhabomyosarcoma of the female genital tract. Cancer 2001;91;2454.

Ellen S. Rome, MD, MPH
Section of Adolescent Medicine, Cleveland Clinic, A120
9500 Euclid Avenue
Cleveland, OH 44195 (USA)
Tel. +1 216 444 3566, E-Mail romee@ccf.org

Sultan C (ed): Pediatric and Adolescent Gynecology. Evidence-Based Clinical Practice. 2nd, revised and extended edition. Endocr Dev. Basel, Karger, 2012, vol 22, pp 84–100

Clinical Expression of Precocious Puberty in Girls

Charles Sultan[a,b] · Laura Gaspari[a,b] · Nicolas Kalfa[b,c] · Françoise Paris[a,b]

[a]Unité d'Endocrinologie-Gynécologie Pédiatriques, Département de Pédiatrie, Hôpital A. de Villeneuve, [b]Service d'Hormonologie (Développement et Reproduction), Hôpital Lapeyronie, CHU Montpellier et Université Montpellier 1, et [c]Service de Chirurgie Pédiatrique, Hôpital Lapeyronie, CHU Montpellier, Montpellier, France

Abstract

Premature development of breast and/or pubic hair in a prepubertal girl used to raise questions and concerns from the families. There is actually a wide range of clinical expressions of precocious puberty in girls and not all presentations are considered to be true precocious puberty. Central precocious puberty occurs in 10–20% of girls, but beside the typical forms other clinical presentations have been identified. In 50–60% of the cases, only one secondary sex characteristic shows premature development and raises the diagnosis of premature thelarche, premature pubarche or isolated metrorrhagia. In 10% of the cases, autonomous ovarian overproduction of estrogens causes peripheral precocious puberty. Lastly, hyperestrogenism may have exogenous causes, such as exposure to environmental chemical pollutants. A decision on therapeutic management is based on clinical, biological and radiologic examinations, and LHRH analogous treatment should be limited to central precocious puberty before the age of 8 years.

The premature appearance of secondary sexual characteristics like breast development and pubic hair is upsetting and prompts many families to consult in pediatric endocrinology. Yet the management of precocious puberty is not always straightforward, especially given the unusually wide range of clinical expression: not all presentations of precocious puberty are true precocious puberty [1]!

- Ten to twenty percent of all cases are instances of central precocious puberty (CPP) [2]. The course of its development needs to be carefully assessed and a central tumor must be eliminated. In its typical form, CPP progresses rapidly and the accelerated bone maturation leads to early fusion of the bone plates, thus compromising final adult height. Other clinical presentations have been identified and will be discussed further on.
- In 50–60% of the cases, only one secondary sexual characteristic shows premature development and the diagnosis is premature thelarche (breast development) [3],

Table 1. Mean ages for normal pubertal development stages in girls, based on Tanner stages for breast development (B) and pubic hair (P)

Pubertal stage	Age, years
Breast buds (B2	10.1
Sparse pubic hair growth (P2)	11.2
Darker, coarser pubic hair growth (P3)	12.2
Growth spurt	12.2
Menarche	12.7
Adult pubic hair in type and quantity (P5)	14
Mature breast (B5)	14

premature pubarche (appearance of pubic hair) [4] or metrorrhagia. In these cases, the etiology should be sought, and clinical, biological and radiographic management is devoted to preventing the precocious onset of puberty.

- In 10% of the cases, the development of secondary sexual characteristics has an adrenal or ovarian cause, with an autonomous hyperproduction of estrogens causing precocious pseudopuberty independently of gonadotropin activation. In these cases, it has become increasingly evident that the hyperestrogenism may have an exogenous cause, such as environmental chemical pollutants in the air, water, and food chain. These xenoestrogens have a chemical structure that mimics the actions of natural estrogens by stimulating the activity of target tissues.

In all cases, the initial step is to evaluate the level of estrogen secretion, in terms of both its impact on target organs (breasts, growth rate, bone maturation, etc.) and its course over time. A good understanding of the various ways that precocious puberty clinically presents in girls is vital for the decision on therapeutic management, as the optimal treatment is often not evident during the initial evaluation.

Evaluation of the Pubertal Stage

One of the first steps in diagnosis is the estimation of pubertal stage. The Tanner stages have been the reference for many years, as they are very well codified (table 1). In routine clinical practice, this relatively precise staging is complemented by examination of the sesamoid bone of the hand. This marker of bone maturation appears toward 11 years and signals the start of puberty.

The Tanner stages have been the reference for generations of pediatric endocrinologists. In an American study of a very large cohort of girls examined between the ages of 3 and 11 years [5], most of the girls appeared to enter puberty at a younger age (9.9 years for B2 and 10.5 years for P2). This drop in the age of puberty onset was most evident in black girls. The authors attributed their findings to the impact of environmental factors (chemical pollution). The findings that most of the girls entering puberty at the youngest ages (between 6 and 8 years) do not present with short adult height [6] and that the duration of puberty (tempo) is inversely linked to the age of onset (timing) should be considered as relevant to clinical practice, especially to any decision about therapeutic management. The prediction of adult height based on bone age, according to the method of Bayley-Pineau [7], is one of the most reliable parameters in this regard [8].

These works as a whole have done much to elucidate the development of secondary sexual characteristics and the normal course of puberty in girls [9, 10].

The activation of the gonadotropic axis is marked by a peak in LH above 5 μIU/ml and an LH/FSH ratio above 1 during LHRH testing [11]. Conversely to the assertions of other groups, we do not accept the basal values of LH (whatever the standard used) as a marker of pubertal onset.

The measurement of plasma estradiol by radioimmunology is not a reliable method to evaluate the onset of puberty because of its low specificity and high fluctuations. Only the analysis of the biological activity of estrogens using ultrasensitive methods is able to provide useful information on pubertal onset.

Last, pelvic ultrasonography with measurement of the uterus should be systematically performed: onset of puberty shows an increase in ovarian volume (>1.5 cm^3) and uterine size, with length exceeding 3.5 cm. The finding of an increased diameter of the uterine fundus and a uterine vacuity line reflects significant estrogenization.

Clinical, biological, anthropometric and radiographic evaluations are all helpful in distinguishing normal puberty from precocious puberty, which may have important clinical, psychological and therapeutic implications [12, 13].

Puberty Onset

A substantial number of clinical, biological and experimental studies has demonstrated that the onset of puberty is a central process [14]: the activation of the GnRH pulse generator [15], which is modulated by peripheral signals (intrauterine and postnatal growth, fat mass, insulin sensitivity, gonadal steroid levels) and environmental signals (light, stress and environmental pollution) (fig. 1). The essential role of the GnRH pulse generator in puberty onset (which is part of the global process of maturation) was confirmed by the recent identification of key genes whose natural or experimental loss of function abolished GnRH production [16].

These genes were essentially IAP, TTF1, Nell-2, GPR-54 and FGF-Rc, all of which regulate the processing or secretion of GnRH either directly or through its glutamatergic regulation. Moreover, at the level of the astroglia, TGF-α and the neuroregulins are able to stimulate GnRH production via the Erb β-4 receptor. Although

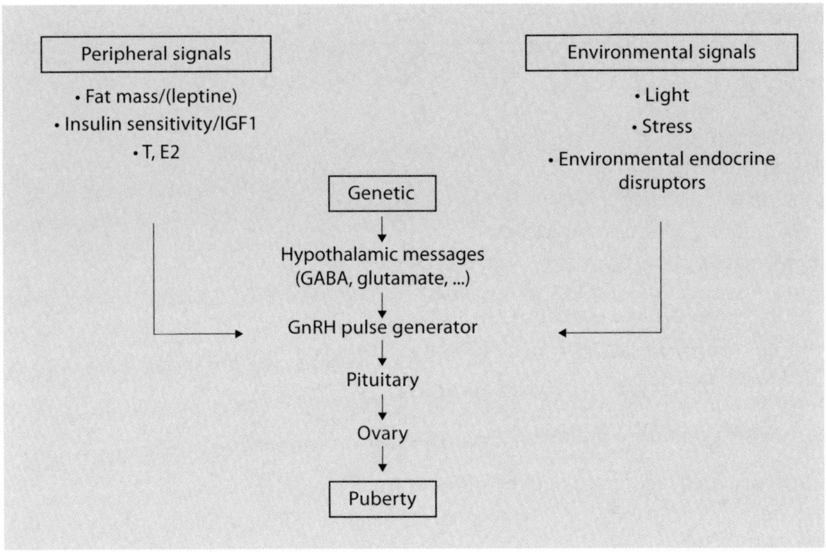

Fig. 1. Onset of puberty.

a hyperproduction caused by TGFα has been associated with CPP, it is also possible that the hyperexpression of one of the genes regulating glutamate production or GnRH itself is a cause of CPP. In fact, the high frequency of the familial form of CPP supports the major role of a genetic factor in gonadotropic activation [17, 18].

Clinical Expression of Precocious Puberty

Precocious puberty is eight times more frequent in girls than in boys [19]. Premature breast development, pubic hair and growth acceleration should prompt several questions (table 2), the answers to which will provide clues as to the best adapted treatment strategy [20, 21].

1. Did puberty clinically begin before 8 years?
2. What has been the progression of the clinical symptoms?
3. Are there biological or radiographic signs of exaggerated maturation?
4. How is predicted adult height affected?
5. What are the psychological consequences?
6. Is the hormonal secretion gonadotropin-dependent or gonadotropin-independent?
7. In the case of central gonadotropin activation is it due to a tumor or is it idiopathic?

Table 2. Clinical forms of precocious puberty

Central precocious puberty	
	Typical form
	Extremely precocious puberty
	Slowly progressing puberty
	Spontaneously regressive puberty
	Central precocious puberty in adopted children
	Familial central precocious puberty
	Central precocious puberty and genetic abnormality
Advanced puberty	
	Simple advanced puberty
	Advanced puberty and growth retardation
	Advanced puberty after premature pubarche
Incomplete, partial or dissociated precocious puberty	
	Premature thelarche
	Premature pubarche
	Isolated metrorrhagia
Peripheral precocious puberty: precocious pseudopuberty	
Ovarian autonomy	
	McCune-Albright syndrome, ovarian cyst
	Granulosa cell tumor
Adrenal tumor (feminizing)	
Environmental pollution (pesticides)	

Central Precocious Puberty

Typical Form

The simultaneous development of breasts >B3 and pubic hair >P3 in a girl younger than 8 years suggests CPP when growth rate is also accelerated (>2 SD of the mean for chronological age). When the medical history is taken, the family should be questioned about past head X-rays, brain trauma, and neonatal infection of the central nervous system (meningitis, encephalitis) [22]. In addition, the impact on the child's psychological health or well-being should be assessed [23].

The clinical examination will reveal a modification in the orientation of the vulva, development of the labia majora, and vaginal secretion. The weight curve should be systematically analyzed. The child should be examined for scoliosis or body asymmetry, as this is a constitutive element of a syndrome associated with CPP. Once this initial clinical step is concluded, it is important to confirm the diagnosis of a central cause and to determine the etiology. The hormonal work-up is limited to LHRH testing and a predominant LH response signals central gonadotropin activation [24].

Table 3. Etiology of central precocious puberty

Idiopathic (75%)
Sporadic
Familial
Secondary to a brain tumor (15–20%)
Hypothalamic hamartoma
Optic chiasm glioma
Astrocytoma
Secondary to central nervous system damage (5–10%)
Malformation: hydrocephalus
Arachnoid cyst
Brain irradiation
Head injury
Secondary to the removal of a peripheral inhibition
Late-onset congenital adrenal hyperplasia, after treatment
McCune-Albright syndrome, after treatment
Adopted child
Associated with a genetic disease

In CPP, X-ray of the left wrist and elbow always reveals advanced bone maturation and bone age is often greater than chronological age. This sign is fundamental. In certain forms of explosive precocious puberty, however, clinical expression may precede the accelerated bone maturation, which only occurs some months later.

Pelvic ultrasonography is indispensable. Uterine length greater than 35 mm indicates puberty onset. Multifollicular ovaries reflect central stimulation. Girls differ from boys in that CPP in the former is more frequently idiopathic (75% of the cases) (table 3), although brain MRI should still be systematic [25]. A central nervous system tumor (hypothalamic hamartoma, optic chiasm glioma, etc.) is found in 10–15% of the cases. Moreover, central structures can be affected secondary to infection (meningitis, meningoencephalitis), radiation, or brain trauma.

Other Clinical Forms

In addition to the typical presentation of CPP, which usually occurs between 5 and 8 years, several other forms have been identified and can be distinguished by their etiology, progression, and therapeutic indications (table 3).

Extremely Precocious Puberty

Extremely precocious puberty occurs between 1 and 4 years: the clinical progression is rapid and more anarchic, and menstruation occurs. The search for a cerebral tumor should be particularly painstaking.

Slowly Progressing Puberty

Slowly progressing puberty was defined by Rappaport [26] as moderate breast enlargement, E2 concentration less than 25 pg/ml, an advance in bone maturation of less than 2 years, and a ratio of LH peak over FSH peak less than 1. Moreover, the circulating concentration of IGF-1 is prepubertal. If the clinical picture remains stable after 6 months of observation, treatment to stop puberty is not indicated [27].

Spontaneously Regressive Puberty

Cases of spontaneously regressive puberty have long been a subject of discussion: these are authentic cases of CPP in which the signs of estrogenic secretion spontaneously and completely regress in the 12 months following the consultation for precocious puberty [28]. In our experience, no clinical, biological or radiologic element predicts this particular course. This rare form requires no treatment but points to the need for systematic follow-up over 6–12 months for all cases of sexual precociousness.

Central Precocious Puberty in Adopted Children

Central precocious puberty in adopted children is seen almost exclusively in girls between 4 and 8 years, whatever the country of origin, and its occurrence is variable after arrival in the country of adoption. This form is characterized more by the rapidity of the acceleration in growth velocity and maturation than by the clinical signs, and it evokes the relationship of denutrition/inadequate caloric intake → renutrition → rapid rise in IGF-1 → precocious onset of puberty [29]. According to Bourguignon's group [30], these children have been contaminated by pesticides: the plasma concentration in DDT is unusually elevated. They hypothesize that the cessation of environmental contamination after adoption removes the inhibition of the GnRH pulse generator and favors the premature entry into puberty.

Familial Central Precocious Puberty

Routine clinical experience has shown that the age of menarche has remained remarkably consistent across generations and that in certain families puberty onset has always been more or less precocious. A recent study from the group of Philips [17] reported a high proportion (27.5%) of the familial form of CPP. Analysis indicated autosomal-dominant transmission with weak penetrance. These data suggest the need to pay particular attention to the girls in these families, especially since in this study the girls with familial CPP were evaluated later than the girls with sporadic forms. This clinical form of CPP is a remarkable illustration of the implication of genetic factors in puberty onset.

Advanced Puberty

Advanced puberty is the situation most often encountered in clinical practice [31, 32].

Simple Advanced Puberty

Simple advanced puberty refers to pubertal advance that remains within 2 SD of the norm, generally appearing between 8 and 10 years of age. This type is often the reason for short adult height, because the acceleration of bone maturation is more rapid than statural growth. It is particularly seen in girls of Mediterranean background and a girl showing this simple advance of puberty often has a mother who experienced the same advance (genetic character).

Some authors [33, 34] have tried to delay puberty in order to increase the growth period and thus improve the final adult height. In fact, LHRH analogues did not improve the predicted final height.

Simple Advanced Puberty and Growth Retardation

In many cases, a simple advance of puberty occurs in girls showing growth delay ≤-2 SD, especially those who presented intrauterine growth retardation. The prognosis for final height is affected, with adult height of 145–150 cm. In these cases, treatment to stop puberty can be considered, such as the association of an LHRH analogue and growth hormone [35].

Advanced Puberty after Premature Pubarche

At a chronological age of 8–10 years, some girls have presented with premature pubarche and gonadal onset of puberty at a bone age of 10–11 years. Some of these girls, especially the obese, are at risk of developing polycystic ovarian disease in adolescence [36]. They require close clinical, biological and radiologic follow-up throughout the adolescent period.

'Incomplete' Puberty

Incomplete puberty refers to the premature and often isolated development of a secondary sexual characteristic: the breast (premature thelarche) or pubic hair (premature pubarche). Occasionally isolated metrorrhagia is seen. These situations are very frequently observed in daily practice and are difficult to diagnose. Incomplete puberty is usually considered to be a variant of normal puberty, but it may be caused by an underlying pathology that should be sought or it may be the only current sign of a CPP that will develop in the future.

Premature Thelarche (fig. 2)

Premature thelarche refers to isolated breast development in girls between 2 and 7 years, which differs from the genital crisis of the newborn whose breast development (associated with strong estrogenization and even milk production) may last for the first 18 months of life. This premature breast development is bilateral in half the cases, unilateral, or, less frequently, asymmetric. Volume varies: 60% at B2, 30% at B3, and 10% at B4. The breast is often tender and palpation is sometimes painful. There is no discharge.

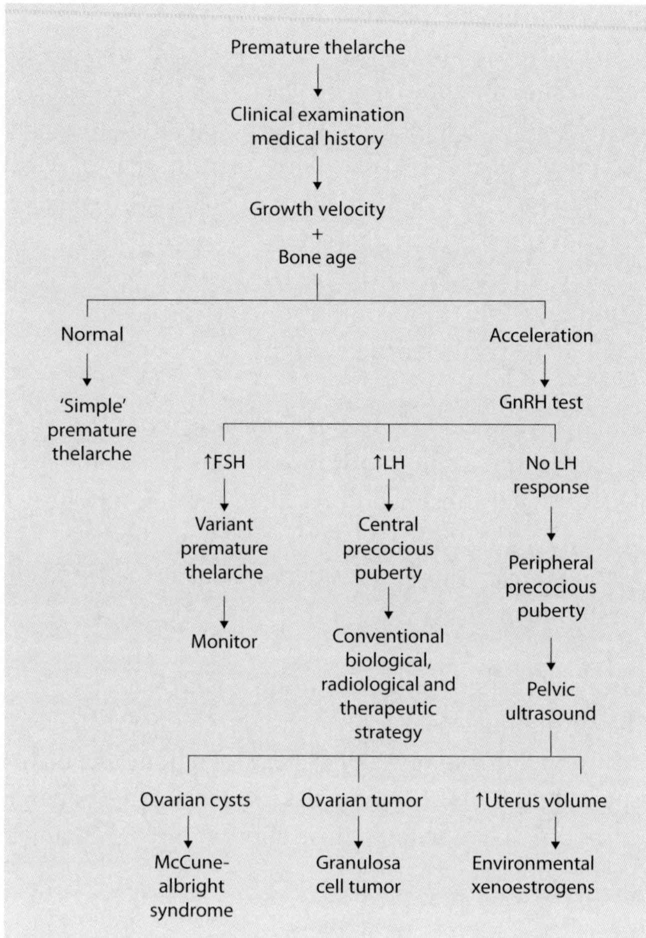

Fig. 2. Decision tree for premature thelarche.

In persistent or marked forms of thelarche, the hormonal work-up should be limited to the LHRH test to confirm a predominant FSH response [37]. Bone maturation is rarely accelerated. The progression is characterized by fluctuations over time: spontaneous remission, persistence, and aggravation of breast volume, which should evoke the possibility of puberty onset [38–40]. In this case, pelvic ultrasound can provide useful information.

When estrogen secretion if patent (simultaneous increase in uterine volume), contamination by products with estrogen-like activity should be considered and sought (soy-rich foods, environmental pesticides, etc.). In its usual form, premature thelarche requires no treatment.

Premature Adrenarche/Pubarche (fig. 3)
Premature pubarche refers to the appearance of pubic hair before 8 years. It is usually isolated although axillary hair is occasionally observed. The clinical examination

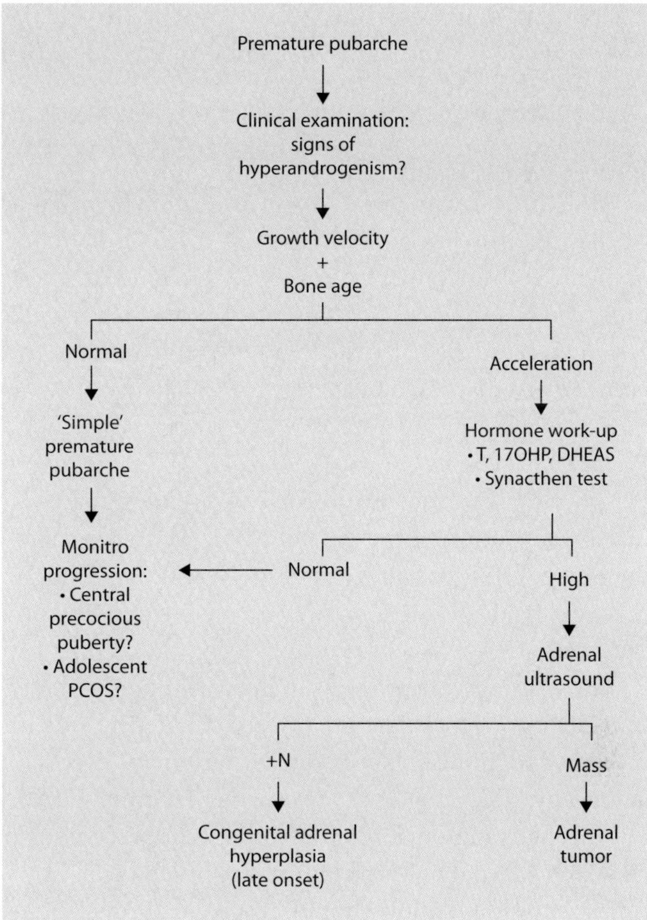

Fig. 3. Decision tree for premature pubarche.

is centered exclusively on the detection of other signs of hyperandrogenism, such as acne, abnormal perspiration, and clitoral hypertrophy. Growth velocity and bone maturation are usually only slightly accelerated.

Depending on the clinical picture, an androgen work-up (testosterone, 17OH-progesterone, DHEAS and possibly a synacthen test should be done.

In most situations, the maturation of the adrenal function that precedes puberty is accelerated or early, although the reason remains unknown. The 'physiological' character of adrenarche cannot mask the authentic forms of secondary congenital adrenal hyperplasia, during the course of which the precocious puberty reveals a deficiency in 21-hydroxylase (21OH). The finding of a homozygous mutation of the 21OH gene (or a double heterozygous mutation) requires specific treatment, but the efficacy of treatment for heterozygous forms has not been determined.

Last, precocious puberty in the context of intrauterine growth retardation and insulin resistance should be followed closely for several years, according to some [36]:

it is thought that precocious puberty might provide the conditions for CPP, PCOS in adolescence [41] and adult metabolic syndrome, which has become a serious management problem in public health.

Isolated Metrorrhagia

Several clinical manifestations of transitory ovarian activity have been observed in isolated metrorrhagia: menstruation that is isolated or associated with breast development, with inconsistent response to the LHRH test and the frequent presence of functional ovarian cysts. Menstruation may recur cyclically. These rises in estrogenization increase the risk of accelerated bone maturation, and treatment to stop puberty is thus often discussed but rarely undertaken.

Peripheral Precocious Puberty: Precocious Pseudopuberty

Peripheral precocious or precocious pseudopuberty is not characterized by the premature activation of the gonadotropic axis: it is caused by an abnormally high production of estrogens and, more rarely, androgens because of a 'tumor' on the ovary or adrenal glands. It is iso- or heterosexual depending on the whether the excess steroid hormone strengthens or transforms the child's phenotype.

The considerable progress in determining the molecular mechanisms of hormone transduction signals has greatly contributed to our understanding of the physiopathology and clinical expression of peripheral precocious puberty caused by ovarian autonomy. This progress may one day culminate in a specific treatment for this rare but incapacitating disorder. Heterosexual precocious pseudopuberty secondary to a virilizing adrenal or ovarian tumor is much rarer.

Increasing attention should be given to precocious pseudopuberty secondary to environmental contamination by chemical products such as pesticides, herbicides, and fungicides. Endocrine disruptors with the capacity to mimic estrogens are able to generate estrogen secretion, resulting in simple thelarche to veritable menstruations.

Peripheral Precocious Puberty Caused by Ovarian Autonomy

McCune-Albright Syndrome

McCune-Albright syndrome (MAS) is a sporadic disorder characterized by the classic triad of precocious puberty, fibrous bone dysplasia, and café-au-lait spots. Diverse endocrine abnormalities can also be associated: somatotrophic pituitary adenomas, hypothyroid goiter, and adrenal hyperplasia.

Precocious Puberty. MAS affects girls almost exclusively and is characterized by its extreme precociousness and the gravity of the immediate clinical picture: isolated menstruation as early as the first months or first years of life. The full clinical picture will develop later, with breast enlargement and pubic hair. The often voluminous ovarian cysts discovered by ultrasound are cyclic and are difficult to treat: cystectomy or ovariectomy is often necessary when all other treatments fail. The acceleration of growth velocity is considerable (+2, +3 SD) and constant, on the order of 9–10 cm per year. Bone maturation is also accelerated and will thus compromise the prognosis for final adult height.

The biological work-up will show very high plasma estradiol associated with dramatically low plasma gonadotropins and no response to GnRH stimulation. This indicates LH/FSH-independent precocious puberty and situates this type of precocious puberty within the context of the ovarian-autonomous syndromes.

Café-au-Lait Spots. The café-au-lait spots of MAS are hyperpigmented, typically light brown or brown, with irregular borders ('coast of Maine') that distinguish them from the smooth-bordered spots observed in neurofibromatosis. The spots are usually unilaterally distributed, on the same side as the bone lesions. The size and number are variable but may increase with the patient's age. When associated with precocious puberty, they are an essential diagnostic element.

Fibrous Bone Dysplasia. Fibrous bone dysplasia is the third element in the classic triad. This bone abnormality may remain silent for many years, only to be revealed by a spontaneous fracture or on the occasion of a slight injury. X-rays reveal pseudocysts of the bone cortex that rapidly invade the entire skeleton.

Other Endocrine Pathologies. Other endocrine pathologies are seen to varying degrees: hyperthyroidism, acromegaly, gigantism, hypercorticism, hyperprolactinemia, and hyperparathyroidism. These types of endocrine hyper-functioning are also caused by autonomous hormonal hyperproduction.

The hyperproduction of growth hormone is much greater than that which is seen in CPP: generally, it is due to a pituitary tumor, hyperplasia or adenoma, and both medical and surgical treatment are difficult. Hyperprolactinemia is frequently noted: it is usually due to the same mechanism as involved in GH hypersecretion. It does not modify the course of precocious puberty. Hypercorticism is also observed in some cases. It is autonomous and ACTH levels are always low. In certain cases, hyperfunctioning of the thyroid gland is seen with goiter and low TSH. Hyperparathyroidism associated with high levels of calcium and alkaline phosphatase has been reported in patients presenting bone lesions and spontaneous fracture.

Molecular Bases of McCune-Albright Syndrome. The specific location of the skin lesions and the sporadic character of MAS (no documented cases of hereditary transmission) suggest that this disorder is due to a somatic mutation that occurs early in development. The result is a mosaic distribution of abnormal cells. The appearance and the severity of the bone, skin and endocrine abnormalities thus depends on the number of cells carrying the mutation.

Moreover, the diverse endocrine hyperfunctioning syndromes observed in the course of MAS have in common the presence and activation of cells that respond to extracellular signaling by activation of the adenyl cyclase system. The growth and activity of gonads, thyroid, adrenal cortex, certain pituitary cells, melanocytes and osteoblasts are stimulated by an increase of intracellular AMPc under the dependence of adenyl cyclase membrane.

The hypothesis of local hyperproduction of AMPc was confirmed several years ago: MAS is caused by a genetic abnormality that causes a constitutive activation of adenyl cyclase. The evidence of activating Gαs mutations in various tissues of MAS patients [42] further supports this mechanism.

Granulosa Cell Tumors

Although rare (10% of the ovarian tumors in children), granulosa tumors are expressed in early childhood by strong estrogen secretion that results in marked breast development, accelerated growth velocity, and by menstruation. These ovarian tumors are discovered in a wide variety of circumstances:

- Endocrine disturbances:
  - The hormonal activity of the tumor explains why 80–90% of the girls under 8 years present isosexual precocious pseudopuberty. This pubertal advance induced by the estrogen secretion of the tumor cells is independent of the low levels of GnRH and prepubertal gonadotropins. On clinical examination, breast development is frequently noted but this is variable, metrorrhagia, accelerated growth velocity and sometimes advanced bone age are also noted. The preoperative plasma estrogen concentration is almost always elevated. Virilization with precocious pubarche, acnea, hirsutism and rarely clitoromegaly is related to aromatase deficiency inside the tumor.
  - Endocrine symptoms may also be present in cases of ovarian granulose cells in the post pubertal period. Symptoms are more difficult to detect, such meno-metrorragia and hyperandrogenism.
  - Precocity of diagnosis and an early recognition of endocrine signs from ovarian granulosa cell tumors significantly improves its prognosis with a lower risk of peritoneal extension [43].

  In most patients, the levels of inhibin and AMH are elevated and return to normal postsurgery. The level of inhibin is correlated with tumor extension and eventual relapse. If the estradiol level is initially high, this too can be useful for follow-up. However, its interest is limited because (1) 30% of granulosa tumors are nonsecreting, (2) its level depends on the surrounding theca cells and is thus variable, and (3) physiological puberty can interfere with measurement.
- During emergency surgery (10% of the cases) for acute abdominal pain and vomiting that is mistakenly diagnosed as acute appendicitis. These symptoms are due to torsion of the ovary or more rarely tumor rupture.
- An abdominal-pelvic mass that may be quite voluminous. This mass is frequently asymptomatic and it is discovered by the parents. It may also cause compression of the urinary tract (lumbar pain, colic nephritic, urinary infection) or the intestine (constipation, incomplete occlusion syndrome).
- As a fortuitous discovery during surgical intervention for other reasons.
- By discovery of an ovarian cyst during prenatal diagnosis, which is an exceptional situation.

Surgery is the treatment of choice for a granulosa cell tumor. A careful preoperative evaluation is necessary to preserve fertility and future hormonal functioning. Staging includes peritoneal cytology and exploration of the abdominal cavity. Limited tumors can be treated by salpingo-ovariectomy, as the rate of relapse is minimal. For bilateral tumor, a conservative treatment of the contralateral ovary should be discussed. In stages with extraovarian extension, chemotherapy is recommended. Follow up includes careful clinical, hormonal and ultrasonographic evaluation.

Due to its excellent prognosis and the often complete recovery after initial surgery, juvenile OGCT has usually been considered as benign condition. Survival of the patients with stage Ia tumors is around 90%, the overall survival in the whole group approximating 85%. However, the minority of tumors that have spread within the abdomen or recurred after initial therapy have a much poorer prognosis and OGCT should be considered a ovarian cancer of good prognosis rather than a benign condition. It is still not possible to identify those patients who will relapse in the future, and the mechanism of this relapse remains to be elucidated. Nevertheless, molecular biology [44] has identified 2 markers of prognosis:

- Mutations of the Gs alpha protein – a protein included in the transduction of the FSH signal – have been found in hot spot position 201 in 30% of patients' DNAs [45]. The oncologic stages were significantly different according to the gsp oncogene status. Patients with a hyperactivated Gαs exhibited a significantly more advanced tumor ($p < 0.05$). Gsp oncogene is indeed implicated in cell proliferation level and cell invasion capacity.
- Another prognostic factor of OGCT could be the level of the differentiation of the tumoral cell. One of the earliest differentiating genes of granulosa cell in the fetus is FOXL2. FOXL2, a forkhead transcription factor, is a regulatory element of the organogenesis of the mammalian ovary. The patients with no or reduced expression of FOXL2 in thei tumor exhibit significantly more advanced oncologic staging. All patients requiring complementary treatment (chemotherapy or complementary surgery) showed reduced FOXL2 expression in the tumor. The extinction of this gene implicated in granulosa cell differentiation is compatible with an uncontrolled proliferation of these cells [46].

Feminizing tumors of the adrenal gland are relatively rare causes of precocious pseudopuberty.

Precocious Pseudopuberty and Environmental Pollution

The lower age for onset of puberty is thought to be due to environmental contamination by pesticides [5]. Moreover, European pediatric endocrinology groups unanimously agree that the frequency of premature thelarche has clearly been rising over the past several years.

Several reports have detailed veritable epidemics of precocious pseudopuberty. In Italy, 21% of the girls in preschool classes presented with premature thelarche in association with poultry intake. More recently, the high frequency of premature thelarche before 7 years (34%) in Puerto Rico was associated with phthalates levels three times higher than that seen in controls [47].

Many experimental data indicate the impact of chemical contamination (pesticides) during gestation on the timing and tempo of puberty, and these data have been extensively reviewed [48]. The growing recognition of the potential impact of endocrine disruption on the timing of puberty should prompt in-depth investigation of the environmental conditions of a child's development [49] when conventional etiologies prove negative.

Conclusions

Daily clinical practice reveals a wide diversity in the clinical expression of precocious puberty in girls. Pubertal development seems to occur along a continuum from normal to advanced to precocious, which reinforces the importance of an etiological approach to these increasingly frequent situations, through clinical, biological and radiologic examinations. A better understanding of the clinical presentation should improve the therapeutic indication, especially concerning the use of LHRH analogues, which should be limited to CPP before the age of 8 years as this particular situation is liable to compromise final adult height, according to the clinical, biological and radiologic data [50].

References

1 Kaplowitz P: Update on precocious puberty: girls are showing signs of puberty earlier, but most do not require treatment. Adv Pediatr. 2011;58:243–258.

2 Mogonsen SS, Aksglaede L, Mouritsen A, Sørensen K, Main KM, Gideon P, Juul A: Diagnostic work-up of 449 consecutive girls who were referred to be evaluated for precocious puberty. J Clin Endocrinol Metab. 2011;96:1393–1401.

3 de Vries L, Guz-Mark A, Lazar L, Reches A, Phillip M: Premature thelarche: age at presentation affects clinical course but not clinical characteristics or risk to progress to precocious puberty. J Pediatr 2010;156:466–471.

4 Paris F, Tardy V, Chalançon A, Picot MC, Morel Y, Sultan C: Premature pubarche in Mediterranean girls: high prevalence of heterozygous CYP21 mutation carriers. Gynecol Endocrinol. 2010;26:319–324.

5 Herman-Giddens ME, Slora EJ, Wasserman RC, et al: Secondary sexual characteristics and menses in young girls seen in office practice: a study from the pediatric research in office setting networks. Pediatrics 1997;99:505–512.

6 Marti-Henneberg C, Vizmanos B: The duration of puberty in girls is related to the timing of its onset. J Pediatr 1997;131:618–621.

7 Bayley N, Pinneau SR: Tables for predicting adult height from skeletal age: revised for use with Greulich Pyle hand standards. J Pediatr 1952;50:432–441.

8 Bar A, Linder B, Sober EH, Saenger P, Dimartino-Nardi J: Bayley-Pinneau method of height prediction in girls with central precocious puberty: correlation with adult height. J Pediatr 1995;126:955–958.

9 Kaplowith PB, Oberfield SE: Reexamination of the agent limit for defining when puberty is precocious in girls in United States: implications for evaluation and treatment. Pediatrics 1999;104:936–41.
10 Sultan C, Paris F, Jeandel C, Attal G, Lumbroso S, Dumas R: L'âge de la puberté et de la ménarche. Gynécologie Pratique, Hors-Série, 2001.
11 Lighetti L, Predieri B, Ferrari M, Gallo C, Livio L, Milioli S, Forese S, Bernasconi S: Diagnosis of central precocious puberty: endocrine assesment. J Pediatr Endocr Metab 2000;13:709–15.
12 Soriano-Guillén L, Corripio R, Labarta JI, Cañete R, Castro-Feijóo L, Espino R, Argente J: Central precocious puberty in children living in Spain: incidence, prevalence, and influence of adoption and immigration. J Clin Endocrnol Metab 2010;95:4305–4313.
13 Cohen D, Janfaza M, Klein KO: Importance of leuprolide acetate variable dosing for precocious puberty: a range of acceptable suppression. J Pediatr Endocrinol Metab. 2009;22:629–634.
14 Terasawa E, Fernandez DL: Neurobiological mechanisms of the onset of puberty in primates. Endocr Re. 2001;22:111–151.
15 Parent AS, Teilmann G, Juul A, Skakkebaek NE, Toppari J, Bourguignon JP: The timing of normal puberty and the age limits of sexual precocity: variations around the world, secular trends, and changes after migration. Endocr Rev 2003;24:668–693.
16 Seminara SB, Messager S, Chatzidaki EE, et al: The GPR54 gene as a regulator of puberty. N Engl J Med 2003;349:1614–1627.
17 de Vries L, Kauschansky A, Shohat MPM: Familial central precocious puberty suggests autosomal dominant inheritance. J Clin Endocrinol Metab 2004;89:1794–1800.
18 Palmert MR, Boepple PA: Variation in the timing of puberty : clinical spectrum and genetic investigation. J Clin Endocrinol Metab 2001;86:2364–2368.
19 Wheeler MD, Styne MD: Diagnosis and management of precocious puberty, current issues in pediatric and adolescent endocrinology. Pediatr Clin N Am 1990;37:1255–1271.
20 Brauner R: Pubertà precoce centrale: trattarla sistematicamente. La pubertà femminile ed i suoi disordini. Naples, Guiseppe de Nicola, 2003, pp 109–112
21 Rosenfield RL: Selection of children with precocious puberty for treatment with GnRH analogs. J Pediatr 1994;124:989–91.
22 Cisternino M, Arrigo T, Pasquino AM, Tinelli C, Antoniazzi F, Beduschi L, Bindi G, Borelli P, De Sanctis V, Galluzzi F, Gargantini L, Lo Presti D, Sposito M, Tato L: Etiology and age incidence of precocious puberty in girls: a multicentric study. J Pediatr Endocrinol Metab 2000;13:695–701.
23 Baumann DA, Landolt MA, Wetterwald R, Dubuis JM, Sizonenko PC, Werder EA: Psychological evaluation of young women after medical treatment for central precocious puberty. Horm Res 2001;56:45–50.
24 Iughetti L, Predieri B, Ferrari M, Gallo C, Livio L, Milioli S, Forese S, Bernasconi S: Diagnosis of central precocious puberty: endocrine assessment. J Pediatr Endocrinol Metab 2000;13:709–715.
25 Cassio A, Cacciari E, Zucchini S, Balsamo A, Diegoli M, Orsini F: Central precocious puberty: clinical and imaging aspects. J Pediatr Endocrinol Metab 2000;13:703–708.
26 Fontoura M, Brauner R, Prévot C, Rappaport R: Precocious puberty in girls: early diagnosis of a slowly progressing variant. Arch Dis Child. 1989;64: 1170–1176.
27 Palmert T, Malin HV, Boepple PA: Unsustained or slowly progressive puberty in young girls: initial presentation and long-term follow-up of 20 untreated patients. J Clin Endocrinol Metab 1999; 84:415–23.
28 Lyon AJ, De Bruyn R, Grant DB: Transient sexual precocity and ovarian cysts. Arch Dis Child 1985;60: 819–822.
29 Kiess W, Muller G, Galler A, et al.: Body fat mass, leptin and puberty. J Ped Endocrinol Metab. 2000; 13:717–722.
30 Krstevska-Konstantinova M, Charlier C, Craen M, et al: Sexual precocity after immigration from developing countries to Belgium: evidence of previous exposure to organochlorine pesticides. Hum Reprod 2001;16:1020–1026.
31 Brauner R: Variantes de la puberté normale. Rev Prat 1992;1397–1399.
32 Mul D, Oostdijk W, Drop SLS: Early puberty in girls. Best Pract Res Clin Endocrinol Metab 2002;16:153–163.
33 Cassio A, Cacciari E, Balsamo A, et al: Randomised trial of LHRH analogue treatment on final height in girls with onset of puberty aged 7.5–8.5 years. Arch Dis Child 1999;81:329–332.
34 Mul D, Wit JM, Oostdijk W, Van den Broeck J: The effect of pubertal delay by GnRH agonist in growth hormone deficient (GHD) children on final height. J Clin Endocrinol Metab 2001;86:4655–4656.

35 Mul. D, Oostdijk W, Waelkens JJJ, Drop SLS: Gonadotrophin releasing hormone agonsit (GnRHa) treatment with or without recombinant human growth hormone (GH) in adopted children with early puberty. Clin Endocrinol (Oxford) 2001; 55:121–129.
36 Ibanez L, Potau N, Virdis E, et al: Postpubertal outcome in girls diagnosed of premature pubarche during childhood: increased frequency of functional ovarian hyperandrogenism. J Clin Endocrinol Metab 1993;76:1599–1603.
37 Traggiai C, Stanhope R: Disorders of pubertal development. Best Pract Res Clin Obstet Gynaecol 2003; 17:41–56.
38 Pasquino AM, Pucarelli F, Segni M, Mancini MA, Municchi G: Progression of premature thelarche to central precocious puberty. J Pediatr 1995;126:11–14.
39 Stanhope R, Brook CGD: Thelarche variant: a new syndrome of precocious sexual mauration? Acta Endocrinol (Copenh) 1990;123:481–486.
40 Stanhope R, Traggiai C: Precocious puberty (complete, partial); in Sultan C (ed): Pediatric and Adolescent Gynecology: Evidence-Based Clinical Practice. Endocr Dev. Basel, Karger, 2004, vol 7, pp 57–65.
41 Ibanez L, Virdis R, Potau N, et al: Natural history of premature pubarche: an auxological study. J Pedoiatr Endocrinol Metab 1992;74:254–257.
42 Lumbroso S, Paris F, Sultan C: McCune-Albright syndrome: molecular genetics. J Pediatr Endocrinol Metab 2002;15:875–882.
43 Kalfa N, Patte C, Orbach D, Lecointre C, Pienkowski C, Philippe F, Thibault E, Plantaz D, Brauner R, Rubie H, Guedj AM, Ecochard A, Paris F, Jeandel C, Baldet P, Sultan C: A nationwide study of granulosa cell tumors in pre- and postpubertal girls: missed diagnosis of endocrine manifestations worsens prognosis. J Pediatr Endocrinol Metab 2005;18:25–31.
44 Kalfa N, Veitia RA, Benayoun BA, Boizet-Bonhoure B, Sultan C: The new molecular biology of granulosa cell tumors of the ovary. Genome Med 2009;1: 81.
45 Kalfa N, Ecochard A, Patte C, Duvillard P, Audran F, Pienkowski C, Thibaud E, Brauner R, Lecointre C, Plantaz D, Guedj AM, Paris F, Baldet P, Lumbroso S, Sultan C: Activating mutations of the stimulatory g protein in juvenile ovarian granulosa cell tumors: a new prognostic factor? J Clin Endocrinol Metab 2006;91:1842–1847.
46 Kalfa N, Philibert P, Patte C, Ecochard A, Duvillard P, Baldet P, Jaubert F, Fellous M, Sultan C: Extinction of FOXL2 expression in aggressive ovarian granulosa cell tumors in children. Fertil Steril 2007;87: 896–901.
47 Colon I, Caro D, Bourdony C, Rosario O: Identification of phtalate esters in the serum of young Puerto Rican girls with premature breast development. Environ Health Perspect 2000;108: 895–900.
48 Sultan C, Jeandel C, Paris F, Balaguer P, Audran F, Sampaio D, Trimeche S, Daurès JP, Nicolas JC: Conséquence endocriniennes de la pollution environnementale chez l'enfant. In Mises au point cliniques d'Endocrinologie, Nutrition et Métabolisme. Editions de Médecine Pratique, 2003, pp 109–124.
49 Mazur W: Phytoestrogen content in foods. Baillière's Clin Endocrinol Metab 1998;12:729–742.
50 Orio F, Paris F, Jeandel C, Sultan C: Pubertà precoce centrale ed analoghi de l'LHRH: indicazioni e resultati. La pubertà femminile ed i suoi disordini. Naples, Guiseppe de Nicola, 2003, pp 101–108.

Prof. Charles Sultan, MD, PhD
Unité d'Endocrinologie-Gynécologie Pédiatriques
Département de Pédiatrie
Hôpital A. de Villeneuve
FR–34295 Montpellier cedex 5 (France)
Tel. +33 467 33 86 96, E-Mail c-sultan@chu-montpellier.fr

Sultan C (ed): Pediatric and Adolescent Gynecology. Evidence-Based Clinical Practice. 2nd, revised and extended edition. Endocr Dev. Basel, Karger, 2012, vol 22, pp 101–111

Ovarian Cysts in Prepubertal Girls

C. Pienkowski[a] · A. Cartault[a] · L. Carfagna[b] · P. Ernoult[a] · J. Vial[c] · F. Lemasson[b] · A. Le Mandat[b] · P. Galinier[b] · M. Tauber[a]

[a]Unité d'Endocrinologie, Génétique et Gynécologie Médicale, [b]Unité de Chirurgie Viscérale et [c]Service d'Imagerie Pédiatrique, Hôpital des Enfants, Toulouse, France

Abstract

Visualization of follicles is perfectly physiological during childhood, their diameter generally does not exceed 10 mm. Ovarian cyst in childhood is well defined for a fluid image >20 mm. Generally mild and asymptomatic, ovarian cysts are fluid formations usually discovered incidentally by ultrasound. Some are hormonally active and cause the development of sexual characteristics. The natural history of functional cysts is eventual regression, and persistence is suggestive of organic tumor. The onset of pain is a sign of complication, and an abrupt sharp pain with vomiting is suggestive of ovarian torsion, in which case surgical intervention is urgent. In all cases, the diagnosis is based on pelvic ultrasound. MRI and tumor marker assays are required to determine the nature of an organic cyst before proceeding to surgery. These cysts may appear functional from the fetal period onward and will require management from the first days of life. Certain endocrine disorders such as precocious puberty, hypothyroidism, and aromatase deficiency cause functional cysts in girls. Recurrent bleeding is due to hormonally active cysts and suggests McCune-Albright syndrome. Although the persistence of a cyst suggests a neoplasm, a fluid character indicates benignity. Imagery is a useful aid in the diagnosis of epithelial tumors (cystadenomas) or teratoma (dermoid cyst).

Childhood ovarian cysts can occur in the first decade but are more common in the neonatal and adolescent periods: the frequency of functional cysts decreases in early childhood and then increases as puberty approaches. During childhood, most large banal cysts are derived from degenerated follicular cysts and, in addition to functional cysts, cystic neoplasms may be encountered [1]. Moreover, hormonally active cysts cause rapid pubertal development or precocious pseudopuberty [2, 3]. In these cases, the possibility of an autonomous ovarian cyst due to a G protein mutation in McCune-Albright syndrome [4, 5] should be considered. Ultrasonography is an excellent tool for detecting the presence of banal cysts in young children and no malignancy has yet appeared as banal on ultrasonography or computed tomographic scan. Management of ovarian cysts depends on the clinical signs, the sonographic appearance and volume of the mass, and its persistence.

Clinical Presentations

Most cysts develop without any pain, are completely asymptomatic, and are discovered incidentally on ultrasonography performed for other reasons. The onset of pain is often a sign of complication. In the case of a painful syndrome, pelvic ultrasonography confirms the diagnosis. In the case of an endocrine syndrome, hormonal investigations are necessary and complete the ultrasound findings.

Painful Abdominopelvic Syndrome

Painful abdominopelvic syndrome can be acute or subacute, and it may be associated with various nonspecific signs (nausea, vomiting, or urinary disorders). Sometimes, a recent history of intermittent abdominal pain is reported by the patient. The syndrome can be extremely painful with associated vomiting. In the series of Galinier et al. [6], 44/45 patients presented with an abrupt onset of abdominal pain, and in 60% of the cases, vomiting was concomitant with pain onset. When an ovarian complication such as torsion or hemorrhage is feared, emergency surgical treatment is required to preserve the ovary. The family and physician should be attentive to repeated manifestations as they may signal recurrence; emergency ultrasonography should always be performed.

The patient may also present vague pelvic pain associated with palpable abdominopelvic mass. Low abdominal or pelvic pain and an abdominopelvic mass strongly suggest ovarian torsion. In this case, a blood sample is drawn for tumor marker evaluation and surgery should be carried out without waiting for the results.

'Endocrine' Signs

The 'endocrine' syndrome is marked by precocious development of sexual characteristics. Rapid breast development followed by metrorrhagia suggests precocious pseudopuberty due to hormonally active cysts. Metrorrhagia often consists of recurrent red blood loss lasting 2–3 days. When looking for an etiology, skin pigmentation should be taken into account, as the association of precocious puberty, 'café-au-lait' skin spots, and polyostotic fibrous dysplasia characterizes the McCune-Albright syndrome [5].

Diagnostic Tools

Pelvic Ultrasonography

Pelvic ultrasonography is central to the management of ovarian cysts. Classically, it is carried out by the suprapubic approach with a full bladder, which allows study

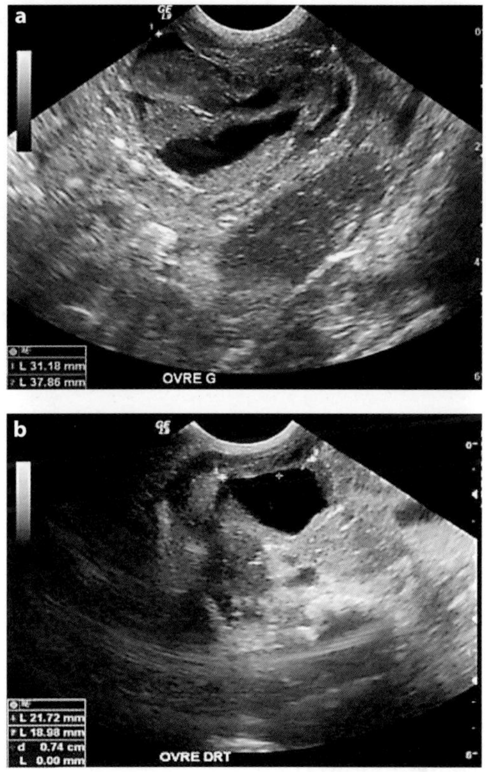

Fig. 1. Neonatal ovaries with bilateral cyst. **a** Complex heterogenous left ovary (ovarian torsion). **b** Simple fluid right ovarian cyst.

not only of the cyst but of all the internal genital organs. It is quite common to note the presence of 1 or 2 small images fluid on ovarian ultrasound of a young girl. Visualization of follicles is perfectly physiological during childhood and their diameter generally does not exceed 10 mm. The definition of an ovarian cyst is to clarify, generally defined for a fluid image >20 mm. An analysis of the cyst itself indicates the size, shape and even volume by measurement of the three diameters, the thickness and regularity of the wall, and the nature of the cyst content. An anechogenic, purely liquid image with a thin, regular wall is in favor of a functional cyst. Volume measurement provides a basis for surveillance and for the decision of possible needle aspiration [7]. Ultrasonography is then indispensable for topographic localization to guide aspiration. An image that is not purely liquid raises problems of differential diagnosis. If the child is symptomatic, there may be a cystic complication such as hemorrhage or ovarian torsion. The mass may be a tumor with a cystic component, raising the problem of its benign or malignant nature. Certain morphological signs are informative: volume of the tissue component, wall thickness, growths, and rigid septations with angulated junctions. Morphological color Doppler and pulsed Doppler spectral imaging studies may also be useful [8], since these techniques provide information on the vascularization of the mass, for example, by differentiating the avascular but echogenic content of a hemorrhagic cyst from hypervascularized tumoral tissue. At a later stage, ultrasonography is used to investigate the condition of the contralateral ovary and the appearance of the uterus, its dimensions and endometrium. This information is indispensable for therapeutic management.

In the child, ultrasonography is limited by the impossibility of a vaginal approach. However, suprapubic sonography is generally sufficient for accurate diagnosis and therapeutic management of ovarian cysts. Recourse to other imaging techniques (CT, MRI) is justified essentially in two circumstances: confirmation of the multitissular nature (fat, calcification) of a dermoid cyst and assessment of the extent of a mass that is tissular rather than liquid and suspected of being malignant [9].

Hormonal Investigation

Plasma measurement of sex steroids (estradiol, testosterone and androgens levels) and basal or stimulated levels of the gonadotropins LH and FSH must be done in any endocrine syndrome. Estradiol hypersecretion, associated with undetectable levels of LH and FSH that do not respond to stimulation after an LH-RH test, confirms the peripheral origin of the autonomous independent gonadotropin secretion and suggests a secretory ovarian tumor [10]. It is also useful to assess the hormonal activity of a cyst by measurement of the estrogens and androgens in the cyst fluid.

Tumor Markers

Tumor marker measurement is a useful aid for diagnosing lesions with a solid component that are difficult to analyze by ultrasonography and for surveillance after tumor removal [11]. Certain markers are specific for tumors with an embryonic component, such as alpha-fetoprotein in embryonic carcinomas and immature teratomas. Beta-human chorionic gonadotropins are more specific markers of choriocarcinomas and dysgerminomas. Elevated levels in pseudocystic tumors indicate a neoplastic component secreting various protein markers according to tumoral origin. CA 19.9 is a useful tool for the diagnosis of mature cystic teratoma of the ovary. Elevated CA 19.9 levels appear to correlate with larger tumor diameter and a higher rate of ovarian torsion [12].

The Various Etiologies

Functional Ovarian Cyst

Functional cysts can occur at any time. These cysts can be discovered from the fetal period and during childhood.

Fetal Ovarian Cyst/Neonatal Management

Follicular ovarian cysts in fetuses and neonates increase in frequency with advancing gestational age and certain maternal complications, such as diabetes mellitus, preeclampsia, and rhesus isoimmunization. Among live births, the best estimate of

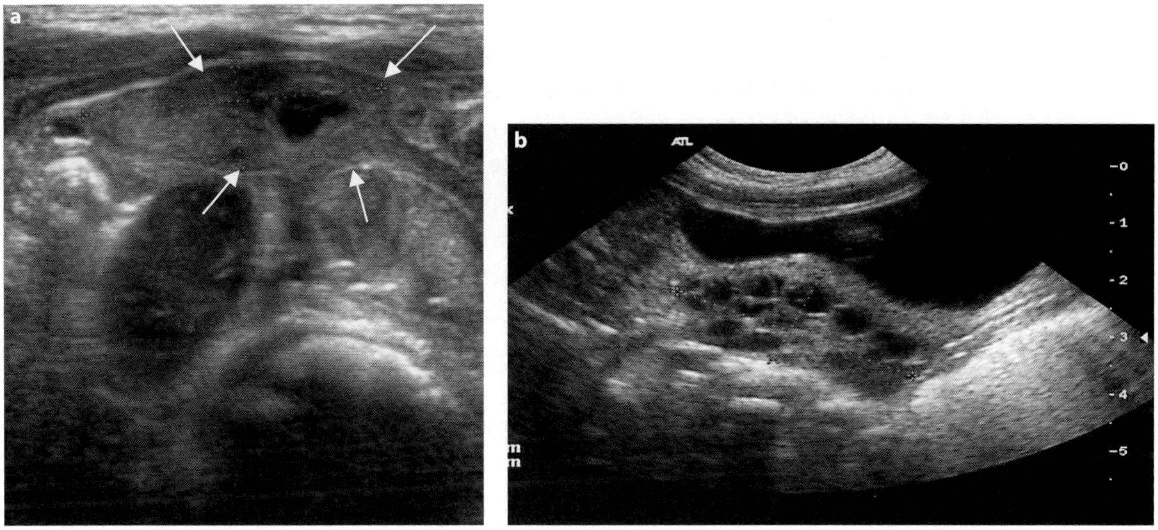

Fig. 2. Ultrasonographic monitoring of right ovarian cyst. **a** Four days after cyst aspiration. **b** Two months later follicles are well visible.

the incidence of clinically significant ovarian cysts is 1 in 2,500. Simple or complex, before or after birth, the cyst is usually asymptomatic, but it may be complicated by intracystic hemorrhage (complex cyst), which is often secondary to ovarian torsion, raising the risk of ovarian loss. The management of the fetal ovarian cyst is highly debated, and prenatal and postnatal management of ovarian cysts has not yet been clearly defined [13, 14].

Treatment options include conservative management, antenatal or neonatal cyst aspiration, laparoscopic cystectomy or laparotomy. Both surgery and simple ultrasonographic monitoring while waiting for spontaneous resolution are acceptable, keeping in mind that preserving the ovarian parenchyma is the main objective.

After birth, simple cysts are generally monitored and can be punctured if they are voluminous (diameter >50 mm) and easy to reach. When there are very recent signs of intracystic hemorrhage on the first day of life, conservative surgery is justified with the aim of detorsion [14]. Surgical teams are more or less interventionist. The benefit of surgery for a complex cyst has not been clearly demonstrated. When a cyst is complicated by a history of adnexal torsion (i.e. more than a week ago), the chance of preserving the ovary is slim as it is likely to be necrotic. In this case, some teams prefer not to operate but rather to monitor the ovary by sonography [13].

Central Pituitary Involvement: Transient or Persistent Activation?

Small asymptomatic cysts are a common finding in young girls. Large cysts, although less common, may not always be associated with abnormal sexual development. Occasionally, these cysts may enlarge and continue to produce estrogen, resulting in pubertal development. The incidence of ovarian cysts is very low, <5% in females between birth and age 8, and small cysts are more frequent than large cysts. In a retrospective analysis [15], 1,818 ultrasound studies in prepubertal girls were examined: only 99 patients (4.5%) presented ovarian cysts. Small visible follicles <10 mm (average 2–3 mm) were found in 82 of these patients (83%), large cysts of >20 mm were found in 17, and only 5 of these 17 patients presented pubertal development. The appearance of pubertal signs can be transient, with breast development increasing during ovarian cyst formation and decreasing with spontaneous resolution. Unilocular cysts <50 mm may be followed conservatively with ultrasonography until regression. The risk of torsion increases with a diameter >50 mm and with rapid progression.

On the other hand, in premature thelarche, FSH-predominant pulses increased the prevalence (2- to 3-fold) of detectable ovarian microcysts of small diameter, <10 mm [16]. Therefore, when larger cysts are due to persistent precocious puberty, ultrasonographic measurement of uterine and ovarian volume offers a reliable means of distinguishing between isolated premature thelarche and central precocious puberty [17]. In precocious puberty, clinical signs such as breast development and pubic pilosity, accelerated growth velocity and advanced bone maturation are evident. This situation is rare and the ovarian cyst must be removed, with hormonal investigations programmed a few weeks later to evaluate hormonal status and differentiate between transient pseudopuberty, which is generally gonadotropin-independent, and the true onset of central precocious puberty [3, 18]. These investigations associate an LH-RH test and sampling for estradiol measurement [18]. At the present time, if the hormonal results confirm the onset of central pubertal activity with an LH peak after LH-RH stimulation, we propose cerebral pituitary MRI and treatment with GnRH analog.

Pseudopuberty due to an Autonomous Cyst

McCune-Albright Syndrome

The best known type of precocious pseudopuberty with recurrent ovarian cysts is McCune-Albright syndrome, which occurs in early childhood [4]. It is manifested by metrorrhagia and rapid breast development in small girls aged between 2 and 5 years. On questioning, it is not rare to learn of an identical but briefer episode in the preceding months [19]. Pelvic ultrasonography establishes the diagnosis by identifying an ovarian cyst and signs of estrogen impregnation of the uterus. This is peripheral or pseudopuberty, which is confirmed by hormone measurements (elevated estradiol and undetectable LH and FSH levels that do not react to an LH-RH test). These cystic lesions may persist, exposing the child to recurrent metrorrhagia; they may also resorb within a few weeks or become complicated by adnexal torsion or hemorrhage [20]. The decision to intervene using ultrasound-guided percutaneous aspiration or surgically by laparoscopy is made according to the individual case.

McCune-Albright syndrome is a sporadic disorder, characterized by diffuse anomalies all due to constitutional activation of the Gs-adenylate cyclase-cAMP transduction system [5]. When the ovary is affected, recurrent episodes of metrorrhagia due to the development of an ovarian cyst are strongly indicative of this etiology [19, 20]. The difficulty lies in confirming the diagnosis when the cysts remain isolated, with no bone involvement, café-au-lait spots or other endocrine disorder. These other manifestations may appear several years later. It is thus important to confirm the diagnosis by molecular studies to search for activating mutations of Gs alpha proteins, which can be negative in blood samples [21]. These studies can be carried out on all affected tissues and on ovarian cell samples obtained after cyst fluid aspiration or directly from the cell wall [19, 21]. Discovery of this mutation in patients with isolated recurrent ovarian cysts raises the dual problem of treatment in the child and long-term surveillance. This is a gonado-independent form of puberty and the usual puberty-inhibiting treatments are ineffective; only aromatase inhibitors seem to have a certain efficacy [18].

Other Endocrine Affections

Aromatase Deficiency. Nineteen cases of aromatase (*CYP19*) deficiency have been reported. Aromatase is a cytochrome P450 enzyme (CYP19) that catalyzes the formation of aromatic C18 estrogens from C19 androgens. cP450arom appears to be the product of a single gene, *CYP19*, located on chromosome 15q21.1. Placental aromatization of androgens protects the female fetus against the virilizing action of fetal androgens. After birth, the dual effect of aromatase deficiency, excessive androgens and insufficient estrogens, is a cause of virilization in girls. In the prepubertal period, high levels of ovarian androgens and gonadotropins facilitate the formation of large hemorrhagic cystic follicles. Both serum basal and GnRH-induced FSH levels remain clearly elevated. Serum basal LH levels are normal but a hyper-response after GnRH stimulation is observed. Therefore, to prevent the risk of torsion of enlarged ovaries and ovarian cysts during infancy and early childhood, long-term treatment with a GnRH analog may be considered as a therapeutic option [22].

Acquired Infantile Hypothyroidism. The onset of signs of hypothyroidism may be very insidious in childhood, and may follow their course for several months before diagnosis. Some pictures are atypical. Gordon et al. [23] described the case of a girl with metrorrhagia associated with rapid pubertal development. Pelvic ultrasonography showed large polycystic ovaries. Percutaneous aspiration of the ovarian cysts together with the institution of thyroid replacement therapy led to the regression of both the cysts and the pubertal signs. The same anomalies have been described in the adult with bilateral ovarian cysts. In this case, the cysts are due to interaction between elevated TSH levels and the ovarian FSH receptor.

Adrenal Disorder. Excessive steroid production by the adrenal glands may stimulate small ovarian cysts to develop into large cysts capable of causing gonadotropin-independent precocious puberty, as has been reported in young girls with rapid sexual development. The signs decrease with cyst removal. However, serum 17-hydroxyprogesterone responses to ACTH seem to be in favor of nonclassical forms of 21-hydroxylase deficiency [24]. The pathogenic hypothesis is that the adrenal gland might be the source of the increase in steroid sulfates (SDHA). In turn, these steroids could be converted into estrogens by the small follicular cysts that occur as a normal developmental process. Estrogen could stimulate cyst growth and increased gonadotropin-independent estrogen production.

Ovarian Neoplasms

In addition to simple functional cysts, there are organic cysts. Some neoplasms have a predominantly cystic appearance [9]. The absence of a solid component is a criterion of benignity.

A benign epithelial tumor is suggested in the presence of a cystic tumor with homogeneous signal intensity and no solid component [9]. Benign serous tumors are usually cystic (cystadenomas) but may also present as half-solid, half-cystic (cystadenofibroma) or, more rarely, mainly solid (adenofibroma). Bilateral tumors suggest serous tumors; serous cystadenomas are uni- or bifocal, with thin walls of less than 3 mm. The mucinous cystadenoma is a larger-sized cystic tumor that is usually unilateral and multifocal. The cystadenofibroma associates a cystic component that is often multifocal and a solid fibrous portion. This tumor is difficult to diagnose because of the irregular presence (50% of the cases) of a solid component (which resembles a cystadenoma) and, in certain cases, the latter can mimic a malignant form of the disease on imaging. Cystadenofibromas are rare (2% of ovarian tumors), essentially serous, and more rarely mucinous or even endometrioid. Adenofibromas are white fibrous microcystic tumors. In all cases, cystectomy is indicated, with the entire wall of the cyst removed while preserving the healthy ovary.

Dermoid cysts are the most frequent neoplasms in childhood, with the mean age of diagnosis being 10 years. They are benign germinal tumors that develop slowly but they may become very large. Ultrasonography shows their heterogeneous appearance with a solid cystic component containing ectodermal tissue (skin, hair, dentin) and calcifications that are also clearly visible on plain radiographs. Treatment consists of cystectomy and careful examination of the contralateral ovary. Monitoring by ultrasonography is continued for several years.

Juvenile granulosa cell tumors are tumors that develop during childhood; they derive from granulosa cells and tend to be of low malignity. These neoplasms manifest by precocious pseudopuberty and most of them have mixed components, both solid and liquid. Purely cystic tumors are principally virilizing granulosa cell tumors. They secrete estrogens or androgens, which accounts for the rapid appearance of pubertal signs and metrorrhagia. They are generally benign and treatment is surgical excision. Postoperative follow-up consists of ultrasonography and measurement of anti-Müllerian hormone and inhibin, which are specific markers of this type of tumor. Greatly decreased postoperative levels are a criterion of cure, whereas an increased level raises the fear of recurrence.

Other tumors such as sex cord-stromal and mixed germ cell tumors are very rare in childhood. They have been reported in girls with isosexual precocity, but the ultrasonographic appearance is very different, with heterogeneous and solid components.

Proteus Syndrome (OMIM 176920)
Proteus syndrome is a rare, sporadic disorder that causes postnatal overgrowth of multiple tissues in a mosaic pattern. The gene is localized on 10 q23–31. Characteristic manifestations include overgrowth and hypertrophy of limbs and digits, connective tissue nevi, epidermal nevi and hyperostoses. Various benign and malignant tumors and hamartomas may complicate the clinical course of patients with the syndrome. Commonly encountered tumors include hemangiomas, lymphangiomas and lipomas. Tumors of the genital tract occur less often. Bilateral ovarian cystadenomas are regarded as having diagnostic value in Proteus syndrome when they occur within the first two decades of life.

Management

The management of an ovarian cyst in prepubertal girls depends on the clinical manifestations and cyst appearance on ultrasound examination [25, 26].

If a cyst is totally anechogenic, all teams agree that the patient should be monitored for a period ranging from 4 weeks to 3 months. Control ultrasound studies done 2 weeks after diagnosis and then at monthly intervals enable assessment of any change in volume. If there is any clinical or ultrasonographic change or if the cyst persists for more than a reasonable period of observation, excision must be planned as it may be an organic, fluid cyst such as a serous cystadenoma or a dermoid cyst.

If adnexal torsion is suspected or if the cyst is heterogeneous, emergency surgery should be performed (see chapter on 'Ovarian masses in adolescent girls'). Ovarian masses associated with torsion are usually benign. Galinier et al. [6] described 45 cases of ovarian torsion in 40 girls. The ovarian mass was benign in 22 cases and low-grade malignancy in 2 cases.

If acute rupture with hemorrhage occurs, it is important to determine whether the bleeding is self-limited or associated with hemodynamic instability. In the latter case, the child should be stabilized and then taken to surgery, which can usually be performed by laparoscopy or laparotomy. A hemoperitoneum is not a contraindication to laparoscopy. Free blood and clots are aspirated and hemostasis assured by fulguration of the areas of bleeding.

The presence or recurrence of a secretory cyst suggests McCune-Albright syndrome and every effort must be made (aspiration or surgery) to obtain diagnostic evidence by molecular biological analysis; long-term surveillance is also necessary in this case (bone and other endocrine expression). Granulosa cell tumors are very rare and the initial presentation associates precocious pseudopuberty with a heterogeneous mass. Treatment is surgical with ovariectomy.

Conclusion

Cysts in the prepubertal period are rarer than in the neonatal and pubertal periods. When found, small cysts (<10 mm) without pathological significance are most common. The persistence of a cyst suggests a neoplasm; benign epithelial tumors have a cystic appearance. Radiologic data confirm the presence of calcifications in benign teratoma. Precocious pseudopuberty with recurrent ovarian cysts evokes the diagnosis of McCune-Albright syndrome and it is necessary to analyze the Gs alpha gene in cystic ovarian tissue. The finding of this mutation is of importance for long-term follow-up.

References

1 van Winter JT, Simmons PS, Podratz KC: Surgically treated adnexal masses in infancy, childhood, and adolescence. Am J Obstet Gynecol 1994;170:1780–1786.

2 Arisaka O, Shimura N, Nakayama Y, Yabuta K, Yoshizawa Y, Hirai Y, Yoshimine T, Kuwabara N: Ovarian cysts in precocious puberty. Clin Pediatr 1989;28:44–47.

3 Kosloske AM, Goldthorn JF, Kaufman E, Hayek A: Treatment of precocious pseudopuberty associated with follicular cysts of the ovary. Am J Dis Child 1984;138:147–149.

4 McCune DJ: Osteitis fibrosa cystica: the case of a nine year old girl who also exhibits precocious puberty, multiple pigmentation of skin and hyperthyroidism. Am J Dis Child 1936;52:743–744.

5 Weinstein LS, Shenker A, Gejman PV, Merino MJ, Friedman E, Spiegel AM: Activating mutations of stimulatory G protein in the McCune-Albright syndrome. N Engl J Med 1991;325:1688–1695.

6 Galinier P, Carfagna L, Delsol M, Ballouhey Q, Lemasson F, Le Mandat A, Moscovici, Guitard J, Pienkowski, C, Vaysse P: Ovarian torsion – management and ovarian prognosis: a report of 45 cases. J Pediatr Surg 2009;44:1759:1765

7 Caspi B, Goldchmit R, Zalel Y, Appelman Z, Insler V: Sonographically guided aspiration of ovarian cyst with simple appearance. J Ultrasound Med 1996;15: 297–300.

8 Brown DL, Doubilet PM, Miller FH, Frates MC, Laing FC, DiSalvo DN, Benson CB, Lerner MH: Benign and malignant ovarian masses: selection of the most discriminating gray-scale and Doppler sonographic features. Radiology 1998;208:103–110.

9 Bouic-Pagès E , Perrochia H, Mérigeaud S, Giacalone PY, Taourel P. MR Imaging of primary ovarian tumors with pathologic correlation. J Radiol 2009; 90:787–802

10 Low LC, Wang Q: Gonadotropin independent precocious puberty. J Pediatr Endocrinol Metab 1998; 11:497–507.

11 Schwartz PE: Ovarian masses: serologic markers. Clin Obstet Gynecol 1991;34:423–432.

12 Hong H, Kim HS: Elevated CA19.9 levels in mature cystic teratoma of the ovary. Int J Biol Markers 2009; 24:52–56
13 Galinier P, Carfagna L, Juricic M, et al: Fetal ovarian cysts management and ovarian prognosis: a report of 82 cases. J Pediatr Surg 2008;43:2004–2009
14 Monnery-Noché ME, Auber F, Jouannic JM, et al: Fetal and neonatal ovarian cysts. Prenat Diagn 2008; 28:15–20.
15 Millar DM, Blake JM, Stringer DA, Hara H, Babiak C: Prepubertal ovarian cyst formation: 5 years' experience. Obstet Gynecol 1993;81:434–438.
16 Freedman SM, Kreitzer PM, Elkowitz SS, Soberman N, Leonidas JC: Ovarian microcysts in girls with premature thelarche. J Pediatr 1993;122:246–249.
17 Haber HP, Wollmann HA, Ranke MB: Pelvic ultrasonography: early differentiation between isolated premature thelarche and central precocious puberty. Eur J Pediatr 1995;154:182–186.
18 Carel JC, Leger J: Precocious puberty. N Engl J Med 2008;358:2366–2377.
19 Pienkowski C, Lumbroso S, Bieth E, Sultan C, Rochiccioli P, Tauber M: Recurrent ovarian cyst and mutation of the Gs alpha gene in ovarian cyst fluid cells: what is the link with McCune-Albright syndrome? Acta Paediatr 1997;86:1019–1021.
20 Rodriguez-Macias KA, Thibaud E, Houang M, Duflos C, Beldjord C, Rappaport R: Follow up of precocious pseudopuberty associated with isolated ovarian follicular cysts. Arch Dis Child 1999;81:53–56.
21 Lumbroso S, Paris F, Sultan C: Activating Gsa mutations: analysis of 72 patients (104 DNA) presenting with signs of McCune-Albright syndrome. An international collaborative study. 82nd US Endocrine Society Meeting, Toronto, 2000.
22 Belgorosky A, Guercio G, Pepe C, Saraco N, Rivarola MA: Genetic and clinical spectrum of aromatase deficiency in infancy, childhood and adolescence. Horm Res 2009;72:321–330.
23 Gordon CM, Austin DJ, Radovick S, Laufer MR: Primary hypothyroidism presenting as severe vaginal bleeding in a prepubertal girl. J Pediatr Adolesc Gynecol 1997;10:35–38.
24 Uli N, Chin D, David R, Geneiser N, Roche K, Marino F, Shapiro E, Prasad K, Oberfield S: Menstrual bleeding in a female infant with congenital adrenal hyperplasia: altered maturation of the hypothalamic-pituitary-ovarian axis. J Clin Endocrinol Metab 1997;82:3298–3302.
25 Murray S, London S: Management of ovarian cysts in neonates, children and adolescents. Adolesc Pediatr Gynecol 1995;8:64–70.
26 Kanizsai B, Orley J, Szigetvari I, Doszpod J: Ovarian cysts in children and adolescents: their occurrence, behavior and management. J Pediatr Adolesc Gynecol 1998;11:85–88.

Catherine Pienkowski
Unité d'Endocrinologie, Génétique et Gynécologie Médicale, Hôpital des Enfants
330, avenue de Grande Bretagne, TSA 70034
FR–31026 Toulouse Cedex (France)
Tel. +33 534 558 556, E-Mail pienkowski.c@chu-toulouse.fr

Sultan C (ed): Pediatric and Adolescent Gynecology. Evidence-Based Clinical Practice. 2nd, revised and extended edition. Endocr Dev. Basel, Karger, 2012, vol 22, pp 112–137

Sexual Abuse in Prepubertal Children and Adolescents

B. Herrmann[a] · F. Navratil[b]

[a]Pediatric Department, Klinikum Kassel, Kassel, Germany; [b]University of Zürich Children's Hospital, Zürich, Switzerland

Abstract

Medical involvement in the diagnosis and treatment of child sexual abuse (CSA) has a well-defined role within a multidisciplinary concept. Due to the increasingly high rate of normal anogenital findings in victims of CSA, forensic aspects are of limited value in establishing the diagnosis. In selected cases however, medical findings may play an important role in corroborating a child's history. Correct evaluation of normal and abnormal findings, normal variations and several differential diagnoses requires sound knowledge in pediatric gynecology. In some cases, physical consequences of CSA (injuries, infections, and pregnancy) need to be diagnosed and treated (prevented) accordingly. The majority of abused children have an altered and distorted body image. It is of paramount importance to reassure the child that its body is normal, physically undamaged, intact or that it will heal ('primary therapeutic aspect of the medical examination'). Thus, the medical examination has an enormous potential to incorporate a therapeutic message into the diagnostic procedure if performed in a qualified and sensitive manner. By communicating with the psychosocial und jurisdictional systems, physicians may initiate proper child protection and therapy. Therefore, medical evaluation of sexually abused children must always be integrated into a multiprofessional concept of child protection.

Child sexual abuse (CSA) has been and continues to be a diagnostic challenge. For nearly three decades has medicine been involved in the diagnosis, treatment and management of sexually abused children and adolescents. CSA is no longer 'another hidden pediatric problem' as Kempe (1978) stated more than 30 years ago. In the United States of America and – to a lesser extent – in Great Britain, many physicians have integrated knowledge about the recognition of CSA into their medical education and practice. A great number of specialized referral centers evolved and developed a significant expertise in evaluating abused children in a qualified and nontraumatizing manner.

A number of reports have summarized the results of numerous studies and research and of the accumulating clinical experience and have described the shortcomings and limitations of our current knowledge and outlined the emphasis on further research [1–7]. The American Academy of Pediatrics has published and recently revised guidelines to facilitate the management of CSA for health care providers [8, 9]. A couple of handbooks and a very instructive CD-ROM atlas give an excellent overview of all aspects of medical involvement in CSA evaluation [10–14].

The situation in most countries in Europe seems to be far less satisfying. We feel an urgent need for all physicians caring for children to develop a basic understanding of behavioral and physical indicators of CSA. Furthermore, the need for specialized referral centers is evident. Child abuse examinations should preferentially be performed by specialists in pediatric and adolescent gynecology. Nevertheless, even those specialists will need supplementary qualification and training in the evaluation of sexually abused children and adolescents. The same goes even more for general pediatricians and gynecologists who engage in this specialty. Given the inherent risk of both under- and overdiagnosis of CSA, both with devastating consequences for children and their families, a thorough understanding of the medical approach is crucial. Performing medical examinations requires sound knowledge about the specifics of anogenital findings in abused and nonabused children as well as knowing the potentials and limitations of medical diagnosis in CSA. This knowledge needs to be contributed and blended into a multiprofessional approach. Especially in Europe, physicians frequently are just beginning to find and define their role within the child protection system. In contrast to the emotional and often unqualified public debate on CSA, medical professionals have a significant responsibility to contribute a rational and objective approach to the multidisciplinary assessment, diagnosis, management and treatment of sexually abused children and adolescents ('Cool science for a hot topic' – [15]). Nevertheless, CSA is an emotionally disturbing and troubling event even for medical professionals and requires emotional balance and commitment. The first step to the diagnosis of CSA and of utmost importance is being aware and acknowledging that the problem exists. Recognition of sexual abuse requires a high index of suspicion and familiarity with the historical, physical, and behavioral indicators of abuse.

General Considerations on Child Sexual Abuse

Although there is no universal definition, sexual abuse is generally defined as the involvement of developmentally immature children or adolescents in sexual activities that they do not fully comprehend, to which they are unable to give informed consent and that violate social taboos of family or other adult-child relationships. Adults take advantage of the power and age differential which removes meaningful consent. The adult's intention to use children for his (or her) sexual arousal and gratification is an important element of the definition. Other definitions describe the unwanted, manipulative, and exploitative character of the interaction and recognize the importance of age difference (mostly 4–5 years). Developmental asymmetry and the use of coercion differentiate abuse from normal sexual play [16, 17].

Sexual abuse includes a spectrum of sexual activities ranging from nontouching to invasive penetrative abuse. In contrast to general public opinion, CSA is mostly a chronic sexualized relationship over months and years between fathers, step-fathers, other relatives or known individuals and the child. Abuse may start in early childhood and continue into adolescence.

Strangers as offenders make up approximately 10% of all cases. These occurrences tend to be rather single events and often are more accurately characterized as 'sexual assault'. Most of sexual abuse is committed by men (approximately 90%), with higher numbers of female perpetrators when boys are victimized (up to 25%). At least 20–25% of the perpetrators are juveniles. This underscores the importance of early intervention including perpetrator treatment. Probably this is the most effective measure of prevention of further abuse of other children. Offenders appear to be 'normal', socially well-adapted people essentially from all social backgrounds. Many, but not all, have been sexually abused as children, and many abuse more than one child.

Victims are girls in 70–80% of the subjects including all age groups, peaking in the prepubertal school age. Adolescents make up at least 25% of sexual abuse victims and tend to be victimized by peers ('date rape'). Lower socioeconomic status is not consistently demonstrated in the research and may be caused by assessment bias. However, unstable social conditions may predispose a child to sexual abuse. Single-parent homes and step-parents seem to be significant risk factors [18, 19].

Although not reported in all studies, developmentally disabled or handicapped children appear to be at higher risk for sexual abuse particularly when the disability affects communication [20].

Current research indicates a prevalence of CSA way in the percent range. That makes CSA for example far more prevalent than all malignancies in childhood together (approximately 0.2%). Finkelhor [18] summarized 19 prevalence studies and concluded that a prevalence of 15–20% of women and 5–10% of men having experienced sexual abuse as children would be a reasonable conservative estimate. Incidence studies do not report the true occurrence, but only those cases that are recognized. Substantiated reports of CSA to US American Child Protection Agencies increased dramatically from 6,000 to 132,000 from 1976 to 1986, being relatively stable until 1994 and declining since then for unknown reasons [4, 19].

Because of possible devastating short- and long-term effects CSA has marked but varying effects on children's health and well-being. A large variety of short-term behavioral abnormalities and symptoms have been reported as indicators and presenting symptoms of CSA. They include nearly all emotional, psychosomatic, self-destructive and antisocial behaviors in children and adolescents, focusing on age inappropriate sexualized behavior, especially when coercive. However there is no single diagnostic criterion or specific syndrome within the variety of symptoms which proves CSA by itself. A basic understanding of normative sexual behavior is important to distinguish normal and abnormal sexual play and activity. Inadequate sexual behavior should be interpreted as indicator but not as proof of CSA and its absence does not rule out abuse [17, 20, 21].

Masked presentations of CSA are common and include the whole range of psychosomatic disorders, with gastrointestinal complaints being most prevalent in younger and chronic pelvic pain in older victims. Feelings of guilt, shame, isolation, lowered self-esteem, criminal behavior and self-injuring behaviors are prevalent among victims of abuse [23–25]. The abnormal behavior frequently is an important coping mechanism of the victim, well described by Summit [26] as 'child sexual abuse accommodation syndrome'. The difficulty in evaluating a history and the nonspecific complaints of an individual has been widely discussed in the psychosocial literature [27].

CSA is associated with substantial increased risk of subsequent psychopathology. Several factors contribute to the great variety of long-term outcomes of victims of former CSA from severe to asymptomatic. Sexual abuse varies significantly in severity and extent, the amount of physical force used, the relationship with the offender, frequency and duration of the abuse, the age of the child, preexisting psychosocial problems and positive or negative effects of professional intervention. Other important factors that influence the outcome are preexisting adverse psychological circumstances, co-existing physical abuse or neglect in terms of additional vulnerability potentially compensated by resilience factors (intra- or extrafamilial support).

A variety of reports have highlighted mental health problems (e.g. depression, suicide, multiple personality disorders, post-traumatic stress disorder, eating disorders, anxiety disorders, substance abuse), physical health problems (e.g. functional gastrointestinal disorders, chronic pelvic pain, dysmenorrhea), and psychosexual dysfunction (e.g. sexual dysfunction, promiscuity, adolescent pregnancy, re-victimization, prostitution). Interpersonal, close relationships are often difficult for abuse victims. They tend to have problems with issues of control, anger, shame, trust, dependency and vulnerability [24].

General Considerations on Medical Aspects of Child Sexual Abuse

The majority of abused children show no physical evidence. The frequency of normal findings varies from 23 to 94%, based on differences in definition of abuse and findings [1, 28]. A meta-analysis by Bays and Chadwick [1] in the early 1990s reported normal findings in more than 50% of abuse victims. In a study by Adams et al. [28] with the subtitle 'It's normal to be normal', they examined 236 children with perpetrator conviction for sexual abuse who had normal genital examination findings in 28%, nonspecific in 49%, suspicious in 9%, and abnormal findings in 14%. In cases of perpetrator confession of penile-vaginal penetration, it is noteworthy that 39% of the victims presented with normal findings in another report [29]. In a study by Berenson et al. [30] only 2% of 192 girls between 3 and 8 years who reported digital-vaginal or penile-vaginal penetration had hymenal transections, perforations or deep posterior notches. The majority of girls were not examined acutely however. Heger et al. [31] examined 2,384 children and found normal examinations in 95% of children who had disclosed and in 92% in girls who reported penetration. Another study from New Zealand reports 5% diagnostic findings and 90% normal findings in 2,134 victims of CSA [32]. In a retrospective case review of 36 pregnant adolescent girls by Kellog et al. [33] who presented for sexual abuse evaluations only 2 of the 36 subjects had definitive findings of penetration. Nowadays, it is generally accepted that 90–95% of abused children have normal findings on examination [7, 16, 34, 35].

The most important reason for the paucity of abnormal findings is the nature of the abuse itself. Frequently, it does not involve physical contact sufficient enough to produce physical sequelae (fondling, oral abuse, masturbation, pornographic photography and others). Therefore, the 'absence of evidence is no evidence of absence' (of abuse). Furthermore, smaller children often do not have sufficient knowledge about their anatomy in order to appropriately describe what exactly has occurred. They may interpret any diffuse pain in the anogenital area as invasive or penetrative. There are no data at which age children are developmentally capable of differentiating 'on' from 'in'. Medically, 'penetration' is defined as the introduction of an object beyond the hymenal membrane into the vagina. In a jurisdictional view, however, even slight penetration between the labia majora constitutes the legal term 'penetration'. Finally, the outcome and traumatizing nature of CSA is not primarily affected by the fact if penetration has occurred or if medical signs of trauma are evident [11].

A significant difference exists between CSA and rape and contributes to the diagnostic difficulties. Especially prepubertal children are seldom forcibly raped and in the majority of cases force and restraint are not used. Therefore, only some children have obvious physical sequelae caused by more serious injuries. Those victims, who sustain physical injury from the abuse, seldom present acutely so that the retrospective interpretation of healed trauma constitutes the major difficulty in evaluating these findings. Those children and adolescents who are victims of stranger assaults or rape will rather present acutely with evident findings, due to familial support and immediate action taken. Acute findings are easier to document but children seldom disclose in this phase.

Another significant factor contributing to the frequent absence of physical findings is the enormous potential of rapid and often complete healing of most anogenital injuries. In selected cases even transections of the prepubertal hymen have been demonstrated to heal to integrity. A single incomplete hymenal rupture may heal as early as 9 days after trauma. More typically though, complete transections to the base of the hymen lead to permanent disfigurations of the hymenal membrane in form of a cleft or concavity [12, 13, 36–38].

The frequency of findings related to abuse will also depend on variables inherent to the health care system: qualification and willingness of the examiner to acknowledge CSA as a possible differential diagnosis, the timing of the examination, qualified and empathetic preparation of the child (in order to obtain consent and cooperation), a good lighting source, good documentation for peer-review or second opinion and to a smaller amount the availability of technical support (generally a colposcope for magnification, lighting and documentation).

Potentials and Limitations of the Medical Approach

As a normal physical examination is frequent in victims of CSA, the forensic aspect of the evaluation cannot be the primary or exclusive goal. A medical approach to CSA has to reflect the potentials but also the limitations and possible risks of the medical evaluation. It is crucial that the needs of the child have absolute priority over the desire to collect forensic evidence. Especially in referring nonmedical child protection professionals there is some concern that the physical examination of sexually abused children may further traumatize the child, as it is believed to be a emotional invasive and distressing procedure, potentially causing a 're-victimization'. Although scientific data to support this view is lacking, the possibility is evident. Possibly this may influence referral patterns and selection of patients for the medical evaluation. This again underscores the paramount importance of interprofessional communication and cooperation. An essential prerequisite of examining possibly abused children in a nontraumatizing manner is to avoid any force or coercion and to communicate this principle to other professionals. The experience of specialized child protection centers and a number of reports indicate that well documented examinations help to avoid repetitive examinations and thereby may prevent further potential trauma.

The emotional response to the medical examination is probably not only influenced by factors inherent to the examination situation itself, but also by multiple other variables, such as pre-existing factors (e.g. general anxiety, previous experiences with the medical system, the age and developmental status of the child) and on the other hand the characteristics and severity of the abuse [39]. Several studies with small samples and the impression of experienced experts in the field indicate that most children seem to cope well with the examination. Children who have disclosed sexual abuse should be evaluated for injuries, anogenital infections, sexually transmitted diseases or pregnancy and treated accordingly. Because a majority of abused children appear to have an altered and distorted body image, it is of paramount importance to reassure the child that its body is normal, physically undamaged, and intact or that it will heal. Doctors, especially pediatricians, who define disease or well-being in other medical settings, are powerful authorities in this respect. They can help to relieve feelings of physical abnormality and initiate the process of recovery ('primary therapeutic aspect of the medical examination'). Thus, the medical examination has an enormous potential to incorporate a therapeutic message into the diagnostic procedure [40, 41]. A prospective study using questionnaires and the Genital Examination Distress Scale found that parents and children found the medical examination significantly less stressful than they had anticipated. They highlighted the importance of being involved in the process, the child's reaction, staff attitudes and the doctor's explanations. Increased parental distress was linked with lack of knowledge about the medical examination, and with the child being 12 years old or older, but not with type (severity) of abuse. Both parents and children emphasized the importance of staff attitudes, explanations offered and the relationship between the doctor and the child. This has implications for clinician training and practice [42, 43].

In cases of suspected CSA, the cooperation with other professions is crucial. The medical examination may contribute valuable aspects to a multidisciplinary approach. Due to evident reasons mentioned above, however, a medical examination can never exclude the possibility of CSA. Therefore, child protection professionals need to know each other and cooperate in mutual respect. They also need to know their respective potentials and limitations. Medical involvement in CSA cases does not only depend on the clinician's engagement and skills but also in the confidence the child-protection and law-enforcement systems develop in the clinician.

History

History-taking should avoid further trauma to the child and still gain a maximum of information. Depending on a possible previous historical evaluation it is not always necessary to repeat questioning on all details of the abuse, which is often difficult and embarrassing for the child. In some cases, however, information on the specifics of what has happened will contribute to interpret physical signs in the light of history [12]. It is advisable to take a separate history from the child and the caretaker if possible. A gentle and open attitude of the examiner and a quiet and accepting atmosphere are essential. The use of anatomically correct dolls is controversial and should be reserved only to very experienced examiners in this field.

History taking should also be interjected with certain therapeutic messages like 'it was good to tell', that many children experience abuse, and that children are never responsible for the abuse. Questions directed to the child should be simple, nonleading and not suggestive of the answer. Scrupulous and verbatim documentation is crucial for further court proceedings and the credibility of the child. In selected cases children may disclose sexual abuse during the medical examination, for instance if they are asked if someone has ever touched them 'in this area' while the anogenital examination is performed [44].

Physical Examination

The preparation and conduct of the physical examination of sexually abused children requires 'time, patience and a gentle manner. . .' [45] and formal medical education in the field. Appropriate timing of the examination is the first step. Most examiners agree to perform immediate examinations if the alleged contact took place less than 72 h ago. The same goes for acute bleeding anogenital injuries. Recent studies indicate that forensic findings in prepubertal girls are unlikely to be found after 24 h, suggesting an urgent forensic examination only within this time frame [46]. Other studies have shown that many subtle genital injuries will disappear within a few days, so the examination should be timed accordingly [38, 47, 48]. Due to typically delayed disclosure most examinations are non-emergency though. Often a perceived 'emergency aspect' rather reflects panic on the side of the referring party, being care-givers as well as non-medical professionals. In most cases the examination can and should be scheduled according to the needs of the child as well as those of the examining institution. This also avoids confronting a frightened child with an untrained (and maybe also frightened!) examiner in the emergency department in the middle of the night.

The issue of sedation or anesthesia for the examination remains controversial. Although some argue in favor because of a reduction of immediate stress, it is not routinely warranted. General anesthesia is usually required in cases of acute bleeding anogenital injuries.

Anticipating and addressing children's fears concerning the medical examination are crucial for a successful examination. Younger children rarely have problems with issues of shame. They rather are fearful of painful and unknown procedures. Any form of force or coercion is strictly contraindicated.

The child should be given as much choices as possible in the procedure to ensure a sense of control. It is important to explain all steps of the examination in an age appropriate terminology. The child should be reassured that the purpose of the examination is to check if everything is 'alright', that it is healthy and 'okay'. Clinical experience indicates that at least for prepubertal children the style and gentleness of the examination are far more important factors for the emotional impact than the gender of the examiner [41].

The sense of control may be enhanced by examining a 'fearful' doll which expresses all the potential fears which children might have in this situation. Asking the child to help the doctor examine the doll lets them anticipate their own examination, gain a sense of control and power and actively cope with their own fears by comforting the doll [11].

Even for nonpediatricians, a complete head-to-toe examination is mandatory. It should always precede the anogenital examination in order not to focus on the anogenital area (like the abuser has done). The implicit message is that the whole child is important. It also allows estimating the developmental stage and avoids missing extragenital signs of sexual or physical abuse.

The anogenital examination in cases of suspected sexual abuse of the prepubertal child is principally an external visualization by varying techniques of separation, traction and positioning. It does not require anal or vaginal palpation or the use of specula. In adolescents, the use of a speculum is appropriate but not mandatory. Stirrups may be used in older consenting children, while often increasing unfamiliarity and fear in younger children.

The genital examination begins in the most comfortable and least frightening position, the supine position with abducted legs ('frogleg position'). Especially younger children may prefer to be examined on the caretaker's lap. The separation technique of the labia majora allows an overview over the external genital structures. The traction technique is the mandatory next step and markedly improves visualization and opening of the hymenal orifice, especially when redundant hymenal tissue is present. In this technique the labia majora are grasped between thumb and index finger exerting slight traction down and outwards. Meanwhile, most examiners agree to routinely include the prone knee-chest position into the examination except in those cases when visualization in the supine position is complete and satisfactory. In cases with unclear or suspicious findings in the supine position the knee-chest position is invaluable as it markedly improves unfolding of the hymen due to gravity. The examiner's hands rest on the buttocks with thumbs pointing inwards and slightly pulling upwards and laterally. The persistence of suspicious findings in the knee-chest position improves their validity. Also, the visualization of the inner vagina up to the cervix can be achieved without specula in a significant number of cases. Children who have experienced anal penetration may feel uncomfortable and frightened in this position. The response and affect of the child have to be carefully monitored when requesting this position.

The inspection of the anus is mandatory and can be performed in the prone knee-chest position or in the left lateral decubitus position. The latter is preferable in boys who tend to be abused anally.

Pubertal children are preferably examined in the lithotomy position. Visualization of the redundant pubertal hymen can be difficult. Running behind the inner aspect of the membrane circumferentially with a moistened cotton swab can help to identify traumatic changes of the hymenal rim.

A recent study compared the effectiveness of different examination techniques and found prone knee chest position to be the most successful method for detecting hymenal injuries in both pubertal and prepubertal girls. The authors recommend to routinely use a multimethod approach. Current guidelines require verification of significant findings by all three examination techniques [11, 12, 14, 49, 50].

Explaining each step of the examination and talking with the child throughout the examination on non-abuse-related issues, or motivating the child to tell a story, allows the child to relax. This enhances cooperation and improves visualization by less muscular tension to the genital tissues. Generally, all visualization and photo documentation should be done before taking swabs. The unestrogenized prepubertal hymen is very sensitive. In cases when screening for sexually transmitted diseases is indicated the use of small urethral swabs which are moistened with sterile saline helps to avoid a potentially painful contact with the hymen. Large cotton swabs should be avoided in prepubertal children. Alternatively, a small urethral catheter can be used to irrigate the posterior portion of the vagina with a small amount of saline which then is aspirated again for further processing.

The colposcope is nowadays frequently used for the external visualization of the anogenital area of possibly abused children and adolescents. Nowadays mostly equipped with a digital camera or a video system it enhances visualization by incorporating a powerful lighting source, fixed or variable magnification and the possibility of accurate documentation. Photo or video documentation of all abnormal findings allow preservation of visual evidence, later detailed reviewing and discussion of findings, peer-review and a second opinion. The latter is required before labeling a finding as 'diagnostic' according to recent guidelines [50]. It also lays the foundation of any research and is an excellent tool for education of students, residents and colleagues. Documented visual evidence may be presented in court and may help to avoid potential further emotional trauma by repeated examinations. Although colposcopy improves the incidence of positive findings only slightly and the unaided examination is sufficient in most cases it has become a valuable tool in the evaluation of possibly abused children [51].

Forensic Evidence Collection and Interpretation

Forensic evidence is infrequently found in CSA cases due to reasons discussed earlier (delayed disclosure, etc.). However, in selected cases the medical expert in child abuse may be asked for a competent forensic work-up in an acute assault which is usually done at the same time as the physical examination. This requires coordinating specific details of collection, labeling, and packaging with the forensic laboratory. Handling of the specimens must be documented with scrutiny to maintain the chain of evidence. Pregnancy and sexually transmitted diseases have forensic significance but are usually not classified in this category.

The decision to perform a forensic examination mainly depends on the time of presentation after the assault. The recommendation of a 72-hour time frame is based on experience in adult victims that semen, seminal fluid and other products are rarely recoverable after this time. A study by Christian et al. [46], however, did not find any positive swabs for sperm or semen later than 9 h postcontact in 273 children. No forensic evidence was collected after 24 h except for the clothing or linen of the children. They concluded that guidelines for forensic evaluation of adult victims may not be appropriate for children. The impression that acute forensic examinations should be restricted to a 24-hour time frame in prepubertal victims is discussed as a future recommendation in recent guidelines. Further studies confirm this aspect but have also shown that many subtle genital injuries will disappear within a few days, so the examination should be timed accordingly [46–48, 52].

Sperm may be present on a wet mound for only 30 min, in the adult vagina for 12–20 h, rarely up to 48–72 h, in the cervix up to 5 days. Survival time of sperm in the prepubertal vagina is significantly shorter. Dead or immotile sperm is detectable longer. Dry specimens, however, are quite stable and sperm in stains has been detected up to 12 months [12].

The Wood's lamp or ultraviolet light has traditionally been recommended to identify semen on a victim's skin. Research has shown significant limitations and shortcomings: semen and urine were not distinguishable, urine fluoresces considerably longer, and a number of child care products will equally fluoresce undistinguishable from semen. Keeping these limitations in mind, the Wood's lamp may serve as a screening aid where to take swabs from a victim's body [53].

The marked elevation of acid phosphatase in the vagina indicates sexual contact within 24–48 h, but it may also turn to normal within 3 h in some cases. p30, a semen glycoprotein of prostatic origin and MHS-5, an antibody against a vesicle protein, are male specific and improve sensitivity markedly. Negative results of all tests do not exclude sexual abuse however.

Semen, blood, saliva, body hair and other materials found on the victim may help to prove the identity of the offender by several methods. They include ABO blood group antigens, subtypes of the enzyme phosphoglucomutase, the enzyme peptidase A and most sensitive DNA profiling. Bite mark identification by a forensic odontologist may also determine the offending person by analysis of good quality photographs taken with a ruler. Swabs from acute bite marks may be analyzed for genetic markers [54].

Anogenital Findings

Normal Findings – Anatomy and Terminology

For professionals involved in the evaluation of children for possible sexual abuse it is crucial to develop a thorough understanding of the appearance of the anogenital anatomy both in abused and nonabused children. It is difficult to describe a finding as abnormal without fully understanding the range of normal at each developmental level. The increasing knowledge on medical diagnosis in sexual abuse has gone from early imprecise and misleading work to detailed macrophotographic analysis of subtle anogenital findings. As a result of this evolution, the range of findings now interpreted as normal or unspecific (abnormal but not related to abuse) has continuously increased while the number of findings which clearly indicate abusive trauma has decreased [3, 37, 55]. In the first decade of medical CSA research many previously undescribed findings were interpreted as related to trauma in the light of a child's history suggesting abuse. Many of these findings later were demonstrated in studies of nonabused children, mainly by the groups of McCann and Berenson [56–63]. Although there are methodological considerations and limitations to nonabuse studies, their work has greatly enhanced our knowledge. A main concern is the question if the screening tools are specific enough to exclude undisclosed sexual abuse (for discussion of limitations and methods of research, see Berenson [55]).

The evaluation and description of anogenital findings should be done on the basis of a descriptive and standardized terminology of normal structures. Clinicians involved in describing findings of abused children should speak the same language and describe normal variations and pathologic changes in the same terminology. Although specialists in pediatric and adolescent gynecology are expected to be familiar with the specific terminology it is worthwhile to have a look at the concepts developed in the recent child abuse literature [11–14]. The documentation in the medical record should be as specific as possible and avoid general terms as 'normal genitalia', not reflecting the great variety of normal. 'Vulva' and 'pudenda' also lack specificity. 'Virgo intacta', 'virginal introitus', 'marital hymen', 'gaping vulva' or 'enlarged vaginal opening' are insufficient, imprecise and not descriptive terms and should be strictly avoided.

The term 'posterior fourchette' may not be familiar in Europe. It describes the posterior joining of the labia minora (frenulum labiorum pudendi minorum), an area which is especially vulnerable to trauma by attempted penile penetration. The description of genital findings should begin with the external, superficial structures and move on to the inner structures according to the conduct of the examination.

Much of medical research on genital changes in CSA has focused on the hymen. This was especially true in the first decade of research in the 1980s, when considerable efforts were made to attribute the probability of sexual abuse according to measurements of the hymenal orifice's transverse diameter. Paradise summarized the debate at the end of the decade in a report titled 'Predictive accuracy and the diagnosis of sexual abuse: a big issue about a little tissue'. She pointed out that 'the diagnosis of sexual abuse inevitably rests not on a genital measurement but on descriptive statements made by a child' [64]. The size of the hymenal opening increases with age and depends on a wide variety of factors like examination position, examination technique, amount of traction used and the degree of relaxation of the child, thus potentially varying within the same examination. Genital measurements have lost any significance in the evaluation of children for possible sexual abuse and are no longer used in current guidelines [65, 66]. Two reports described post-traumatic scarring leading to entirely closing off the hymnal opening, resembling an imperforate hymen [67, 68]. With the exception of complex genital abnormalities all girls are born with a hymen – several studies have failed to document a single case of an absent hymen at birth in more than 25,000 newborn girls. Thus, an entity known as 'congenital absence of hymen' does not exist as a sole congenital abnormality [3].

The appearance of the hymenal membrane is quite variable and is strongly influenced by the factors mentioned above but also by age and hormonal factors. The whitish-pink hymen of newborn girls is mostly annular, rather thick and redundant due to maternal estrogen influence. The appearance changes markedly due to withdrawal of estrogen thus creating the typical and most prevalent crescentic, semilunar configuration mostly found in children over 3 years of age. The hymen becomes a thin, more translucent and reddish membrane due to vascularization until pubertal raise of estrogen again creates a paler, redundant and fimbriated appearance. Hymenal configurations observed in children are:

- Annular (circumferential, concentric) – mostly in newborns and infants.
- Crescentic (semilunar, posterior rim type) – most frequent in prepubertal girls.
- Fimbriated (denticular) – mainly in newborns, small infants and puberty.
- Normal variants include: sleeve-like (hymen altus), septate, microperforate (= cribriform) or imperforate hymen. An asymmetric appearance is frequent, not abnormal and often results from asymmetric traction [55–63].

The hymen is an elastic tissue, unlike the common lay misconception of a piece of paper irrevocably 'broken' by penetration or the idea of an impermeable membrane. The degree of elasticity is difficult to quantify, although penetration of a digit may occur without sequelae. The use of tampons may cause enlargement of the hymenal opening but no disruption of its integrity. Masturbation in prepubertal girls is clitoral and does not cause injury of the hymen, especially because the prepubertal hymen is well innervated and quite pain susceptible. Also, physical activities like gymnastics, running, jumping or splits do not lead to hymenal damage [3, 69].

Among the hymenal variations a '*notch*' is an angular or v-shaped indentation on the edge of the hymenal membrane. It is referred to as '*concavity*' when its appearance is curved or u-shaped. Superior (also referred to as 'anterior') notches in the supine position are common in nonabused children. The withdrawal of estrogen in infants and resulting involution of tissue in the periurethral area may lead to formation of new superior notches. Posterior notches that extend to the vestibular or vaginal wall have only been reported in abused children and have then been referred to as '*transections*'. No transections between 4 and 8 o'clock have been found in nonabused children, making it a finding consistent with penetrating trauma [12, 38, 50].

Other hymenal variations include 'external ridges' on the external surface of the hymen. They are frequently found in newborns and tend to resolve in most children until 3 years of age. They have previously been misinterpreted as new scar formation. 'Longitudinal intravaginal ridges' or columns were reported in 25–89%, a variance maybe reflecting age or racial differences in the studies. 'Bumps' or 'mounds' (also referred to as 'projections') mostly occur when an intravaginal ridge attaches to the hymenal rim, but may also exist as isolated finding. They have been found in 7–34% of the nonabused population and also are no indicators of abuse as misconceived in earlier studies. 'Tags' or elongated projections of the hymenal rim are often incorrectly referred to as polyps. The latter are benign mucosal tumors growing into a lumen, while tags may result from previous vaginal septa or intravaginal ridges protruding from the hymenal rim. Their prevalence ranges from 2 to 25%. Vestibular and periurethral supporting bands also have been misinterpreted as scar formation while being found in 50 to 90% of non-abused girls. Other variations of normal described in McCann's study were erythema of the vestibule (56%), labial adhesions (39%), lymphoid follicles in the fossa navicularis (34%), and urethral dilatation with labial traction (15%). A posterior fourchette midline avascular area also called 'linea vestibularis' is found in up to 25% and has the potential to be confused with scar tissue [55–63].

Normal perianal findings in both sexes include erythema (41%), increased pigmentation (30%), venous congestion (73%), midline skin tags (11%), and smooth midline wedge shaped areas referred to as 'diastasis ani' (26%). The latter results from a congenital anomaly of external sphincter muscle fibers. This finding also has a considerable potential for misinterpretation as scar tissue [62]. A recent study found significant differences in perianal anatomy between boys and girls as well as between different examination positions. The authors interpret the differences as a result of of anatomical and muscular differences between boys and girls [70].

Findings in Abused Children

The reasons for the paucity of specific findings in sexual abuse victims have been discussed earlier in this text, the abusive physical contact producing no injury being the most prominent reason. The timing of the examination crucially determines the frequency of abnormal findings in those cases where injury has occurred, mainly because of the rapid and often complete healing of anogenital injuries and typically delayed disclosure. The kind of findings vary considerably with the nature of the abuse, hereby involved objects, the degree of force used, the age of the child and the frequency of the abuse. The time since last incidence and a history of pain and/or bleeding increase the likelihood of detecting abnormal physical findings. The range of findings varies considerably, involving superficial mucosal abrasions and scratches to clear transecting lacerations of anogenital tissues. As the offender frequently uses little physical force, many resulting injuries tend to be superficial and heal rapidly. Most of these findings resolve within 2–3 days after trauma, which is consistent with the characteristics of wound healing. A recent study has shown scars to be infrequent in genital trauma. Healing of hymenal injuries does not leave scarring at all [36]. Up to 2007, there has been very limited evidence on the healing patterns following acute trauma [38, 71–73]. A recent retrospective multicenter study by McCann et al. [38, 52] significantly adds to the current knowledge by contributing longitudinal data of acute and healing genital trauma. Their final sample included 113 pubertal and 126 prepubertal girls and confirms much of the previous reports on the characteristic of healing genital trauma. Hymenal abrasions, petechiae, mild submucosal hemorrhages and hematomas healed completely in 2–3 days in most cases and were rarely identified up to 15 days, when rated 'moderate' or 'marked'. Complete transections to the base of the hymen left a permanent defect or gap. Partial thickness tears may heal completely or leave a partial notch. Except in rare cases of supposedly non abused adolescents, complete transections of the hymen have only been observed following penetrating trauma, which may be abuse or accident in selected cases. In McCann's study on nonhymenal findings, similar to the hymenal findings, abrasions resolved within 2–3 days, petechiae within 24 h and submucosal hemorrhages and hematoma within 7–14 days. Blood blisters were observed up to 31 days [52].

Female Genitalia

The majority of studies describe findings of female genitalia. Minor trauma is frequently caused by genital fondling, rubbing or vulvar coitus (rubbing of the penis between the labia). It mostly leads to unspecific changes like erythema or superficial abrasions of the inner aspects of labia minora, periurethral area, vestibule or the clitoris which heal to integrity within a few days. In cases of digital manipulation these findings are frequently found in the superior-anterior region in supine position (between 9 and 3 o'clock). A history of dysuria is a valuable corroborating history of this type of sexual abuse. Dysuria may also follow coitus however. Penetration of the hymenal orifice with a small object like a finger may possibly leave no physical sequelae due to the elastic nature of the hymenal tissue [12].

When an object forcefully penetrates into the vagina residual signs are obvious when examined acutely. The extent of injury increases with lower age. The majority of abuse related findings are found in the posterior area involving the posterior part of the hymen, fossa navicularis, posterior fourchette, the posterior commissure and the lateral walls of the vagina. A penile penetration causes disruption of the hymenal rim especially between 5 and 7 o'clock but can be found anywhere between the 3 and 9 o'clock position. This results in incomplete or complete transections and v-shaped notches or clefts of the hymenal membrane. Within a few weeks, the notches lose their clear-cut and sharp appearance and develop into a smoother, u-shaped aspect, referred to as concavities. In some cases, a narrowing of the posterior rim develops. The edges of the hymenal rim may become thickened or rolled and intravaginal structures may be more readily exposed. Even if repeated penetration may lead to an enlargement of the hymenal transverse diameter it is no longer considered to be diagnostic sign [7, 8, 34, 64].

Repeated irritation of genital mucosa may result in chronic inflammation (recurring vulvovaginitis) or in labial agglutination (labial synechia) as an acquired post-inflammatory condition. Both findings may gain significance with a corroborating history [74]. Due to their unspecific nature and prevalence in the prepubertal child caution should be used when they present as supposed isolated and sole indicators of possible sexual abuse.

Male Genitalia

Even less findings than in girls have been reported in sexually abused boys. Very rarely acute abrasions, hematoma and petechiae occur in abused boy's genitals.

Anal Findings

The interpretation of anal signs of abuse (sodomy) in boys and girls is far more controversial than genital signs of trauma. The frequency and significance of findings are subject to substantial disagreement in the literature [62, 75]. The ability of the external sphincter to dilate considerably when passing large bolus of fecal matter without any injury to the anal tissues is a major contributing factor. Variables influencing the presence of physical signs include the size of the object introduced, the amount of force used, the age of the victim, the use of lubricants, frequency of episodes and time elapsed since the last episode.

Again, acute and extensive findings are not very problematic to interpret. Deep lacerations and significant trauma to the anus are obvious results of anal penetration. In these cases anoscopy may be helpful for identification of internal injuries like bruising, petechiae, or lacerations and for collection of seminal products [76]. In the absence of acute findings anoscopy is not indicated. The significance of chronic anal signs remains more problematic. High numbers of abnormal anal findings in children evaluated for sexual abuse in British studies [75] have not been replicated in US and other studies and many have been demonstrated to occur in nonabused populations [50, 77].

Anal fissures may result from constipation, and are not considered suspicious for abuse per se. Flattened anal folds, hyperpigmentation, perianal grooves, anal dilatation less than 2 cm and anal skin tags are frequently seen in nonabused children [50]. Special controversy has evolved about the sign of 'reflex anal dilatation' (RAD). Mainly earlier British studies had confidence about the significance of this finding ('dilatation over 0.5 cm') [75]. The paucity of studies to date does not allow final conclusions on the significance of chronic anal findings. In the opinion of the authors they may be overestimated in British studies and underestimated in American reviews. As an isolated sign RAD should not be interpreted as diagnostic of CSA. A dilatation more than 2 cm without visible stool is currently classified as an 'indeterminate finding' and warrants further evaluation [50].

Extragenital Signs of Sexual Abuse

Those signs are infrequent and rather seen in the context of rape: hematomas and bite marks in the so called erogenous zones, especially the inner thighs, breasts, neck and buttocks; bruising, hematomas and strangulation marks of the neck, the extremities or the flank in the kidney region (due to forceful sodomy); petechiae of the sclerae caused by strangulation; petechiae of the soft palate or tear of the labial frenulum due to forceful oral penetration [12].

Classification of Findings

In order to categorize anogenital findings different authors developed classification scales which intend to relate the findings to the probability of their abusive origin. Several revisions of a scale developed by Adams have been popular as a comprehensive categorization schema for analyzing and interpreting findings. In a review of former version of Adam's paper, Ricci cautioned the use of the schema as '. . .it is important to recognize however, that this schema is a suggestion, a way of organizing one's thoughts about a constellation of findings. Although. . . in line with much of the current research. . . it is important to recognize that any schema must be interpreted within the context of each individual case' [12]. Finally, a major revision by an outstanding expert panel has been developed between 2003 and 2008 after a rigorous revision process, considering the scope and limitations of current research. The guidelines were published 2005 and 2007 and updated 2008 (table 1). The word 'classification' was finally removed. The participants cautioned the use of the schema by stating that 'the revised document should be used solely as a tool to assist medical providers in making clinical determinations of the possible significance of medical findings in children they evaluated for suspected sexual abuse'. The historical part was removed due to insecure data and misuse as a 'checklist' and the findings section was restricted to three major groups: normal, indeterminate and definite evidence [50].

Guidelines for decision making, especially in respect to mandated reporting of sexual abuse have been published by the Committee on Child Abuse and Neglect of the American Academy of Pediatrics [8]. Classification scales help to assess probabilities but must never be misinterpreted as rigid instructions how to interpret anogenital findings. The current state of knowledge and its limitations have to be kept in mind and updated continuously as in all other medical disciplines.

Sexually Transmitted Diseases

Sexually transmitted diseases (STD) are discussed in a different chapter of this book. We only refer to a few important characteristics with regard to CSA.

STD may be the only medical indicator of sexual abuse in selected cases. The American Center for Disease Control (CDC) states that the diagnosis of a sexually transmitted disease in a child beyond the neonatal period suggests sexual abuse [79]. The interpretation differs according to the respective disease. STD are diagnosed in

Table 1. 2005–2008 guidelines for medical care of children evaluated for suspected sexual abuse: consensus statement and revision of the former 'Adams classification' (detailed references in the original article: [50])

I. Findings Documented in Newborns or Commonly Seen in Nonabused Children
(the presence of these findings generally neither confirms nor discounts a child's clear disclosure of sexual abuse)

Normal variants

1. Periurethral or vestibular bands
2. Intravaginal ridges or columns
3. Hymenal bumps or mounds
4. Hymenal tags or septal remnants
5. Linea vestibularis (midline avascular area)
6. Hymenal notch/cleft in the anterior (superior) half of the hymenal rim (prepubertal girls), patient supine
7. Shallow/superficial notch or cleft in inferior rim of hymen
8. External hymenal ridge
9. Congenital variants in appearance of hymen, including crescentic, annular, redundant, septate, cribiform, microperforate, imperforate
10. Diastasis ani (smooth area)
11. Perianal skin tag
12. Hyperpigmentation of the skin of labia minora or perianal tissues in children of color
13. Dilation of the urethral opening with application of labial traction
14. 'Thickened hymen' (estrogen effect, folded edge of hymen, swelling from infection, or swelling from trauma; compare to follow-up examination)

Findings commonly caused by other medical conditions

15. Erythema of the vestibule, penis, scrotum or perianal tissues (irritants, infection, or trauma*)
16. Increased vascularity of vestibule and hymen (due to local irritants, or normal pattern in the nonestrogenized state)
17. Labial adhesion (may be due to irritation or rubbing)
18. Vaginal discharge (various infectious and noninfectious causes; cultures must be taken)
19. Friability of the posterior fourchette or commisure (irritation, infection, or by examiner's traction on the labia majora)
20. Excoriations/bleeding/vascular lesions (lichen sclerosus, eczema or seborrhea, vaginal/perianal group A streptococcus, urethral prolapse, hemangiomas)
21. Failure of midline fusion (perineal groove)
22. Anal fissures (usually due to constipation, perianal irritation)
23. Venous congestion, or venous pooling in the perianal area (usually due to positioning of child; also seen with constipation)
24. Flattened anal folds (may be due to relaxation of the external sphincter or to swelling of the perianal tissues due to infection or trauma*)
25. Partial or complete anal dilatation less than 2 cm (anterior-posterior), with or without stool visible

* Follow-up examination is necessary before attributing these findings to trauma

Table 1. Continued

II. Indeterminate findings: insufficient or conflicting data from research studies
(May require additional studies/evaluation to determine significance; these physical/laboratory findings may support a child's clear disclosure of sexual abuse, if one is given, but should be interpreted with caution if the child gives no disclosure; report to Child Protective Services may be indicated in some cases)

Physical examination findings

26. Deep notches or clefts in the posterior/inferior rim of hymen, in contrast to transections [see 41]
27. Deep notches or complete clefts in the hymen at 3 or 9 o'clock in adolescent girls
28. Smooth, noninterrupted rim of hymen between 4 and 8 o'clock, appearing less than 1 mm wide; examined in the prone knee-chest position, or using water to 'float' the edge of the hymen, child in supine position
29. Wart-like lesions in the genital or anal area (biopsy and viral typing may be indicated in some cases)
30. Vesicular lesions or ulcers in the genital or anal area (infectious and noninfectious causes, cultures, serology, and/or nucleic acid amplification tests should be done)
31. Marked, immediate anal dilation to AP diameter of 2 cm or more; absence of other predisposing factors such as chronic constipation, sedation, anesthesia, neuromuscular conditions

Lesions with etiology confirmed: indeterminate specificity for sexual transmission

32*. Genital or anal condyloma accuminata in child; absence of other indicators of abuse

33*. Herpes type 1 or 2 in the genital or anal area in a child with no other indicators of sexual abuse

* Report to child protective services is recommended by AAP Guidelines 2005; in contrast to the 2005–2007 version of the 'Guidelines' not recommended in the 2008 version

III. Findings diagnostic of trauma and/or sexual contact
The following findings support a disclosure of sexual abuse, if one is given, and are highly suggestive of abuse even in the absence of a disclosure, unless a clear, timely, plausible description of accidental injury is provided by the child and/or caretaker
It is recommended that diagnostic quality photodocumentation of the examination findings be obtained and reviewed by an experienced medical provider before concluding that they represent acute or healed trauma
Follow-up examinations are also recommended

Acute trauma to external genital/anal tissues

34. Acute lacerations or extensive bruising of labia, penis, scrotum, perianal tissues, or perineum (may be from unwitnessed accidental trauma or from physical or sexual abuse)
35. Fresh laceration of the posterior fourchette, not involving the hymen (must be differentiated from dehisced labial adhesion or failure of midline fusion; also caused by accidental injury or consensual sexual intercourse in adolescents)

Residual (healing) injuries
These findings are difficult to assess unless an acute injury was previously documented at the same location

36. Perianal scar (rare; may be other medical conditions: Crohn's disease, accidental injuries, or previous medical procedures)
37. Scar of posterior fourchette or fossa (pale areas in the midline may also be due to linea vestibularis or labial adhesions)

Table 1. Continued

Injuries indicative of blunt force penetrating trauma (. . .or from abdominal/pelvic compression injury, if such history is given) 38. Laceration (partial or complete tear) of the hymen, acute 39. Ecchymosis (bruising) on the hymen (absence of a known infectious process or coagulopathy) 40. Perianal lacerations extending deep to the external anal sphincter (not to be confused with partial failure of midline fusion) 41. (Healed) hymenal transection An area between 3 and 9 o'clock on the rim of the hymen where it appears to have been torn through, to or nearly to the base, so there appears to be virtually no hymenal tissue remaining at that location Must be confirmed using additional examination techniques, such as a swab, prone knee-chest position, Foley catheter balloon (adolescents only), or water to float the edge of the hymen This finding has also been referred to as a 'complete cleft' in sexually active adolescents and young adult women 42. Missing segment of hymenal tissue Area in the posterior (inferior) half of the hymen, wider than a transection, with an absence of hymenal tissue extending to the base of the hymen, which is confirmed using additional positions/methods Presence of infection confirms mucosal contact with infected and infective bodily secretions, contact most likely to have been sexual in nature 43*. Positive confirmed culture for gonorrhea (from genital area, anus, throat) beyond neonatal period 44*. Confirmed diagnosis of syphilis, if perinatal transmission is ruled out 45. *Trichomonas vaginalis* infection in a child older than 1 year of age; organisms identified by culture or in vaginal secretions by wet mount examination (by an experienced technician or clinician) 46*. Positive culture from genital or anal tissues for Chlamydia, if child is older than 3 years at time of diagnosis and specimen was tested using cell culture or comparable method approved by the Centers for Disease Control 47*. Positive serology for HIV, if perinatal transmission, transmission from blood products and needle contamination has been ruled out * Considered diagnostic of sexual transmission by AAP guidelines 2005
Diagnostic of sexual contact 48. Pregnancy 49. Sperm identified in specimens taken directly from a child's body

1–5% of abused children. The differences result from factors like type and frequency of the abuse, the age of the victim, the methods for testing and varying regional prevalence. Cultures and smears for STD should only be obtained in selected cases as the yield of positive cultures is very low in asymptomatic children [8, 80]. Proposed selection criteria for STD screening include genital discharge at examination or in the recent history, a perpetrator with a known or suspected STD or with high risk behavior, anogenital findings indicating penetrative abuse, a history of genital-to-genital (or genital-to-anal) contact or penetration, concern of the patient or it's caretakers or specific genital lesions. The screening includes vaginal and anal cultures for gonorrhea and Chlamydia and a vaginal smear for *Trichomonas vaginalis*. Prepubertal gonorrhea and chlamydial infections are localized vaginal infections. Swabs should be taken from the vaginal wall beyond the hymen. Cervical swabs are not indicated before adolescence. Extending the screening to syphilis, hepatitis B and HIV should be done on a case to case decision. Adequate and optimal technique of obtaining specimens, choice testing methods and cultures are of paramount importance due to the forensic implications of positive results. Recently, the use of nucleic acid amplification methods has become increasingly popular in testing for STDs. Specific considerations and limitations have to be kept in mind when used for possible prepubertal sexual abuse [79].

Except in documented congenital infections confirmed positive cultures for *Neisseria gonorrhea* in a prepubertal child or serologic proof of an acquired syphilis are definite evidence of sexual abuse. Perinatally acquired infections with *Chlamydia trachomatis* have been demonstrated to persist as long as 2 years in the genital area and up to 3 years in the pharynx. Infections appearing after the first two years of life are strong indicators of CSA. Infections with *T. vaginalis* should raise the suspicion of sexual abuse and warrant further screening. *Herpes genitalis* and *Condylomata accuminata* have lost specificity as indicators of sexual abuse in the last decade and are classified as 'indeterminate findings' in 2010 guidelines. Recent reports suggest a significant number of transmissions through non sexual household contacts [8, 12, 50, 82].

Differential Diagnosis

Beside the normal findings, normal variants and unspecific findings there are a number of important differential diagnoses to consider when evaluating children with abnormal anogenital findings for possible sexual abuse.

One of the frequent areas of concern is accidental genital injuries. The pattern of injury and accompanying history however generally provide sufficient information for differentiating them from abusive trauma. Most accidents result from straddling, referring to children falling on hard objects like a bicycle bar or a furniture arm with their genital area. Usually this causes an injury of the external genital structures which are crushed between the object and the underlying bones. The injuries involve the labia majora and minora and the clitoral hood and rarely involve the deep and protected structures like the hymen and the posterior fourchette. Published reports regarding accidental genital injuries describe them to be mostly minor and superficial, located anterior, external and unilateral. In most cases of accidental injuries the hymen is not involved [83, 84]. Exceptions are rare cases of accidental penetrating injuries [85]. Other types of injury reported in the literature include a case of posterior vaginal laceration near the hymen by a water slide accident, seat belt injuries in motor vehicle accidents, hymenal tears resembling penetrating trauma in girls run over in motor vehicle accidents and midline splitting injuries with and without hymenal involvement due to inline skating accidents [86, 87]. All reports stress the overwhelming importance of the history which tends to be spontaneous, acute and dramatic. It is consistent with the injuries and does not change over time or between different caretakers or between caretakers and child. Also the immediate consultation of medical help favors the diagnosis of accidental trauma.

Dermatologic conditions which need to be differentiated from sexual abuse include erythema and excoriations in unspecific skin irritation or infection, diaper dermatitis, lack of hygiene, irritant substances (bubble bath, cosmetic care products), moniliasis, genital varicella and oxyuriasis. Recurrent vaginitis is often an area of concern especially when expressed in the context of custody debates. The child returning from the separated father after a weekend visit with red genitals may as well have experienced a paternal lack of hygiene, or his aversion to properly clean the genital area because he fears allegations of sexual abuse. Although abuse is possible and parental separation may result from nondisclosed abusive family constellations research indicates much lower numbers of abused children in this context as commonly thought [88]. Vaginitis is the most prevalent pediatric gynecology health problem and requires a systematic approach and broad differential diagnosis. Unclear and recurring vaginitis should warrant concern and further evaluation but is never diagnostic per se [86].

An infection caused by group A β-hemolytic streptococci (GABHS) may cause a fiery red, edematous and tender vaginal or perianal inflammation, sometimes accompanied by various forms of discharge: thin, thick, serous, blood tinged, creamy, white, yellow or green. Cultures have to be specifically requested as streptococci do not grow on routine media. Treatment is according to pharyngeal infections with a 10-day course of oral penicillin [89].

A frequently mistaken diagnosis of CSA occurs in children who present with anogenital lichen sclerosus et atrophicus. After initial white papules that form to white plaques, the skin becomes delicate and atrophic. It is extremely susceptible to minor trauma like wiping with toilet paper, causing fissuring or alarming subepidermal hemorrhages and spontaneous bleeding. The typical presentation is an 'hourglass' or 'figure of eight' configuration of decreased pigmentation around the labia majora and the anus [90, 91].

Cutaneous bleeding in the anogenital area may be caused by leukemia, disseminated intravascular coagulation, purpura fulminans and other coagulation disorders. Urethral bleeding is rather caused by urethral prolapse (more prevalent in African-American girls), polyps, hemangioma, or papilloma than by sexual abuse. Vaginal bleeding requires careful evaluation of the underlying causes, primarily by vaginoscopy. Most frequently it is caused by vaginitis (approximately 70%). Other less frequent causes include precocious puberty, sarcoma botryoides (embryonal rhabdomyosarcoma), internal or external application of hormones, or unspecific, idiopathic bleeding [86].

Congenital conditions mistaken for sexual abuse include hemangioma of the hymen, vagina and labia. They may bleed or ulcerate. Failure of midline fusion is a congenital defect resembling scar tissue. Sometimes it is combined with an anteriorly located anus and also frequently creates confusion and misinterpretation as an abuse related finding. Anal findings to be differentiated from abuse are fissures in chronic obstipation, morbus Crohn, rectal prolapse or a streptococcal-A cellulitis [12].

Overall Assessment

In spite of an abundance of data on medical findings in CSA victims and their differentiation from normal, normal variants and other differential diagnoses, the medical proof of abuse remains the exception when evaluating suspected sexual abuse cases. This would be the case in acute anogenital trauma in the absence of a convincing history of accidental trauma, proof of gonorrhea or syphilis (after excluding a congenital infection), pregnancy, proof of semen, sperm cells, acid phosphatase or sperm specific glycoprotein p30 in or on the body of a child.

The overall assessment of the likelihood of sexual abuse and the final conclusions have to be done conscientious and need to include all physical findings, possible laboratory results and especially the history obtained from the child. The medical expert contributes a thoughtful and qualified piece of evidence to the multidisciplinary puzzle of evaluating children for possible CSA. Strictly medical interventions in CSA include treatment of injuries, infections, or STDs, and emergency contraception. Reassurance of physical intactness should be an integral part of the medical examination. Furthermore, the physician participates in referral to therapy, emotional guidance of the family, and assisting the legal system in cases with confirmatory findings. It is crucial to develop extensive interdisciplinary and multiprofessional cooperation and consultation in all cases.

Although we are constantly learning more about the role and significance of medical aspects in suspected sexual abuse cases the diagnosis 'CSA' primarily rests on the professionally and qualified obtained descriptive statements made by an abused child.

Terminology

Superior/inferior half of the hymenal rim refers to above/below the 3 o'clock to 9 o'clock line in the supine position.

References

1 Bays J, Chadwick D: Medical diagnosis of the sexually abused child. Child Abuse Negl 1993;17:91–110.

2 Navratil F: The genital examination in suspected child sexual abuse: a diagnostic dilemma. Ann NY Acad Sci 1997;816:414–421.

3 Kerns D: Establishing a medical research agenda for child sexual abuse. Child Abuse Negl 1998;22(special issue):453–660.

4 Atabaki S, Paradise JE: The medical evaluation of the sexually abused child: Lessons from a decade of research. Pediatrics 1999;104(suppl):178–186.

5 Girardet RG, Lahoti S, Parks D, McNeese M: Issues in pediatric sexual abuse –what we think we know and where we need to go. Curr Probl Pediatr Adolesc Health Care 2009;32:216–246.

6 Sapp MV, Vandeven AM: Update on childhood sexual abuse. Curr Opin Pediatr 2005;17:258–264.

7 Berkoff MC, Zolotor AJ, Makoroff KL, Thackeray JD, Shapiro RA, Runyan DK: Has this prepubertal girl been sexually abused? JAMA 2008;300:2779–2792.

8 Kellogg N, Committee on Child Abuse and Neglect: The evaluation of sexual abuse in children: American Academy of Pediatrics Clinical Report. Pediatrics 2005;116:506–512.

9 Kaufman M, Committee on Adolescence: American Academy of Pediatrics: Care of the adolescent sexual assault victim. Pediatrics 2008;122:462–470.

10 McCann J, Kerns D: The anatomy of child and adolescent sexual abuse. A CD-ROM Atlas/Reference. InterCorp, St. Louis, 1999, ww.intercorpinc.com/sabuse.html

11 Herrmann B, Dettmeyer R, Banaschak S, Thyen U: Kindesmisshandlung. Medizinische Diagnostik, Intervention und rechtliche Grundlagen, ed 2, revised. Heidelberg, Springer, 2010.

12 Finkel MA: Medical aspects of prepubertal sexual abuse; in Reece RM, Christian CW (eds): Child Abuse: Medical Diagnosis and Management, ed 3. Elk Grove Village, American Academy of Pediatrics, 2009, pp S269–320.

13 Finkel MA, Giardino AP: Medical Evaluation of Child Sexual Abuse, ed 3. Elk Grove Village, American Academy of Pediatrics, 2009.

14 Kaplan R, Adams JA, Starling SP, Giardino AP: Medical response to child sexual abuse: a resource for professionals working with children and families. St. Louis, STM Learning, 2011.

15 Kerns DL: Cool science for a hot topic. Child Abuse Negl 1989;13:177–178.

16 Kellogg N, Committee on Child Abuse and Neglect: The evaluation of sexual abuse in children: American Academy of Pediatrics Clinical Report. Pediatrics 2005;116:506–512.

17 Friedrich WN: Behavioral manifestations of child sexual abuse. Child Abuse Negl 1998;22:523–531.

18 Finkelhor, D: Current information on the scope and nature of child sexual abuse. Future Child 1994;4:31–53.

19 Leventhal JM: Epidemiology of sexual abuse of children: old problems, new directions. Child Abuse Negl 1998;22:481–492.

20 American Academy of Pediatrics: Committee on Child Abuse and Neglect and Committee on Children with Disabilities: Assessment of maltreatment of children with disabilities. Pediatrics 2001;108:508–512.

21 Kellogg ND, Committee on Child Abuse and Neglect: Clinical report – the evaluation of sexual behaviors in children. Pediatrics 2009;124:992–998.

22 American Academy of Pediatrics, Stirling J Jr; Committee on Child Abuse and Neglect and Section on Adoption and Foster Care; American Academy of Child and Adolescent Psychiatry, Amaya-Jackson L; National Center for Child Traumatic Stress, Amaya-Jackson L: Understanding the behavioral and emotional consequences of child abuse. Pediatrics 2008;122:667–673.

23 Beitchman JH, Zucker KJ, Hood JE, DaCosta GA, Akman D: A review of the short term effects of child sexual abuse. Child Abuse Negl 1991;15:537–556.

24 Beitchman JH, Zucker KJ, Hood JE, DaCosta GA, Akman D, Cassavia E: A review of the long-term effects of child sexual abuse. Child Abuse Negl 1992;16:101–118.

25 Drach KM, Wientzen J, Ricci LR: The diagnostic utility of sexual behavior problems in diagnosing sexual abuse in a forensic child abuse evaluation clinic. Child Abuse Negl 2001;25:489–503.

26 Summit RC: The child sexual abuse accommodation syndrome. Child Abuse Negl 1983;7:177–193.

27 Everson MD: Understanding bizarre, improbable and fantastic elements in children's accounts of abuse. Child Maltreatment 1997;2:134–149.

28 Adams JA, Harper K, Knudson S, Revilla J: Examination findings in legally confirmed child sexual abuse: it's normal to be normal. Pediatrics 1994;94:310–317.

29 Muram D: Child sexual abuse: relationship between sexual acts and genital findings. Child Abuse Negl 1989;13:211–216.

30 Berenson A, Chacko M, Wiemann C, et al.: A case-control study of anatomic changes resulting from sexual abuse. Am J Obstet Gynecol 2000;182:820–824.

31 Heger A, Ticson L, Velasquez O, Bernier R: Children referred for possible sexual abuse: Medical findings in 2384 children. Child Abuse Negl 2002;26:645-659.

32 Kelly P, Koh J, Thompson JM: Diagnostic findings in alleged sexual abuse: Symptoms have no predictive value. J Pediatr Child Health 2006;42:12–117.
33 Kellogg ND, Menard SW, Santos A: Genital anatomy in pregnant adolescents: 'Normal' doesn't mean 'nothing happened'. Pediatrics 2004;113:e67-e69.
34 Pillai M: Genital findings in prepubertal girls: what can be concluded from an examination? J Pediatr Adolesc Gynecol 2008;21:177–185.
35 Slaughter L, Henry T: Rape: when the exam is normal. J Pediatr Adolesc Gyn 2009;22:7–10.
36 McCann J, Voris J, Simon M: Genital injuries resulting from sexual abuse: a longitudinal study. Pediatrics 1992;89:307–317.
37 McCann J: The appearance of acute, healing, and healed anogenital trauma. Child Abuse Negl 1998; 22:605–616.
38 McCann J, Miyamoto S, Boyle C, Rogers K: Healing of hymenal injuries in prepubertal and adolescent girls: a descriptive study. Pediatrics 2007;119: e1094-e1106.
39 Britton H: Emotional impact of the medical examination for child sexual abuse. Child Abuse Negl 1998;22:573–580.
40 Hornor G, Scribano P, Curran S, Stevens J: Emotional response to the ano-genital examination of suspected sexual abuse. J Forensic Nurs 2009;5: 124–130.
41 De San Lazaro C: Making paediatric assessment in suspected sexual abuse a therapeutic experience. Arch Dis Child 1995;73:174–176.
42 Gully KJ, Britton H, Hansen K, Goodwill K, Nope JL: A new measure for distress during child sexual abuse examinations: the genital examination distress scale. Child Abuse Negl 1999;23:61–70.
43 Marks S, Lamb R, Tzioumi D: Do no more harm: the psychological stress of the medical examination for alleged child sexual abuse. J Paediatr Child health 2009;45:125–132.
44 Coulborn Faller K: Interviewing the prepubertal child for possible child sexual abuse; in Reece RM, Christian CW (eds): Child Abuse: Medical Diagnosis and Management, ed 3. American Academy of Pediatrics, Elk Grove Village, 2009, pp 257–268.
45 Horowitz DA: Physical examination of sexually abused children and adolescents. Pediatr Rev 1987; 9:25–29.
46 Christian C, Lavelle J, Dejong A, Loiselle J, Brenner L, Joffe M: Forensic evidence findings in prepubertal victims of sexual assault. Pediatrics 2000;106:100–104.
47 Palusci VJ, Cox EO, Shatz EM, Schultze JM: Urgent medical assessment after child sexual abuse. Child Abuse Negl 2006;30:367–380.
48 Young KL, Jones JG, Worthington T, Simpson P, Casey PH: Forensic laboratory evidence in sexually abused children and adolescents. Arch Pediatr Adolesc Med 2006;160:585–588.
49 Boyle C, McCann J, Miyamoto S, Rogers K: Comparison of examination methods used in the evaluation of prepubertal and pubertal female genitalia: a descriptive study. Child Abuse Negl 2008;32: 229–243.
50 Adams JA: Guidelines for medical care of children evaluated for suspected sexual abuse: an update for 2008. Curr Opin Obstet Gynecol 2008;20:435–441.
51 Muram D, Arheart KL, Jennings SG: Diagnostic accuracy of colposcopic photographs in child sexual abuse evaluations. J Pediatr Adolesc Gynecol 1999; 12:58–61.
52 McCann J, Miyamoto S, Boyie C, Rodgers K: Healing of nonhymenal genital injuries in prepubertal and adolescent girls: a descriptive study. Pediatrics 2007b:120:1000–1011.
53 Santucci KA, Nelson DG, McQuillen KK, Duffy SJ, Linakis JG: Wood's lamp utility in the identification of semen. Pediatrics 1999;104:1342–1344.
54 Makoroff K, Desai M, Benzinger E: The role of forensic materials in sexual abuse and assault; in Reece RM, Christian CW (eds): Child Abuse: Medical Diagnosis and Management, ed 3. American Academy of Pediatrics, Elk Grove Village 2009;pp 377–388
55 Berenson AB: Normal anogenital anatomy. Child Abuse Negl 1998;22:589–596.
56 Berenson AB, Heger A, Andrews S: Appearance of hymen in newborns. Pediatrics 1991;87:458–465.
57 Berenson AB, Heger A, Hayes JM, Bailey RK, Emans SJ: Appearance of hymen in prepubertal girls. Pediatrics 1992;92:387–394.
58 Berenson AB: Appearance of hymen at birth and one year of age: a longitudinal study. Pediatrics 1993;91:821–825.
59 Berenson AB, Somma-Garcia A, Barnett S: Perianal findings in infants 18 months of age or younger. Pediatrics 1993;91:838–840.
60 Berenson AB: A longitudinal study of hymenal morphology in the first 3 years of life. Pediatrics 1995;95:490–496.
61 Berenson A B, Grady JJ: A longitudinal study of hymenal development from 3 to 9 years of age. J Pediatr 2002;140:600–607.
62 McCann J, Wells R, Simon M, Voris J: Perianal findings in prepubertal children selected for nonabuse: a descriptive study. Child Abuse Negl 1989;13:179–193.
63 McCann J, Wells R, Simon M, Voris J: Genital findings in prepubertal girls selected for nonabuse: a descriptive study. Pediatrics 1990;86:428–439.

64 Paradise JE: Predictive accuracy and the diagnosis of sexual abuse: a big issue about a little tissue. Child abuse Negl 1989;13:169–176.
65 Berenson AB, Chacko MR, Wiemann CM, Mishaw CO, Friedrich WN, Grady JJ: Use of hymenal measurements in the diagnosis of previous penetration. Pediatrics 2002;109:228–235.
66 Ingram DM, Everett VD, Ingram DL: The relationship between the transverse hymenal orifice diameter by the separation technique and other possible markers of sexual abuse. Child Abuse Negl 2001;25: 1109–1120.
67 Berkowitz CD, Elvik SL, Logan MK: A simulated 'acquired' imperforate hymen following the genital trauma of sexual abuse. Clin Pediatr 1987;6:307–309.
68 Botash AS, Jean-Louis F: Imperforate hymen: congenital or acquired from sexual abuse? Pediatrics 2001;108:e53.
69 Emans SJ, Woods ER, Allred EN, Grace E: Hymenal findings in adolescent women: impact of tampon use and consensual sexual activity. J Pediatr 1994; 125:153–160.
70 Myhre AK, Berntzen K, Bratlid D: Perinanal anatomy in non-abused preschool children. Acta Pædiatr 2001;90:1321–1328.
71 Finkel MA: Anogenital trauma in sexually abused children. Pediatrics 1989;84:317–322.
72 McCann J, Voris J: Perianal injuries resulting from sexual abuse: a longitudinal study. Pediatrics 1993; 91:390–397.
73 Heppenstall-Heger A., McConnell G, Ticson L, Guerra L, Lister J, Zaragoza T: Healing patterns in anogenital injuries: a longitudinal study of injuries associated with sexual abuse, accidental injuries, or genital surgery in the preadolescent child. Pediatrics 2003;112:829–837.
74 Berkowitz CD, Elvik SL, Logan MK: Labial fusion in prepubescent girls: a marker for sexual abuse? Am J Obstet Gynecol 1987b:156:16–20.
75 Hobbs CJ, Wynne JM: Sexual abuse of English boys and girls: the importance of an anal examination. Child Abuse Negl 1989;13:195–200.
76 Ernst AA, Green E, Ferguson MT, Weiss SJ, Green WM: The utility of anoscopy and colposcopy in the evaluation of male sexual assault victims. Ann Emerg Med 2000;36:432–437.
77 Myhre AK, Berntzen, K, Bratlid D: X Genital anatomy in non-abused preschool children. Acta Paediatr 2001;92:1453–1462.
78 Ricci LR: Reviewers note on: Adams JA: Evolution of a classification scale: medical evaluation of suspected child sexual abuse. Child Maltreatment 2001; 6:31–36.
79 CDC: Sexually transmitted diseases treatment guidelines. MMWR 2010;59:RR-12.
80 Siegel RM, Schubert CJ, Myers PA, Shapiro RA: The prevalence of sexually transmitted diseases in children and adolescents evaluated for sexual abuse in Cincinnati: rationale for limited STD testing in prepubertal girls. Pediatrics 1995;96:1090–1094.
81 Hammerschlag MR: Use of nucleic acid amplification tests in investigating child sexual abuse. Sex Trans Infect 2001;77:153–157.
82 Beck-Sague CM, Solomon E: Sexually transmitted diseases in abused children and adolescent and adult victims of rape: review of selected literature. Clin Infect Dis 1999;28:S74–S83.
83 Dowd MD, Fitzmaurice L, Knapp JF, Mooney D: The interpretation of urogenital findings in children with straddle injuries. J Pediatr Surg 1994;29:7–10.
84 Bond GR, Dowd MD, Landsman I, Rimsza M: Unintentional perianal injury in prepubescent girls: a multicenter, prospective report of 56 girls. Pediatrics 1995;95:628–631.
85 Boos SC: Accidental hymenal injury mimicking sexual trauma. Pediatrics 1999;103:1287–1289.
86 Kellogg ND, Frasier L: Conditions mistaken for child sexual abuse; in Reece RM, Christian CW (eds): Child Abuse: Medical Diagnosis and Management, ed 3. Elk Grove Village, American Academy of Pediatrics, 2009, S389–426.
87 Herrmann B, Crawford J: Genital injuries in prepubertal girls from inline skating accidents. Pediatrics 2002;110:e16.
88 Corwin DL, Berliner L, Goodman G, Goodwin J, White S: Child sexual abuse and custody disputes: no easy answers. J Interpers Violence 1987;2:91–105.
89 Mogielnicki NP, Schwartzman JD, Elliott JA: Perineal group A streptococcal disease in a pediatric population. Pediatrics 2000;106:274–281.
90 Warrington S, de San Lazaro C: Lichen sclerosus et atrophicus and sexual abuse. Arch Dis Child 1996; 75:512–516.
91 Herrmann B, Veit S, Neises M: Lichen sclerosus et atrophicus. Wichtige Differentialdiagnose zu sexuellem Missbrauch von Kindern. Pädiatr Prax 1998; 55:319–324.

Bernhard Herrmann, MD
Child Protection Center, Pediatric and Adolescent Gynecology
Kinderklinik des Klinikum (Pediatric Department, Klinikum Kassel)
Mönchebergstrasse 43
DE–34125 Kassel (Germany)
Tel. +49 561 980 3389, E-Mail herrmann@klinikum-kassel.de

Sultan C (ed): Pediatric and Adolescent Gynecology. Evidence-Based Clinical Practice. 2nd, revised and extended edition. Endocr Dev. Basel, Karger, 2012, vol 22, pp 138–159

Delayed Puberty

Patrick Fenichel

Service d'Endocrinologie et Médecine de la Reproduction, Centre Hospitalo-Universitaire de Nice, Hôpital de L'Archet, Nice, France

Abstract

Since puberty is a long ongoing developmental process with significant individual and population differences in timing, the definition of delayed puberty for a given individual needs to rest on simple, though arbitrary criteria based on epidemiological data. Although several genes involved in the hypothalamic-pituitary-gonadal maturation cascade have been characterized recently from familial or sporadic cases of primitive isolated hypogonadotropic hypogonadism, many genes regulating puberty onset remain undetermined. In case of delayed puberty and/or primary amenorrhea, a complete clinical examination including a detailed past history will evaluate the development of secondary sex characteristics, verify the association with a growth delay and look for specific indicative features pertaining to the etiological diagnosis. This clinical check-up completed if necessary with biological, ultrasonographic, radiological and genetic investigations will try to determine which girls will have a permanent sexual infantilism of gonadal, hypophyseal or hypothalamic origin, which girls will undergo spontaneous but delayed puberty and which girls have primary amenorrhea with developed secondary sex characteristics. Therapeutic attitude will have to integrate etiological factors, statural prognosis, bone mass preservation and psychological factors.

Introduction

Developmental changes during puberty in girls occur over a period of 3 to 5 years, usually between 9 and 14 years of age. They include the occurrence of secondary sex characteristics beginning with breast development, the adolescent growth spurt, the onset of menarche, which does not correspond yet to the end of puberty, the acquisition of fertility as well as profound psychological modifications. These events are consecutive to the stimulation of the hypothalamic-pituitary-ovarian axis leading to sex-steroid secretions acting on specific receptors. Even though the reactivation of the LH-RH pulse generator, indeed already functional since the perinatal period, has been considered for 20 years [1] to be the primum movens of puberty, the inhibitory and stimulatory neuromediators controlling this reactivation remain to be fully elucidated [2]. Since puberty is a long ongoing developmental process with significant individual and population differences in timing, the definition of delayed puberty for a given individual needed to rest on simple, though arbitrary criteria based on epidemiological data.

Although several genes involved in the hypothalamic-pituitary-gonadal maturation cascade have been characterized recently from familial or sporadic cases of primitive isolated hypogonadotropic hypogonadism [3], many genes regulating puberty onset remain undetermined [4]. Identification of the Ob gene product and the role of leptin in reproduction [5] have highlighted the influence of nutritional factors illustrated by the frequent association of delayed puberty with systemic diseases and/or with a negative energetic balance. More recently it has been shown that kisspeptins, a series of overlapping peptides encoded by the Kiss 1 gene, are required for central activation of the hypothalamic-pituitary-ovarian axis at puberty and that mutations in the kisspeptin receptor GPR54 is associated with primary hypogonadotropic hypogonadism [94].

In case of delayed puberty and/or primary amenorrhea, a complete clinical examination including a detailed past history will evaluate the development of secondary sex characteristics, verify the association with a growth delay and look for specific indicative features pertaining to the etiological diagnosis. This clinical check-up completed if necessary with biological, ultrasonographic, radiological and genetic investigations will try to determine which girls will have a permanent sexual infantilism of gonadal, hypophyseal or hypothalamic origin, which girls will undergo spontaneous but delayed puberty and which girls have primary amenorrhea with developed secondary sex characteristics. Therapeutic attitude will have to integrate etiological factors, statural prognosis, bone mass preservation and psychological factors.

Physiological Aspects

Increase in the pulsatile release of LH-RH is a necessary condition for the onset of puberty as demonstrated 22 years ago by Knobil et al. [1] in rhesus monkeys. Appropriate intermittent pulsatile secretion of LH-RH stimulates the hypophysal-ovarian axis, controls and maintains the menstrual cycle allowing ovarian sex-steroid secretion and follicular maturation. It is well established that the LH-RH neurosecretory system already works in the neonatal period leading to gonadotropin stimulation and estrogenic secretion during the first 6 months of life [6]. Then it enters a dormant state during childhood with reduced LH-RH pulses, low secretion of gonadotropins and very low estrogenic secretion. The nocturnal increase in pulse frequency, pulse amplitude and baseline level of LH-RH will initiate pubertal maturation followed by increasing amplitude in mid-puberty until the time of the first ovulation. Then, in late puberty, the circadian fluctuation and pulse amplitude will decrease to the adult level [6].

Maturation of the LH-RH neurosecretory system allows during the early pubertal period, an increase of mean FSH levels, followed by an increase in mean LH levels. Basal levels of LH, amplitude and frequency of LH pulses increase with circadian fluctuations with an increasing ratio of basal LH/FSH. The increase in gonadotropins stimulates ovarian estrogen secretion inducing peripheral sexual changes and FSH suppression by a negative feedback effect. Periodic changes of increasing secretion of estrogen will lead to the first vaginal bleeding (menarche) before any LH surge and first ovulation [6]. Ovulatory regular adult cycles will occur more than 1 year after menarche. Adult type of pulsatile LH-RH release is mandatory for the positive feedback effect of estrogen after a priming effect of the gonadotropic cells by both pulsatile LH-RH and increasing levels of estrogen [7].

Increase in pulsatile LH-RH release clearly triggers puberty. However, the precise neuronal mechanisms leading to such a reactivation of the LH-RH pulse generator and to the establishment of the adult type of pulsatile LH-RH secretion remains still incompletely elucidated [2]. A classical hypothesis known as the 'gonadostat theory' has proposed that a differential sensitivity of the hypothlamus to the ovarian steroid negative feedback could explain the onset of puberty. However, even though the estrogen-dependent suppression of gonadotropin secretion is stronger in prepubertal girls than in adults it could not explain why children with ovarian dysgenesis or total ovarian destruction have very low levels of FSH and LH during infancy until the prepubertal period [8]. In fact, one has to consider the hypothesis that sexual quiescence before the onset of puberty is the consequence of a central inhibition of LH-RH release, independent of estrogen-negative feedback and that an autonomous increase in pulsatile LH-RH release triggers puberty. Several studies in female monkeys support the evidence that gamma-aminobutyric acid (GABA) is the predominant inhibiting neurotransmitter during prepuberty that acts directly or indirectly on LH-RH neurons through GABAA receptors [2]. These receptors are present on LH-RH neurons and also on glutamate neurons. Maturation of the hypothalamus and the neurosecretory LH-RH system during development and puberty may involve the decrease of GABA synthesis and secretion, allowing decrease of the direct inhibition on LH-RH neurons and the liberation of the glutamate pathway, able to stimulate indirectly, LH-RH release [2].

Though opioids do not play any inhibiting action on LH-RH release before puberty as they play in the adult during stress, the importance of other inhibitory neurotransmitters before and at the onset of puberty are still under discussion [2]. For example neuropeptide Y (NPY) plays several important roles in regulating brain function, including food intake behaviors. It seems to have an inhibitory action on LH-RH release before puberty and this inhibiting effect decreases during and after puberty [2]. Quantitative or qualitative undernutrition can delay puberty and induce functional amenorrhea [9]. Metabolic factors such as glucose and/or amino acids may act directly by modulating neurons involved in the control of LH-RH release. Rosa Frisch has postulated that a minimal weight, body mass index or, better, body fat mass was necessary for the onset of puberty in girls [10]. In fact, leptin, the product of the Ob gene, secreted by adipose tissue, increases in girls during the pubertal stages [11]. Leptin receptors are present in the hypothalamic centers especially on NPY neurons. Leptin could serve as a link between the reproductive function and the energetic balance [12, 13] and participate in the onset of puberty and the maintenance of the adult hypothalamo-hypophyseal-ovarian axis. Leptin deficiency is associated with primitive hypogonadotropic hypogonadism [5] while puberty can be induced by recombinant leptin [14]. However, this induction cannot be obtained before a critical age which suggests that leptin has to be considered more as a permissive factor for the timing of puberty rather than a trigger of the onset of puberty [15]. Nevertheless, it seems useful to evaluate leptin blood level in all situations of functional delay of puberty associated in girls with negative energetic balance consecutive to general diseases or to intentional or not undernutrition.

The hypothalamic-somatotropic-insulin-like growth factor I axis and the hypo halamic-gonadotropic-ovarian axis undergo striking similarities and relationships during puberty. Both are controlled by a neurosecretory system which includes pulsatile intermittent secretion (LH-RH/GHRH) which will present developmental changes during puberty resulting in an amplification of pulsatile neurohormone secretion. Both are controlled by multiple neural, hormonal and metabolic influences. Interactions between both endocrine systems are not yet well understood but puberty needs a functional GH axis for full gonadal activation and onset of puberty is associated with a dramatic increase in linear height velocity. In girls, but probably also in boys, estrogens are responsible for the amplifying secretory activity of the GH axis during puberty [16, 17]. Estrogens will induce the height velocity spurt and then influence epiphyseal maturation. Estrogens have in fact a biphasic action on longitudinal growth [18]. At first very low levels of estrogens may stimulate bone growth indirectly trough stimulation of the GH-IGF-1 axis without affecting sexual maturation and then higher levels of estrogens stimulate secondary sexual characteristics and epiphyseal fusion [18]. Furthermore, GH secretion will contribute through IGF-1 action to the complete ovarian development.

Epidemiological Aspects

Age at onset of puberty varies greatly among individuals and populations and seems to be influenced both by genetic and environmental factors [3]. It follows approximately a normal or a Gaussian distribution [3]. In girls, the onset of menarche has generally been used as the easiest and most objective indicator for comparative studies. It has been well documented that the average age of menarche has decreased in industrialized northern countries by approximately 2–3 months per decade during the last century [18–20]. This secular trend toward an earlier onset of puberty has been related to an increased socioeconomical level, an improved nutrition and a better health. Nevertheless, this decrease seems to attenuate more recently and to reach a plateau in Europe [20] and in the United States [19] with an average age of menarche between 12.5 and 13 years, and a Tanner stage 5 [21] reached between 14 and 14.5 years. However, the same authors reported that the onset of breast development or Tanner breast stage 2 (B2) seemed to occur earlier than previously thought in the United States [19] even though adequate earlier studies of breast development are not available for objective comparison. Whether environmental factors such as endocrine disrupters with estrogenic effects have any influence on that phenomenon remains to be verified [20]. The mean age of B2 is 9.5 [19] to 10.9 years [22] and it will take 4 years to reach complete breast development (B5). One precocious event of girl puberty is the increase of linear growth and peak of growth velocity (9 cm/year) reached between stages B3 and B4 at an age of 12–14 years. Menarche will occur at 12.7 years and ovulatory cycles at age 14. Based on epidemiological data, delayed puberty in girls has been defined as the failure to manifest the initial signs of sexual maturation which begins in girls with breast development by an age of 13 years (2 SD above the mean for the population) or a girl who does not menstruate within 5 years after the onset of pubertal development with uncompleted development of secondary sex characteristics [6]. Infantilism is defined by a delayed puberty for a bone age of 13 years [6]. Primary amenorrhea is defined by the absence of menstruation in a 15-year-old girl whether secondary sexual characteristics are absent, partially or completely developed [3].

Clinical Aspects

First evaluation based on a detailed history and a complete clinical examination will have to confirm undeveloped, partially or completely developed secondary sex characteristics, precise growth development, look for indicative features concerning the etiological diagnosis and evaluate the degree of anxiety of the patient and her parents. Family history will be studied for consanguinity, delay in the age of onset of puberty in parents or siblings, cases of anosmia, or infertility. The patient history will include possible history of disorders during pregnancy, difficulties during labor and delivery with birth trauma, prematurity or hypotrophy, problem of linear growth, anosmia or inadequate nutritional status during childhood associated or not to a chronic disease of the lungs, the heart, the kidney, the blood or the gastrointestinal tract. This examination will also assess the food behavior looking for selective or inadequate diet, signs of anorexia nervosa, excessive intensive sport practice or psychological, affective, relational troubles.

Physical examination includes breasts (glandular tissue and the alveolar size), pubic and axillary pilosity and external genitalia rated according to the standard stages [21] allowing to discriminate between true infantilism, arrested pubertal development or primary amenorrhea. Determination of height and weight as well as number of standard deviations may differ from the mean value for chronological age and will be included to the chart representation of their evolution since birth and completed by the height velocity curve. Physical examination may find associated signs such as galactorrhea, congenital malformations or neurological signs.

Complementary studies will include first FSH and LH determination to discriminate between a gonadal peripheral origin with high FSH level, a hypogonadotropic deficiency with low FSH and LH levels, and a primary amenorrhea with mature adult gonadotropin secretions. Radiographic bone age determination will help to interpret linear growth in relation to pubertal development while pelvic ultrasound will confirm the presence of the ovaries and the uterus and rate their stage of development.

Etiological Aspects
After the clinical examination and simple complementary investigations, the physician often has come to a presumptive diagnosis. The easiest case is when FSH is elevated (hypergonadotropic hypogonadism). In this case, the work up will be completed with a karyotype. If gonadotropins are low it will be less easy: the physician will have to eliminate an organic disease such as tumor by MRI of the brain, to screen for a negative energetic balance, and to identify genetic causes of isolated hypogonadotropic hypogonadism before being able to diagnose an idiopathic constitutive delay of puberty which remains infrequent in girls.

Hypergonadotropic Hypogonadism

Elevated FSH and/or LH levels reflect a peripheral ovarian disease and invite verification of female phenotype, checking for the presence of ovarian and uterine tissues by ultrasound, and determining the karyotype on peripheral blood lymphocytes before examining the ovaries by coelioscopy and biopsy.

Gonadal Dysgenesis with Chromosomal Abnormalities

Turner's Syndrome and Its Variants
Turner's syndrome, the most frequent cause of primitive ovarian failure, associates in its classical monosomic 45 XO form, female phenotype, short stature, several somatic abnormalities and sexual infantilism. In this form, diagnosis has frequently, but not always, been done during infancy [25]. Any suggestive malformations (webbed neck, nail dysplasia, high palate, short fourth metacarpal and strabismus), growth retardation and/or elevated FSH must lead to the verification of the karyotype. However, in its variant forms with mosaicism, or structural abnormalities of an X chromosome (iso, deletion, translocation X/autosome) there are several phenotypes for pubertal development from infantilism to partial secondary sex characteristics development, primary amenorrhea or even spontaneous puberty. Indeed spontaneous puberty occurs in 10–20% [26, 27] followed by premature ovarian failure especially in case of mosaicism with few 45 X cells or deletion of the X short arm.

Treatment with recombinant GH may be able to accelerate partial pubertal development [28]. In fact, both X chromosomes are necessary for the preservation of ovarian function and oocytes. Specifically, some areas such as the Xq13-q26 region contain genes which are thought to prevent premature follicular atresia. In Turner's syndrome, germinal cells are present and normal until the fourth month of intrauterine life. Regression of gonocytes will then depend on the importance of the X defect. At birth, ovarian morphology can vary from ovarian streaks to macroscopically normal ovaries.

Mosaicism can be associated with the partial presence of a Y chromosome found at cytogenetic analysis. A systematic molecular analysis found it in 1 of 40 cases [29]. If present, castration will prevent the development of gonadoblastoma [30].

Gonadal Dysgenesis with a 46,XY Karyotype

In the Swyer syndrome which associates a female phenotype, a normal or elevated height, nonambigous external genital organs, and normal Müllerian structures, the gonads are often reduced to indifferentiated streaks. They may have some testicular characteristics, carry the risk of neoplastic transformation and must therefore be removed. Mutations of the SRY gene will be found only in 20% of cases [31].

46,XY disorders of sex development (DSD) with various degrees of sexual reversion and genital ambiguity has been related to a large panel of mutated genes involved in sex differentiation:

- WT1 with Wilm's tumor and renal insufficiency in the Drash syndrome [32] and without Wilm's tumor but another renal pathology in the Frasier syndrome [32].
- SOX-9 associated to the campomelic dysplasia [33].
- DAX-1 with duplication of the Xp21 region [34].
- SF1 heterozygous mutations in 46,XY patients with ambiguous genitalia, gonadal dysgenesis but no adrenal insufficiency have been recently reported by several groups and seem to be relatively frequent [35, 36].

Defect in Androgen Action

- Complete androgen insensitivity syndrome.

Mutations of the gene coding for the androgen receptor, located on chromosome X, will lead in boys to various degrees of androgen resistance with in the complete form with female external genitalia [37]. Diagnosis will be made only in the peripubertal period. It will be suggested by a primary amenorrhea with no pubian or axillary pilosity, but a normal breast development. LH level is very high with adult male testosterone level; FSH level is not elevated; estradiol is almost at a follicular phase level allowing breast development. Vaginal cavity is short and closed. Ultrasound will confirm the absence of Müllerian and Wolffian structures and identify abdominal or inguinal testes which will have to be removed. Estrogens will complete the feminization without menstruations by lack of uterus and sterility will be without therapeutic solution.

- 5α-Reductase-2 deficiency.

5α-Reductase isozymes convert dihydrotestosterone, a potent androgen from testosterone. Mutations in type 2 isozyme cause 46,XY DSD with ambiguous external genitalia at birth so that they are believed to be girls and are often raised as such. Virilization occurs at puberty with a gender role change and without breast development. Ectopic testes are present as Wolffian-derivative organs. Plasma testosterone levels are high normal with decreased DHT levels and a high T/DHT ratio [38].

Karyotypically Normal 46XX Ovarian Dysgenesis

Ovarian dysgenesis with a normal 46XX karyotype is defined by reduced or altered ovaries, female phenotype, normal stature without any Turnerian malformations. Diagnosis is suggested by a primitive hypergonadotropic hypogonadism with a normal 46XX karyotype. In some cases, a genetic origin has been identified. For the other cases, unidentified autosomal and gonosomal genes may be involved in the development and maintenance of ovarian function.

Syndromic Hypergonadotropic Hypogonadism

- The Perrault syndrome is an autosomal-recessive ovarian dysgenesis with possible deafness [39]. The defective gene has not been identified yet.
- The type I BPEIS (blepharophimosis psosis epicanthus inversus syndrome) can be associated with delayed puberty or more frequently premature ovarian failure. The mode of inheritance is autosomal-dominant and transmitted by males because the women are always infertile with ovarian streaks. The gene FOXL2 has been identified on the chromosome 3 [40, 41].
- Congenital galactosemia is associated with primary ovarian failure diagnosed mostly at an early age [42]. Metabolic toxicity already impairs follicular cells during fetal life [42].

Inactivating Mutation of the FSH or LH Receptor

An inactivating mutation of the FSH receptor has been described first in Finland [43] and is associated either to primary amenorrhea or premature ovarian failure. The ovaries have normal size and biopsies show the presence of multiple pre-antral follicles. It corresponds to the resistant ovaries to gonadotropin syndrome or Savage syndrome. The gene encoding for the FSH receptor is located on chromosome 2 and the mode of inheritance is autosomal recessive. Two observations have been recently described in France [44]. However, a study from the Unites States failed to find any mutated FSH-R gene among 35 cases of premature ovarian failure [45].

A few observations have been reported [46] with an inactivating mutation of the gene encoding for the LH receptor in homozygotic XX women with primary amenorrhea, developed sex characteristics, high LH level and normal FSH level [46] with normal ovarian follicles but without any luteal corpus.

Isolated or Associated Autoimmune Ovaritis
APECED syndrome or type 2 autoimmune polyendocrinopathy includes an ovarian autoimmune failure which occurs usually after puberty.

Iatrogenic Ovarian Failure
Prepubertal girls treated with radiation therapy or chemotherapy may present gonadal failure with delayed puberty, primary or secondary amenorrhea. In case of abdominal or pelvic radiotherapy ovaries must be surgically removed from the radiation field [47]. Chemotherapy induces follicular atresia especially when alkylant agents are used [48] and in association with radiotherapy. Cryopreservation of ovarian fragments is now available in these cases.

Hypogonadotropic Hypogonadism

Delayed puberty may be related to gonadotropin deficiency: FSH and LH plasma levels are low, as are urinary gonadotropins. This insufficiency may be caused by a hypophyseal defect of the gonadotropic cells, isolated or associated to others pituitary cell deficiencies, by a lesion of the pituitary stalk or the defect of the hypothalamic center with altered pulsatile secretion of LH-RH. Theoretically one may differentiate the origin of the defect by a LH-RH stimulation test (100 μg IVD). However, even in the case of normal gonadotropic function, preliminary priming with pulsatile LH-RH may be necessary to obtain a positive response to LH-RH stimulation. LH-RH pulsatile secretion cannot be explored directly but it can be assessed indirectly by measuring LH pulsatility every 10 min for 6 or 8 h during the night.

Gonadotropin deficiency may be secondary due to a direct organic lesion of the hypothalamo-hypophyseal axis (tumoral, inflammatory, vascular or traumatic origin), or to an indirect functional inhibition of the pulsatile LH-RH secretion (chronic disease, negative energetic imbalance). Gonadotropin deficiency may also be primitive caused by a genetic or developmental defect present at birth but unknown until the age of puberty. Finally in absence of any deficiency delayed puberty may be simply due to a constitutional idiopathic delay of puberty usually associated with growth delay.

Gonadotropin deficiency may be associated to other hypophyseal defects, especially GH secretion. The impaired growth is suggested by a decrease of growth velocity and short stature and confirmed by a negative response to dynamic exploration of the somatotropic axis. In case of isolated gonadotropin deficiency, there is usually a normal height for age but a retarded bone age in accordance with the delayed puberty with a very low or absent response to LH-RH whereas girls with functional delayed puberty or constitutional delay are short for chronological age with a normal growth rate for bone age and plasmatic and urinary gonadotropins not so low [49]. If bone age has reached 11 years gonadotropic deficiency is likely: if not, functional or constitutive delay of growth and puberty is more likely.

Acquired Hypogonadotropic Hypogonadism

Organic Direct Gonadotropin Deficiency

Complete medical history and clinical examination associated with systematic computed tomography (CT) or magnetic resonance imaging (MRI) scans of the hypothalamic and pituitary areas as well as the assessment of the other pituitary hormonal secretions will help establish the etiological diagnosis.

– Tumoral origin.

Central nervous tumors leading to delayed puberty can affect either the intra- or the extrasellar control of gonadotropins and are usually associated to other anterior or posterior pituitary deficiencies.

Craniopharyngioma is the most frequent tumor associated with delayed puberty in girls. It originates from Rathke's pouch, generally with a suprasellar development around the pituitary stalk. Clinical symptoms of compression (headache or visual disturbances) and/or endocrine deficiencies (asthenia, short stature, diabetes insipidus, infantilism) generally lead to diagnosis at between 6 and 15 years of age. Ophthalmological examination finds visual defects such as bilateral temporal field deficit, optic atrophy or papilledema. Full endocrine screening may confirm strong or moderate somatotrope, thyreotrope, corticotrope and vasopressin deficiencies associated to gonadotropin deficiency [50]. Radiographic determination of bone age will verify the presence of bone maturation delay. Supra- and intrasellar calcifications are very much characteristic of such a tumor and are well seen on CT scans. Imaging will look for an abnormal sella, a cystic or solid tumor and the presence or not of hydrocephalus. Treatment associates transsphenoidal microsurgery when possible and radiation therapy. Other endocrine deficiencies are supplemented. It is important for the future fertility prognosis to discriminate between a hypophyseal or suprahypophyseal origin of the gonadotropin deficiency because of the possible administration in suprahypophyseal defects of pulsatile intermittent LH-RH to induce ovulation and pregnancy [51].

Germinomas or germ cell tumors of the central nervous system may cause sexual infantilism with vasopressin and GH deficiency discovered around the second decade of life.CT and MRI are able to show tumors greater than 0.5 cm in diameter. The tumor may be located in the suprasellar hypothalamic region, in the pineal region or another area of the CNS. Radiation therapy is the best treatment.

Hypothalamic and optic gliomas associated or not with a Von Recklinhausen disease or astrocytomas seldom cause delayed puberty.

Hyperprolactinomas can develop during peripubertal period and lead to an arrest of pubertal development with primary amenorrhea. In fact, hyperprolactinemia inhibits pulsatile LH-RH secretion inducing gonadotropin deficiency. Thus, evaluation of the PRL axis is necessary in case of hypogonadotropic hypogonadism.

Irradiation of the head in case of CNS tumors, leukemia or tumors of the head and the face may induce progressive hypothalamopituitary deficiency including gonadotropin deficiency.

– Nontumoral Acquired Organic Lesions of CNS

Histiocytosis X (Hans-Schüller-Christian disease) is characterized by multiple organ infiltration (skin, bone, viscera) by histiocytic cells. Infiltration of the pituitary stalk and hypothalamus is possible with diabetes insipidus, GH and gonadotropin deficiency. Enlargement of the pituitary stalk and diabetes insipidus are very suggestive; however, ar positive diagnosis requires the histological analysis of the lesions that are easy to biopsy [52].

Sarcoid or tuberculous granuloma or secondary hemochromatosis may also but more rarely infiltrate the hypothalamopituitary axis and be associated with delayed puberty in girls.

Hydrocephalus may cause such a condition by compression [53].

Traumatic, inflammatory, post-infectious or vascular lesions of the hypothalamopituitary axis are seldom responsible for such a situation.

Functional Hypogonadotropic Hypogonadism

Any situation with a negative energetic balance may interfere with the pattern of LH-RH pulsatile secretion [9] through the leptin/NPY pathway or other neurotransmitters. So, quantitative and qualitative nutritional status, body mass index, body fat mass and plasma leptin levels are important features to assess in case of severe systemic and chronic diseases or particular nutritional status with a possible negative energetic balance.

– Chronic disorders.

Many chronic diseases are associated with delayed or arrested pubertal development depending on the age of onset. Malnutrition, asthenia, negative energetic balance with reduced body mass index, body fat mass and/or qualitative nutritional deficiency may induce functional hypogonadotropic hypogonadism by impairing pulsatile LH-RH secretion. This must be distinguished from the possible primary effects of the disease.

Digestive disease: celiac disease must be considered in case of unexplained growth retardation and delayed puberty. Digestive manifestations may be absent. Positive diagnosis is made by the detection of specific antitransglutaminase antibodies and the typical aspect with atrophic villosities seen on jejunal biopsies [54].

Inflammatory bowel diseases may also be associated with delayed puberty in case of loss of weight and steroid treatment.

Chronic pulmonary disease such as cystic fibrosis can induce the same deficiency in large part due to malnutrition [55].

Chronic renal disease before transplantation or steroid-sensitive nephrotic syndrome.

Major thalassemia [56] or *sickle cell disease* [57] can impair sexual maturation through the same way or by iron deposition in the pituitary gland.

- Negative energetic balance.

Undernutrition of any origin, intentional or not, delays puberty in girls. The secular trend to decrease of the age of onset of puberty in girls is consecutive to the general nutritional improvement in developed countries [22]. Food restriction, vegetarian diet, food behavior disturbance such as seen in anorexia nervosa can be associated with delayed puberty, and/or primary or secondary amenorrhea. Anorexia nervosa is a severe disease with distorted body image, food avoidance, severe weight loss with hyperactivity, decreased basal metabolic rate, hypothermia, constipation, bradycardia and hypotension and severe metabolic abnormalities leading sometimes to death. Leptin is very low [58] in relation to weight loss and lack of body fat mass while the gonadal axis remains or returns to an infantile state.

Intensive exercise in young girls (ballet dancers, athletes, gymnasts) may be associated with delayed puberty due to a negative energetic balance, special diet, and stimulation of the corticotropic axis (endorphins, ACTH, cortisol) under exaggerated stress leading to impairment of pulsatile LH-RH secretion [59, 60].

Congenital Gonadotropin Deficiency

Primary gonadotropin deficiency is associated with very low levels of FSH and LH. It is a rare disease which may result either from a fetal defect in GnRH neuron migration, a defect of pituitary development or from a functional defect of the hypothalamogonadotropic axis. In girls, the diagnosis will often be considered during adolescence in case of delayed or absent puberty with low levels of FSH and LH, concordant bone age, normal stature, unless multiple hypophyseal deficiencies including GH, are associated, and normal karyotype. Response to LH-RH test and study of LH pulsatility are useful for the diagnosis. Magnetic resonance imaging of the hypothalamic-pituitary regions is necessary, while baseline and reserve testing of the other hypothalamic-pituitary axes are needed to detect possible multiple hypophysal deficiencies. Familial history of consanguinity or of similar cases and/or associated clinical features may sometimes help the diagnosis. Different genes have already been identified [61] and a molecular diagnosis is sometimes possible, following the guide indicated in figure 1. Estrogen therapy will be proposed to induce puberty and for adult hormonal substitution with specific infertility treatment by pulsatile LH-RH delivery when gonadotropic cells are functional.

Isolated Idiopathic Hypogonadotropic Hypogonadism

- Impaired pulsatile secretion of LH-RH.

In the absence of anosmia, familial histories have suggested the role of autosomal genes [61]. G protein-coupled receptor 54 (GPR54) and its ligands the kisspeptins

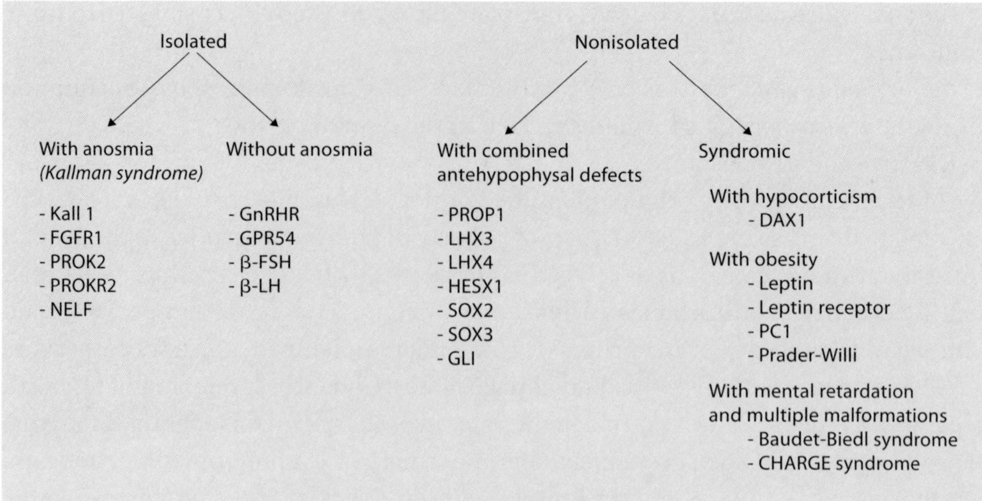

Fig. 1. Etiological guide for congenital hypogonadotropic hypogonadism.

participate in the regulation of LH-RH secretion. Homozygous mutations of GPR54 have been described [62]. In these patients, partial LH-RH neuronal migration is possible leading to partial LH-RH pulsatile secretion [61] and partial pubertal development with primary amenorrhea.

- Mutation of the LH-RH receptor gene.

  In absence of a response to the LH-RH stimulation test and to pulsatile LH-RH administration, a mutation of the LH-RH receptor gene which is located on chromosome 4 can be considered. Several autosomal-recessive forms of congenital isolated idiopathic hypogonadotropic hypogonadism (IHH) have been reported with such mutations. However, the phenotype seems to vary from partial to complete forms and the same molecular defect can exhibit different degrees of hypogonadism [63–65].

- GNRH1 mutation.

  Very recently, a familial mutation of GNRH1 has been reported in a girl [66].

- Inactivating mutation of FSH β-subunit.

  Only a handful of inactivating mutations of the FSH β-gene located on Xp21 in women have been reported: one with partially developed secondary sex characteristics [67] and two with primary amenorrhea [68].

IHH with Anosmia: Kallmann Syndrome

Association of anosmia with IHH is called the Kallmann syndrome (KS). It may be due in boys to the mutated X-linked Kal gene [69]. Indeed, the majority of familial and sporadic cases of KS, including the female cases of KS are caused by defects on autosomal genes (fig. 1) including fibroblast growth factor receptor 1 (FGFR1) [70].

In fact, all these mutations on these different identified genes account for less than 30% of all isolated IHH cases [3]. Additional gene mutations will certainly be identified and help us to elucidate IHH syndromes and control of gonadotropin secretion.

Nonisolated Congenital Hypogonadotropic Hypogonadism

– With combined antehypophysal deficiencies.

Idiopathic dwarfism is associated with delayed puberty. After confirmation of the GH deficiency, treatment with recombinant GH will try to induce pubertal development which needs IGF-1. IGF-1 enhances ovarian stimulation by LH and FSH. Moreover, multiple hypophyseal deficiencies, including thyreotrope, corticotrope and gonadotrope, are possible in case of mutations of developmental genes coding for transcription factors (fig. 1) recently identified such as PROP-1, LHX3, LHX4, HESX1, SOX2, SOX3 or GLI2 [61, 71].

– With obesity.

Prader-Willi syndrome [72] is characterized by massive obesity, infantile hypotonia, mental retardation, short stature, small hands and feet, and a characteristic facies. Delayed puberty is from hypothalamic origin and sometimes improves following weight reduction. A deletion of the long arm of chromosome 15 may be found in some patients.

Laurence-Moon-Biedl syndrome associates obesity, polydactyly, mental retardation and retinitis pigmentosa with delayed puberty [73]. The mode of inheritance is autosomal recessive.

Mutation of the leptin Ob or Ob-R gene is exceptional. Clinical features include morbid obesity with impaired food behavior, decreased basal metabolic rate and hypogonadotropic hypogonadism. Puberty may be induced by recombinant leptin in case of a mutation of the Ob gene [5].

Mutations of the human prohormone convertase 1 (PC1) gene have been reported with obesity, hypogonadotropic hypogonadism, hypocortisolism, abnormal glucose homeostasis due to a very low insulin level and a high proinsulin level [74].

– With hypocorticism.

DAX1 (double-dose adrenal hypoplasia congenital X-linked gene 1) is a transcriptional factor of the orphan nuclear receptor family which is involved in sexual differentiation and development of adrenal gland, hypothalamus, hypophysis and gonads. Mutations of this X-linked gene lead in males to adrenal congenital hypoplasia with neonatal adrenal insufficiency and differed hypogonadotropic hypogonadism revealed at adolescence. However, some cases of isolated IHH have been reported in women, which could represent a mild form of the male HH associated with congenital adrenal hypoplasia. One observation with a homozygotic mutation in a woman with IHH [75] and two other cases have been found by studying families of male cases and represent heterozygotic female forms with delayed puberty [76].

– With mental retardation and multiple malformations.

The CHARGE syndrome associated multiple malformations, mental retardation and HHI and is linked to a heterozygous mutation of the CHD7 gene [77].

Constitutional Delay in Growth and Puberty

Delayed puberty as described earlier has a statistical definition based on epidemiological studies. Onset of development which includes tightly related growth and pubertal development has a variable timing which depends on genetic and environmental factors [2]. This means that some of the girls who present a delayed puberty, generally associated to growth delay and short stature (–2 SD below mean values for height for age) do not have any illness but present a simple variation in the timing of development. In this case, follow-up shows the spontaneous onset of the secondary sex characteristics development and the acceleration of growth velocity.

However, it is sometimes difficult at the beginning, to differentiate between constitutional delay in growth and puberty (CDGP) and true hypogonadotropic hypogonadism. Indeed, some considerations can lead to propose a treatment. Evaluation and follow-up are anyway necessary and the first goal of the clinical, biological and radiological examinations are to eliminate an organic disease. There might be similar cases of CDGP in parents or siblings. First of all, true somatotropic deficiency must be eliminated. In CDGP, short stature and slow growth velocity correlate well with bone age which reflects delayed puberty and not with chronological age. GH secretion may be low on basal levels while stimulation tests are positive, although at a suboptimal level [78], corresponding in fact to a real prepubertal status. There are no real hormonal deficiencies as evidenced by combined pituitary function tests and systematic radiological examination such as MRI do not show any tumoral image or abnormal infiltration.

Medical history does not reveal any known chronic diseases. Celiac disease has been eliminated by negative specific antibodies. Functional delayed puberty with a negative energetic balance must also be eliminated by studying the nutritional, psychological and sportive background. It is particularly important to screen selective food behavior or disorders evocating anorexia nervosa or severe conflicting affective relationships. In fact, the most difficult differential diagnosis is with IHH at the beginning before a regular follow-up. However, in CDGP adrenarche is also delayed but not in IHH. Growth is not delayed in IHH and there is no short stature for age. There are no any associated signs such as anosmia, obesity, or malformations in CDGP and when bone age exceeds 11 years usually pubertal development begins. Biological hormonal data (basal plasma LH, FSH levels, urinary gonadotropins, response to stimulation test with LH-RH or pulsatile LH-RH) are statistically lower for IHH than for

CDPG and become discriminative for a bone age of 11 years. Lack of LH pulses is highly suggestive of IHH but more difficult to study (measured for 24 h at 10-min intervals). The FSH level [79] has been strongly related to lack of LH pulses and LH response to LH-RH agonists [80] seems to be more discriminative than the LH-RH stimulation test.

Primary Amenorrhea with Developed Secondary Sex Characteristics

In case of partially or completely developed secondary sexual characteristics, patients will refer to the physician for primary amenorrhea at an age of 14 or 15 years. Gonadotropin levels are normal and can be stimulated by a LH-RH test. The clinical examination will have to verify the normality of the genitalia using complementary ultrasonography and look for associated clinical and biological hyperandrogenia.

Abnormalities of the Genitalia

- Cyclic pain and hymeneal convexity suggest the hematocolpos of the unperforated hymen. It will be assessed by ultrasound and treated by radial incisions.
- Complete vaginal partition or vaginal aplasia, is visualized using a virgin size speculum. Ultrasound will confirm the presence of uterus and hematometria. The goal of surgical treatment will be to obtain a vaginal cavity connecting with the uterus and allowing sexual intercourse.
- Rokitansky-Kuster-Hauser syndrome [81] associates vaginal aplasia with uterine hypoplasia or aplasia. Ovaries and fallopian tubes are usually preserved. Here again, ultrasonographic evaluation will be of crucial importance and will allow also verification of the renal apparatus because renal abnormalities are frequently associated. Laparoscopy will confirm the diagnosis and help to choose the best surgical treatment. Surgery will consist of creation of a neovaginal cavity by several means to allow sexual intercourse. Nevertheless, pregnancy will not be possible if the uterus is lacking.
- Prepubertal genital tuberculosis with uterine synechia and primary amenorrhea is nowadays exceptional in developed countries.

Hyperandrogenia

Sexual ambiguities have been diagnosed during the neonatal period. However, pubertal development may be associated with progressive hyperandrogenia or virilization including hirsutism, seborrhea, severe acne, alopecia and hyperclitoridism. Clinical hyperandrogenia must be confirmed by biological evaluation with measurement of plasma androgens, LH and FSH, and assessment of the corticotrope axis including basal and ACTH-stimulated 17-hydroxyprogesterone measurement and ultrasonographic ovarian evaluation.

– Mild adrenal hyperplasia with partial enzymatic blockage.

There are other familial cases of hyperandrogenia or known enzymatic deficiency, short stature and mild hyperandrogenia. Elevated basal or stimulated 17-hydroxy-progesterone allows the diagnosis of 21-hydroxylase deficiency. 11β-Hydroxylase or 3β-hydroxysteroid dehydrogenase are less frequently involved.

– Polycystic ovarian syndrome (PCO) with primary amenorrhea.

PCO is suggested by obesity, presence of acantosis nigricans reflecting an hyper-insulinic state, hyperandrogenia, and clinical signs of hyperestrogenia. Hormonal evaluation shows high levels of androgens especially Δ4-androstenedione and total testosterone. The basal level of LH is elevated with a strong response to LH-RH while FSH remains low. Insulin is high as is sex binding globulin too. Ultrasonographic examination shows a typical aspect of the ovaries including enlarged gonads, stromal hypertrophy and multiple peripheral polymicrocysts [82].

– Tumoral syndrome.

Rapid virilization and very high levels of plasmatic androgens must lead to ultra-sonographic and radiologic examination looking for an ovarian or adrenal androgen secreting tumor with a peripubertal development.

Therapeutical Aspects

Treatment of delayed puberty and/or primary amenorrhea necessitates precise etiological diagnosis, determination of bone age and evaluation of psychological consequences on the patient and her family in order to evaluate the most appropriate way to give an explanation, reassurance and information on the prognosis [83].

Specific treatments when possible must be undertaken to improve pubertal development. This includes surgical treatment of tumors or abnormalities of the genitalia, medical treatment of general diseases, correction of the negative energetic balance by improving quantitative and qualitative food intake, body weight and body fat mass and by reducing intensive sport activity. It also includes treatment of endocrine diseases including correction of hypophyseal-associated deficiencies, in particular growth hormone deficiency which will accelerate pubertal maturation or correction of an associated hypothyroidism or inhibition of the corticotropic axis by dexamethasone in case of adrenal hyperplasia.

In the case of polycystic ovarian syndrome, menstruation can easily be obtained by sequential treatment with progesterone: natural micronized progesterone (Utrogestan® 200 mg orally per day 10 or 15 days/month), an isomer of progesterone, dydroprogesterone (Duphaston® 10 mg/day) or a pregnane compound such as chlormadinone acetate (Luteran® 5 mg/day). Weight reduction will also be necessary. If hyperandrogenia is significant and not well accepted; cyproterone acetate, another pregnane compound with high antiandrogenic and antigonadotropic effects can be used (Androcur® 50 mg daily during 15 days associated to estradiol 1 mg daily for 25 days) in pubertal girls with PCO.

Constitutional delay of growth and puberty is classically a situation which necessitates one to wait and observe the evolution until pubertal development occurs spontaneously, but meanwhile parents and patients must be reassured. Nevertheless, some girls will have serious psychological difficulties linked to comparison with their peers and their very low self-esteem regarding their short stature and physical infantile aspect. This can affect success either at school, work or socially [84]. Therefore, estrogen administration may have psychobehavioral benefits for such patients. A short, low-dose estrogen treatment (estradiol 0.5 mg/day orally for 3 months) can be proposed at a chronological age of 14/15 years and repeated to induce the beginning of pubertal development in particular breast development without advancing bone age too much, i.e. up to 13 years bone age [85]. This treatment may help distinguish between isolated gonadotropin deficiency and constitutional delay of puberty and may induce the beginning of spontaneous pubertal development.

A definite lack of pubertal development due to an organic congenital or acquired disease necessitates a protocol of estrogenization [86, 87] that will be performed with several goals: (1) allow the development and maintenance of secondary sex characteristics, (2) induce maturation of the internal genital organs leading to future menstruations and adequate uterine development in order to allow future nidation, (3) induce a correct peripubertal growth spurt without reducing the final height, (4) improve the constitution of the bone mass and prevent accelerated bone loss, and (5) implement a cardiovascular prevention regimen.

Age of treatment has been widely discussed in the past. It depends in fact on the reached height, bone age and in case of Turner syndrome on the associated growth hormone treatment. Estrogen therapy is usually started with a bone age between 12 and 13 years. In case of Turner syndrome growth hormone treatment is systematically proposed. If GH therapy is started early (between 2 and 10 years) estrogen treatment can be initiated at an age-appropriate time (12/13 years) without compromising adult height [88]. If GH is started later estrogen therapy will be delayed; however, the statural gain will be lower [89].

Estrogen therapy will begin with low, continue, and progressively increasing doses, without progesterone during the first year of treatment. Ethinylestradiol, a synthetic estrogen [87] has been widely used (2 μg/day at the beginning to 20 μg at the final adult sequential treatment). Natural estrogens (17β-estradiol) with less metabolic side effects are now frequently used (0.2–2 mg/day) either orally (micronized estradiol) [87] or by transdermic administration (17β-estradiol) [90]. Estrogens are first given alone during 1 year with progressive doses up to 0.5 mg estradiol daily and then accompanied by progesterone. Natural progesterone, 17-hydroxyprogesterone or pregnanes are given in a sequencial mode from day 15 to day 24 of the cycle. After 2 or 3 years, adult doses will be adapted. Follow-up will include clinical signs, bone age, ultrasonographic size of the uterus, bone mineral content evaluated by dual-energy X-ray absorptiometry [91], and psychological evolution and acceptability.

Explanations and information about this chronic hormonal replacement therapy will be given to the patient and her family [92] and the possible future chances of fertility by ovarian stimulation by menotropins or LH-RH pulsatile administration in case of hypogonadotropic hypogonadism [93] will be discussed. Information concerning oocyte donation will also be brought up in case of hypergonadotropic hypogonadism.

References

1 Knobil E, Plant TM, Wildt L, Belchetz PE, Marshall G: Control of the Rhesus monkey menstrual cycle: permissive role of hypothalamic gonadotropin-releasing hormone. Science 1980;207:1371–1373.

2 Terasawa E, Fernandez DL: Neurobiological mechanisms of the onset of puberty in primates. Endocr Rev 2001;22:111–151.

3 Seminara SB, Oliveira LM, Beranova M, Hayes FJ, Crowley WF Jr: Genetics of hypogonadotropic hypogonadism. J Endocrinol Invest 2000;9:560–565.

4 Palmert MR, Boepple PA: Variation in the timing of puberty: clinical spectrum and genetic investigation. J Endocrinol Invest 2001;86:2364–2368.

5 Strobel A, Issad T, Camoin L, et al: A leptin missence mutation associated with hypogonadism and morbid obesity. Nat Genet 1998;18:213–215.

6 Grumbach MM, Styne DM: Puberty: ontogeny, neuroendocrinology, physiology and disorders; in Wilson JD, Foster DW, Kronenberg HM, Larsen PR (eds): Williams' Texbook of Endocrinology, ed 9. Philaldelphia, Saunders, 1998, pp 1509–1625.

7 Fenichel P, Verdino P, Brucker F, et al: Exploration des hypogonadismes d'origine haute par l'association pompe à LH-RH + test à la LH-RH. Rev Fr Endocr Clin 1986;1:27–34.

8 Conte FA, Grumbach MM, Kaplan SL: A diphasic pattern of gonadotropin secretion in patients with the syndrome of gonadal dysgenesis. J Clin Endocrin Metab 1975;40:670–674.

9 Bringer J, Lefebvre P, Boulet F, et al: Deficiency of energy balance and ovulatory disorders. Hum Reprod 1997;12(suppl 1):97–109.

10 Frisch R, Mc Athur JW: Menstrual cycles: fatness as a determinant of minimum weight for height necessary for their maintenance or onset. Science 1974; 185:949–951.

11 Ahmed ML, Ong KL, Morrell J, Cox L, Drayre N, Perry L, Preece MA, Dunger DB: Longitudinal study of leptin concentrations during puberty: sex differences and relationship to changes in body composition. J Clin Endocr Metab 1999;84:899–905.

12 Barash A, Cheung C, Weigle S, et al: Leptin is a metabolic signal to the reproductive system. Endocrinology 1996;137:3144–3147.

13 Foster DL, Nagatani S: Physiological perspectives on leptin as a regulator of reproduction: role in timing of puberty. Biol Reprod 1999;60:205–215.

14 Ahima RS, Dushay J, Flier SN, Prabakaran D, Flier JS: Leptin accelerates the onset of puberty in normal female mice. J Clin Invest 1997;99:391–395.

15 Farooqi IS, Jebb SA, Landmak G, Lawrence E, Cheetham CH, Prentice AM, Hughes IA, McCamish MA, O'Rahilly S: Effects of recombinant leptin therapy in a child with congenital leptin deficiency. N Engl J Med 1999;341:879–884.

16 Veldhuis JD, Metzger DL, Martha PM, Mauras N, Kerrigan JR, Keenan B, Rogol AD, Pincus SM: Estrogen and testosterone, but not a non aromatizable androgen, direct network integration of the hypothalamo-somatotrope (growth hormone)-insulin like growth factor I axis in the human: evidence from pubertal pathophysiology and sex-steroid hormone replacement. J Clin Endocrinol Metab 1997;82:3414–3420.

17 Kerrigan JR, Rogol AD: the impact of gonadal steroid hormone action on growth hormone secretion during childhood and adolescence. Endocrine Rev 1992;13:281–298.

18 Juul A: The effects of estrogens on linear bone growth. Hum Reprod Uptake 2001;7:303–313.

19 Liu XY, Albertson K, Karlberg J: New reference for the age at childhood onset of growth and secular trend in the timing of puberty in Swedish. Acta Paediatr 2000;89:637–643.

20 Fredriks AM, Van Buuren S, Burgmeijer RJF: Continuing positive secular growth change in the Netherlands 1955–1997. Pediatr Res 2000;47:316–323.
21 Tanner JM, Whitehouse RH: Clinical longitudinal standards to height, weight, height velocity, and stages of puberty. Arch Dis Child 1976;51:170–179.
22 Lee PA, Guo SS, Kulin HE: Age of puberty: data from the United States of America. APMIS 2001; 109:81–88.
23 De Muinck Keizer-Schrama SMPF, Mul D: Trends in pubertal development in Europe. Hum Reprod Update 2001;7:287–291.
24 Forest MG: La puberté normale et le retard pubertaire. Reprod Hum Horm 2000;2:109–118.
25 Sävendahl L, Davenoport ML: Delayed diagnoses of Turner's syndrome: proposed guidelines for change. J Pediatr 2000;137:1–8.
26 Rosenfield RL: In Rosenfield RL, Grumbach M (eds): Spontaneous Puberty and Fertility in Turner Syndrome. New York, Marcel Dekker, 1990, pp 131–148.
27 Toublanc JE, Roger M, Chaussain JL: Etiologies of late puberty. Horm Res 1991;36:136–140.
28 Price DA, Albertsson-Wikland K: Demography, auxology, and response to rhGH treatment in girls with Turner's syndrome in the KIGS. Acta Paediatr Suppl 1993;391:69–74.
29 Medlej R, Lobaccaro JM, Berta P, Belon C, Leheup B, Toublanc JE, Weill J, Chevalier C, Dumas R, Sultan C: Screening for Y-derived sex determining gene SRY in 40 patients with Turner syndrome. J Clin Endocrinol Metab1992;72:1289–1292.
30 Krasna TH, Lee ML, Smilow P, Sciorra L, Eierman L: Risk of malignancy in bilateral streak gonads: the role of the Y chromosome. J Pediatr Surg 1992;27: 1376–1380.
31 Vilain E, McElreavey K, Vidaud M, Richaud F, Fellous M: L'analyse de SRY n'explique pas toute la pathologie du déterminisme du sexe. Ann Endocrinol 1991;52:435–436.
32 Little M, Wells C: A clinical overview of WTI gene mutations. Hum Mutat 1997;9:209–225.
33 Wagner T, Wirth J, Meyer J, et al: Autosomal sex reversal and campomelic dysplasia are caused by mutations in and around the SRY-related gene SOX-9. Cell 1994;79:1111–1120.
34 Bardoni B, Zanaria E, Guioli G, et al: A dosage sensitive locus at chromosome Xp21 is involved in male to male sex reversal. Nat Genet 1994;7:497–501.
35 Lin L, Philiobert P, Ferraz-de-Souza B, et al: Heterozygous missense mutations in steroidogenic factor 1 (SF1/Ad4BP, NR5A1) are associated with 46,XY disorders of sex development with normal adrenal function. J Clin Endocrinol Metab 2007;92: 991–999.
36 Köhler B, Lin L, Ferraz-de-Souza B, Wieacker P, Heidemann P, Schröder V, Biebermann H, Schnabel D, Grüters A, Achermann JC: Five novel mutations in steroidogenic factor 1 (SF1, NR5A1) in 46,XY patients with severe underandrogenization but without adrenal insufficiency. Hum Mutat 2008;29: 59–64.
37 Quigley CA, Debellis A, Marschke KB, Elawady MK, Wilson EM, French ES: Androgen recteptor defecs: historical, clinical, and molecular perspectives. Endocr Rev 1995;16:271–321.
38 Imperato-McGinley J, Zhu YS: Androgens and male physiology: the syndrome of 5α-reductase-2 deficiency. Mol Cell Endocrinol 2002;198:51–59.
39 Pallister PD, Opitz JM: The Perreault syndrome: autosomal recessive ovarian dysgenesis with facultative, non sex limited sensorineural deafness. Am J Med Genet 1979;4:239–246.
40 Amati P, Gasarini P, Zlotogora J: A gene for premature ovarian failure associated with eyelid malformation maps to chromosome 3q22-q23. Am J Hum Genet 1996;58:1089–1092.
41 Nicolino M, Bost M, David M, Chaussain JL: Familial blepharophimosis: an uncommon marker of ovarian dysgenesis. J Pediatr Endocrinol 1995;8: 127–133.
42 Dessart Y, Odievre M, Evian D, Chaussain JL: Insuffisance ovarienne et galactosémie congénitale. Arch Fr Pédiat 1982;39:321–322.
43 Huhtaniemi I, Aittomäki K: Mutations of follicle-stimulation hormone and its receptor: effects on gonadal function. Eur J Endocrinol 1998;138:473–481.
44 Touraine P, Beau I, Gougeon A, Meduri G, Desroches A, Pichard C, Detoeuf M, Paniel B, Prieur M, Zorn JR, Milgrom E, Kutten F, Misrahi M: New natural inactivating mutations of the follicle-stimulating hormone receptor: correlations between receptor function and phenotype. Mol Endocrinol 1999;13:1844–1854.
45 Layman LC, Made S, Cohen DP, Jin M, Xie J: The finnish follicle-stimulating hormone receptor gene mutation is rare in North American women with 46XX ovarian failure. Fertil Steril 1998, 69:300–302.

Sultan C (ed): Pediatric and Adolescent Gynecology. Evidence-Based Clinical Practice. 2nd, revised and extended edition. Endocr Dev. Basel, Karger, 2012, vol 22, pp 160–170

Menstrual Disorders

Efthimios Deligeoroglou · George Creatsas

Division of Pediatric-Adolescent Gynecology and Reconstructive Surgery, 2nd Department of Obstetrics and Gynecology, University of Athens, Medical School, 'Aretaieion' Hospital, Athens, Greece

Abstract

Menstrual disorders are very common in adolescence, and can be the cause of a significant amount of stress to both the patients and their parents. Variations of the menstrual cycle in this age are very broad and are mainly caused by the immaturity of the hypothalamic-pituitary-ovarian (HPO) axis. Amenorrhea (either primary or secondary), abnormal uterine bleeding and dysmenorrhea are conditions that require careful evaluation through a stepwise and logical manner. The term primary amenorrhea refers to the condition when menarche fails to occur, while secondary amenorrhea refers to the cessation of menses once they have begun. The occurrence of irregular, prolonged or heavy abnormal uterine bleeding is one of the most urgent gynecological problems in adolescence and the diagnosis of dysfunctional uterine bleeding should be used only when all other organic and structural causes of abnormal vaginal bleeding have been ruled out. Dysmenorrhea refers to painful menstruation and is the most common reason for which a young girl may refer to a gynecologist. It is characterized as primary in the absence of an underlying organic disease, and as secondary when there is evidence of pelvic pathology. Appropriate and early management of the patient is necessary in order to minimize the possibility of future complications regarding woman's reproductive ability.

The Menstrual Cycle in Adolescence

According to World Health Organization, adolescence is defined as the age between 10 and 19 years and is a transitional stage between childhood and adulthood, during which major physical and mental changes occur. The term 'puberty' refers to the sum of all the corporal and psychological changes taking place in adolescence, which lead to sexual maturation. Onset of menses is the milestone of female pubertal development and, despite international variations, usually occurs between the age of 12 and 13 years in well-nourished populations. Age of menarche showed a declining tendency from the start of the 19th century, but since the 1950s it has remained relatively stable. Menarche typically occurs within 2–3 years after thelarche (breast budding) at Tanner stage IV of breast development and is rare before stage III. In 98% of adolescents, menstruation will have started by the age of 15, with the median age being 12.43 years [1]. There appears to be a relationship between body weight and age at the onset of menarche, as earlier menarche has been observed in obese girls. On the other hand, malnutrition, chronic disease, eating disorders and high levels of physical activity are associated with delayed initiation of menstrual periods [2].

During the first gynecologic year (first year after menarche) the mean cycle interval is 32.2 days, varying typically from 21 to 45 days. Normal menstrual flow rarely exceeds 7 days and monthly average blood loss is estimated to 35 ml, ranging from 10 to 80 ml [3]. Early menstrual life is characterized by anovulatory cycles. The frequency of ovulation is related to both time since initiation of menses and age at menarche. Early menarche is associated with early onset of ovulatory cycles and when it occurs before the age of 12, about 50% of cycles are ovulatory in the first gynecologic year. In contrast, it may take 8 to 12 years after the first menstrual period until females with later-onset menarche become fully ovulatory. Long cycles most often occur in the first 3 gynecological years and while the age increases, menstrual cycles tend to become more regular and short. By the third year, 60–80% of menstrual cycles are 21–34 days long, as is typical in adults. An individual's normal cycle length is established around the sixth gynecologic year, at a chronologic age of approximately 19 or 20 years. [4]

Primary and secondary amenorrhea, abnormal uterine bleeding and dysmenorrhea are conditions that can cause significant stress to both the young girl and her parents. Abnormal uterine bleeding (AUB) and especially the subtype of dysfunctional uterine bleeding (DUB) is one of the most urgent gynecological problems during this period, while dysmenorrhea is the most frequent one.

Amenorrhea

Primary amenorrhea is defined as the absence of menstruation in 16-year-old girls who have already developed secondary sexual characteristics, or in 14-year-old girls who have no secondary sexual characteristics development. Especially for the second group (girls with absent secondary sexual characteristics) the term 'delayed puberty' is more appropriate. According to the Practice Committee of the ASRM (American Society for Reproductive Medicine) and due to a trend for earlier age at menarche, adolescent females presenting with amenorrhea and normally developed secondary sexual characteristics should be evaluated by the age of 15 (2 SD above the mean age of 13). Moreover, evaluation is essential for adolescent girls presenting with amenorrhea within 5 years after thelarche – if the latter occurs before the age of 10 –, and amenorrheic girls who are above the age of 13 (2 SD above the mean age of 11) and have not yet developed secondary sexual characteristics [5].

Secondary amenorrhea is the absence of menstruation for 6 months, for adolescents who had previously irregular cycles or for these who are within the first gynecological years. Moreover for adolescents with formerly regular cycles of 21–45 days, it is defined as the absence of 3 or more subsequent menstrual periods. Overall, secondary amenorrhea is defined as the cessation of menses once they have begun.

The term oligomenorrhea (from the Greek word *oligos* meaning few) refers to menstrual cycles longer than 45 days. By far, most cases of oligomenorrhea occur in the first decade after menarche and the most common cause is polycystic ovarian syndrome (PCOS). Oligomenorrhea can be the menstrual disturbance prior to secondary amenorrhea and both can be evaluated following the same algorithm.

The causes of amenorrhea, without including disorders of congenital sexual ambiguity were classified in 2008 by the Practice Committee of the ASRM as follows: (a) anatomic defects of the outflow tract, (b) primary hypogonadism, (c) hypothalamic causes, (d) pituitary causes, (e) other endocrine gland disorders, and (f) multifactorial causes [5].

The problem of amenorrhea should be approached in a logical stepwise manner in order to facilitate the diagnosis. A careful medical history is the starting point of patient's investigation, and should include information about any underlying systemic disease, family medical history and the age of menarche of the girl's mother.

In adolescent patients with primary amenorrhea, the presence of developed secondary sexual characteristics is important and demonstrates that sexual steroids are produced and circulating. During the physical examination particular attention should be paid to signs or symptoms of systemic diseases. Per rectum gynecological examination is essential in order to assess the anatomy of the internal genitalia. Moreover, in case of reproductive tract obstruction it can reveal the presence of hematocolpos and/or hematometra (distension of the vagina and/or uterus due to blood retention within the vaginal canal or the uterine cavity, respectively).

In females with primary amenorrhea and absence of secondary sexual characteristics, measurement of FSH (follicle-stimulating hormone) and LH (luteinizing hormone) levels is recommended. Elevated gonadotrophin levels imply that the cause of the delayed puberty lies within the gonads. On the other hand, low or normal FSH and LH levels point to either constitutional delay of puberty, or hypothalamic/pituitary disorders. Further evaluation of patients with delayed puberty and elevated gonadotrophin levels, requires pelvic ultrasound imaging. This will confirm the findings of the gynecological examination and provide a clear view of the anatomy of internal genitalia (especially the presence, or not of ovarian follicles). The next diagnostic step is a karyotype study which will contribute in the differential diagnosis between ovarian failure (also referred to as ovarian insufficiency), gonadal dysgenesis, Turner syndrome and androgen insensitivity syndrome, as these are the commonest causes of primary amenorrhea in adolescent girls with the aforementioned characteristics.

Progressively deteriorating cyclic abdominal pain combined with primary amenorrhea is a strong indication of genital tract obstruction. In patients with normal pubertal development and primary amenorrhea, rectoabdominal gynecologic examination and pelvic ultrasound are essential since they can reveal the existence of congenital anatomic defects of the outflow tract. When congenital malformations of the genital tract have been ruled out for an adolescent girl with normal pubertal development and primary amenorrhea, further evaluation should be performed following the algorithm for secondary amenorrhea.

The evaluation of an adolescent patient with secondary amenorrhea should begin with pregnancy exclusion, even though a young girl may deny having had sexual intercourse. Further evaluation requires the search for signs of clinical hyperandrogenism, like acne, hirsutism, deepening of voice and clitoromegaly. Should any sign of clinical hyperandrogenism be present, FSH, LH, testosterone and DHEA-S (dehydroepiandrosterone sulfate) must be measured. When a mild to moderate elevation of testosterone levels along with an LH/FSH ratio above 2 is observed, PCOS is the most probable diagnosis. DHEA-S serum levels between 500 and 700 mg/dl require further investigation of the adrenal gland function, with serum 17OH-progesterone concentration measurement. DHEA-S serum levels above 700 mg/dl suggest that the cause of hyperandrogenism is the late onset type of congenital adrenal hyperplasia. In patients with secondary amenorrhea and normal serum androgen levels, despite the presence of clinical hyperandrogenism, progesterone challenge test should be performed in order to assess the levels of circulating estrogens and their effect on the endometrial function.

Secondary amenorrhea along with absence of clinical hyperandrogenism signs requires measurement of FSH, LH, TSH (thyroid-stimulating hormone) and prolactin levels, as amenorrhea may also be the result of hyperprolactinemia or thyroid gland disease. TSH levels that are either lower or higher than normal range indicate that thyroid disease may be the reason of amenorrhea. A significant elevation of PRL levels (>100 ng/ml) suggests the existence of a pituitary adenoma, while mildly elevated PRL is usually the result of dysregulation in secretion inhibition mechanisms (use of antipsychotic drugs, hypothyroidism, pressure effect on the pituitary stalk). Magnetic resonance imaging (MRI) of the pituitary fossa should be performed in patients with persistent, refractory, or excessive (>100 ng/ml) hyperprolactinemia, which is not related to hypothyroidism and antipsychotic drug use, as it can reveal the presence of lesions in the pituitary gland [6]. If FSH and LH levels are above normal range, measurement must be repeated. If elevation is persistent, in several consecutive measurements, along with normal TSH and prolactin levels, the most probable cause of the secondary amenorrhea is ovarian failure [7]. When FSH, LH, TSH and prolactin levels are within the normal range, progesterone challenge test must be performed. If there is no withdrawal bleeding after the test, an estrogen-progesterone challenge test must be performed to ensure the normal endometrial function.

Dysfunctional Uterine Bleeding – Abnormal Uterine Bleeding

DUB refers to endometrial bleeding that is prolonged, excessive, irregular and not attributable to any underlying structural or systemic disease. Bleeding associated with organic causes such as pregnancy complications, clotting abnormalities, systemic diseases, reproductive tract's pathology, endocrine disorders and iatrogenic causes is defined as AUB [8]. In the USA, the definition of DUB refers to anovulatory bleeding. On the other hand, the European Society of Human Reproduction and Embryology (ESHRE) defined DUB as excessive (by means of severity, duration, or frequency) bleeding of uterine origin, which is not due to demonstrable pelvic disease, complication of pregnancy or systemic disease. Therefore, according to ESHRE, DUB can be either ovulatory or unovulatory.

Differential diagnosis of abnormal uterine bleeding during adolescence should firstly exclude pregnancy-related hemorrhage, as it can pose patient's life at risk. Spontaneous, threatened or incomplete abortion, ectopic pregnancy, post-abortion endometritis or hydatidiform mole are possible diagnoses in this category.

Bleeding disorders should also be excluded, especially in patients presenting with AUB during their first menstrual cycles. One of the initial processes to control blood loss during menstruation is the formation of intravascular platelet plug. Thus, quantitative reduction or functional abnormality of platelets can lead to increased menstrual blood loss. Defects in the coagulation cascade can also lead in AUB [9]. Almost 19% of adolescents with persistent menorrhagia requiring hospital admission have coagulation disorder, and more than 50% of these young women have a coagulopathy such as thrombocytopenia, von Willebrand disease or leukemia [10]. Systemic bleeding disorders are found in 7–20% of women of all ages presenting with menorrhagia [11]. von Willebrand factor's deficiency is a common hereditary bleeding disorder associated with AUB. Especially, among women with von Willebrand's disease, 65% report heavy bleeding at menarche. Factor XI deficiency, Glassman's disease (defective platelets) and aplastic anemia are also associated with AUB. Therefore, systemic bleeding disorders must be of primary consideration in adolescents who present with menorrhagia at menarche or who require hospital admission [12].

Chronic diseases affecting renal or liver function may result in AUB especially if end stage. Such diseases are, however, rare in adolescence. Deficiency of vitamin K-dependent (II, VII, IX, X) or other clotting factors (including fibrinogen and plasminogen) are common among patients with liver disease [13]. Abnormal estrogen metabolism may also result from liver disease causing endometrial proliferation and estrogen breakthrough bleeding. Uremic patients suffer from abnormal platelet function which leads to excessive menstrual bleeding.

Abnormal uterine bleeding can also occur due to reproductive tract diseases. Trauma and genital injury due to rape, sexual abuse or consensual sexual intercourse could result in severe bleeding. Self-injury may result when attempting to insert tampons or other foreign objects in the vagina. Endometritis and pelvic inflammatory disease (PID) due to chlamydia and gonorrhea can cause AUB during adolescence in a frequency of less than 10% of all AUBs. Vaginitis, cervical inflammation or erosion have the potential to cause vaginal bleeding that the patient may interpret as irregular menstruation. Finally, partially obstructive congenital anomalies of the genital tract, such as transverse septa or functional communicating rudimentary uterine horn, could manifest with intermenstrual bleeding.

Various clinical manifestations may coexist along with AUB, and usually signal an underlying endocrine disease. Clinical signs of hyperandrogenism like severe acne, facial and other male pattern hair growth and central obesity may suggest polycystic ovarian syndrome. The adrenal glands can also be a source of androgens and diseases like congenital adrenal hyperplasia, Cushing's disease, adrenal insufficiency and adrenal androgen-secreting tumors (when adrenal glands overproduce androgens) may be associated with signs of severe hyperandrogenism and anovulatory cycles. Hypothyroidism is another cause of menorrhagia and is accompanied by thermoregulatory or metabolic symptoms. Ovarian causes of anovulatory AUB include abnormal function of corpus luteum, steroid-secreting ovarian tumors and imminent premature ovarian failure.

Finally AUB can occur due to iatrogenic causes, e.g. administration of hormonal medications, including intramuscular or subcutaneous implants, IUDs, combined oral contraceptives, combined transdermal patches and vaginal rings. Other drugs associated with AUB, include anticoagulants, neuroleptics and chemotherapeutics.

The causes of abnormal uterine bleeding are summarized in table 1.

Clinical evaluation of the patient presenting with AUB should begin with a careful medical history of the patient, as it can reveal any potential underlying condition. Primary target in the diagnostic algorithm of AUB is to locate the source of bleeding and secondary to rule out all the above-mentioned organic causes. It is important to obtain information about patient's menstrual history, and particularly about age at menarche and length of cycles. The patient should also be asked about the duration of bleeding, the quantity and the amount of blood, the presence (or absence) of clots and the possible presence of pain or cramping. The review of systems should specifically address other unusual or abnormal bleeding, psychosocial stressors, recent weight changes, eating and exercise habits, substance use, and signs of hyperandrogenism (acne, hirsutism). The family history should be reviewed for endocrinopathies and hematologic disorders such as thyroid disorders, functional ovarian hyperandrogenism and von Willebrand's disease. The patient should be asked, in private, about sexual activity, use of contraception, and history of sexually transmitted infections. Diagnosis of DUB is established, only when all of the aforementioned organic causes have been ruled out.

AUB and especially the subtype of DUB is one of the most urgent gynecological problems during adolescence. Treatment of patients with DUB should firstly focus to control bleeding and regulating menstruation. Anemia correction and iron stores replenishment is the second goal of the therapeutic strategy. In the majority of the

Table 1. Causes of abnormal uterine bleeding

• Hypothalamic-pituitary-ovarian axis immaturity
• Endocrine disorders – Polycystic ovarian syndrome – Thyroid dysfunction – Congenital adrenal hyperplasia
• Pregnancy complications – Threatened or incomplete abortion – Ectopic pregnancy – Post-abortion endometritis – Hydatidiform mole
• Coagulation disorders – Thrombocytopenia – von Willebrand disease – Factor XI deficiency – Glassman disease – Aplastic anemia
• Reproductive tract diseases – Trauma – Genital injury – Pelvic inflammatory disease – Vaginitis – Partially obstructive congenital uterine anomalies
• Chronic diseases
• Iatrogenic causes – Hormonal medications – Anticoagulants – Neuroleptics– Chemotherapeutics

cases, hormonal treatment is indicated, but the specific kind and way of hormonal therapy will be dictated by the severity of DUB [3].

In patients with mild DUB, menses are slightly prolonged or irregular, with hemoglobulin levels above 12 g/dl. Hormonal therapy is rarely indicated and patient reassurance and education about the normal menstrual cycle are usually sufficient. Careful follow-up along with appropriate education regarding menstrual calendar keeping will make the adolescent feeling safe [14].

Moderate DUB is characterized by prolonged, profuse menses, impeding daily activities, or by a clearly shortened menses interval accompanied by mild anemia (hemoglobulin levels above or equal to 10 g/dl). Treatment of choice includes the administration of low-dose oral contraceptives or cyclic progestogen. Cyclic oral progestogen is administered for the same 10 days of every month in order to stabilize the endometrium, preventing the action of unopposed estrogens. Consistent iron deficiency anemia can be treated with supplemental oral iron therapy. Nonsteroidal anti-inflammatory drugs (NSAIDs) can also reduce the flow by nearly 50%, in patients with uterine bleeding, through inhibition of prostaglandins' synthetase. Treatment with oral contraceptives should be continued for at least 3–6 months [3].

Heavy bleeding and hemoglobulin levels less than 10 g/dl suggest severe DUB and patients usually require hospitalization. In hypovolemic patients, immediate resuscitation with intravenous fluids for volume expansion and possible transfusion are indicated in order to restore hemodynamic balance. Blood samples must be obtained to exclude an underlying bleeding disorder before starting therapy. Intravenous conjugated equine estrogens have been used during the previous years, being highly effective in controlling uterine bleeding, but they are not available any more. Nowadays, intramuscular medroxyprogesterone acetate together with combined oral contraceptives (COCs) can be administered, as they provide faster results in controlling heavy menstrual bleeding. Hemorrhage usually stops within 24 h and continuation of therapy with COCs alone is in most cases recommended. Dilation and curettage, although not usually performed in adolescence, is indicated in the rare cases in which hormonal treatment is unsuccessful.

After hemodynamic stabilization, the adolescent girl can be treated with COCs [3]. A tablet of COCs containing a high dose of estrogen should be taken every 6 h, along with an antiemetic if nausea is present. After a maximum of eight doses during 48 h, the dose must be tapered over 3 days to one pill daily. Patient will then begin a new COCs pack with the same amount of estrogen for the next 21 days taking one pill daily.

Tranexamic acid is a synthetic derivative of the amino acid lysine, which exerts an antifibrinolytic effect through reversible blockade on plasminogen. The drug has no effect on blood coagulation parameters or dysmenorrhea, with one third of women experiencing side effects, including nausea and leg cramps. Administration of 1 g of tranexamic acid every 6 h for the first 4 days of the cycle can reduces menstrual blood loss by up to 40%, as has been demonstrated by 10 randomized placebo-controlled trials. Other therapies, such as high doses of progestogens given per os or intramuscularly, Gn-RH agonists with add-back therapy and levonogestrel impregnated IUDs have little place in adolescent's DUB management [15].

Dysmenorrhea

Dysmenorrhea is the most common problem in adolescence and presents as painful menstruation. The word 'dysmenorrhea' is originated from the Greek language and denotes a difficulty in menses' outflow.

Dysmenorrhea is characterized as primary in the absence of an underlying organic disease, and as secondary when there is evidence of pelvic pathology.

Primary Dysmenorrhea

Primary dysmenorrhea has a high prevalence in adolescence [16], and is usually observed after the first gynecological years along with the onset of ovulatory menstrual cycles.

COCs and NSAIDs are the most frequently used agents in the treatment of primary dysmenorrhea. Combined oral contraceptives have a beneficial effect on dysmenorrhea by inhibiting ovulation, leading to suppression of endometrial tissue growth and, secondary, to reduction of menstrual flow below normal levels. It also seems to result in a concomitant drop of menstrual prostaglandins' levels. Therefore, the lessening of menstrual flow along with the decrease of prostaglandins' reduces uterine motility and ischemia and thus uterine cramping pain [17]. NSAIDs are the most commonly used medical treatment for dysmenorrhea. More research is needed in order to explore whether specific COX-2 inhibitors are effective in treating dysmenorrhea in the adolescent age group.

In case of no response to neither of the aforementioned treatment methods, laparoscopy and/or hysteroscopy are indicated [18].

Secondary Dysmenorrhea

By definition secondary dysmenorrhea implies organic pelvic lesion. As mentioned above any menstrual pain arising more than 3 years after menarche must be considered to be of pathologic origin. Chronic pelvic or low abdominal pain, beginning one or two days prior menses, irregular or heavy menstrual patterns, dyspareunia and bowel symptoms are signs usually associated with an underlying organic pathology. Patients with secondary dysmenorrhea usually outline several different clinical symptoms in their menstrual history rather than the predictable ones typically described by patients suffering from primary dysmenorrhea.

Endometriosis and pelvic inflammatory disease are the most frequent causes of secondary dysmenorrhea in adolescence. Malformations of the Mullerian ducts in this age group must be considered as a distinct option. Other infrequent causes of secondary dysmenorrhea during adolescence are uterine retroversion in fixed position, stenosis of cervical channel, intrauterine devices without progestin-containing system, uterine fibroids, endometrial or endocervical polyps, adenomyosis and pelvic venous congestion [18].

Dysmenorrhea associated with chronic pelvic pain due to endometriosis is less likely to respond to NSAIDs or combined oral contraceptives. If this lack of response to NSAIDs and COCs happens after at least 3 months of therapy, laparoscopy is indicated. Pelvic examination may elicit mild to moderate tenderness. Uterosacral nodules and pelvic masses are rare findings in patients with endometriosis of this age group. Laparoscopy is the single most useful diagnostic procedure because most adolescents

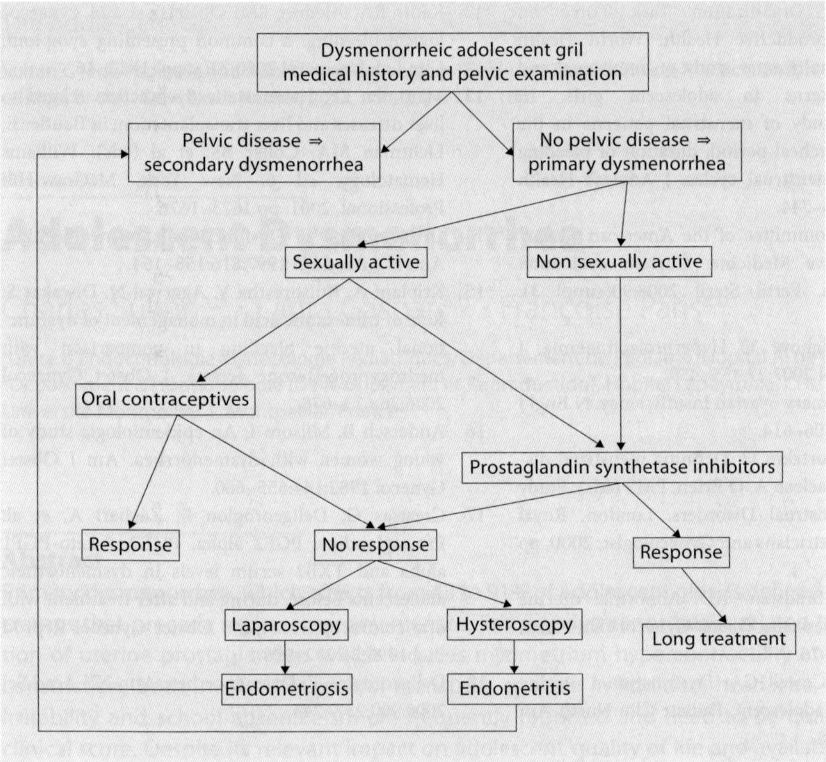

Fig. 1. Evaluation and management of dysmenorrhea.

have minimal or mild stages of endometriosis. Cervical and vaginal cultures, pelvic ultrasonography, magnetic resonance imaging, hysterosalpingography and hysteroscopy can also be helpful in the evaluation of secondary dysmenorrhea. It should be noted that management of secondary dysmenorrhea must target towards the treatment of the underlying organic pathology along with the treatment of pain.

The algorithm of evaluation and management of both primary and secondary dysmenorrhea is demonstrated in figure 1.

References

1 American Academy of Pediatrics Committee on Adolescence, American College of Obstetricians and Gynecologists Committee on Adolescent Health Care, Diaz A, Laufer MR, Breech LL: Menstruation in girls and adolescents: using the menstrual cycle as a vital sign. Pediatrics 2006;118:2245–2250.

2 Ibáñez L, Potau N, Zampolli M, et al: Hyperinsulinemia and decreased insulin-like growth factor-binding protein-1 are common features in prepubertal and pubertal girls with a history of premature pubarche. J Clin Endocrinol Metab 1997;82:2283–2288.

3 Deligeoroglou E, Tsimaris P, Deliveliotou A, et al: Menstrual disorders during adolescence. Pediatr Endocrinol Rev 2006;3(suppl 1):150–159.

37 Freeman EW, Rickels K, Sondheimer SJ: Premenstrual symptoms and dysmenorrhea in relation to emotional distress factors in adolescents. J Psychosom Obstet Gynaecol 1993;14:41–50.
38 Jamieson DJ, Steege JF: The prevalence of dysmenorrhea, dyspareunia, pelvic pain, and irritable bowel syndrome in primary care practices. Obstet Gynecol 1996;1:55–59.
39 Sundell G, Milson I: Factors influencing the prevalence and severity of dysmenorrhea in young women. Br J Obstet Gynec 1990;97:588–594.
40 Teperi J, Rimpela M: Menstrual pain, health and behaviour in girls. Soc Sci Med 1989;29:163–169.
41 Gantt PA, McDonough PG: Adolescent dysmenorrhea. Pediatr Clin North Am 1981;28:389–395.
42 Gidwani GP: Longitudinal study of risk factors for occurrence, duration and severity of menstrual cramps in a cohort of college. Women Health 1998; 37:51.
43 Nabrink M, Birgersson L, Colling-Saltin AS, Solum T: Modern oral contraceptives and dysmenorrhoea. Contraception 1990;42:275–283.
44 O'Connell BJ: The pediatrician and the sexually active adolescent. Treatment of common menstrual disorders. Pediatr Clin North Am 1997;44:1391–1404.
45 Rosenfield RL, Barnes RB: Menstrual disorders in adolescence. Endocrinol Metab Clin North Am 1993;22:491–505.
46 Smith RP: Cyclic pelvic pain and dysmenorrhea. Obst and Gynec Clin North America 1993;20:753–764.

Prof. Charles Sultan, MD, PhD
Unité d'Endocrinologie-Gynécologie Pédiatriques
Département de Pédiatrie
Hôpital A. de Villeneuve
FR–34295 Montpellier cedex 5 (France)
Tel. +33 467 33 86 96, E-Mail c-sultan@chu-montpellier.fr

Sultan C (ed): Pediatric and Adolescent Gynecology. Evidence-Based Clinical Practice. 2nd, revised and extended edition. Endocr Dev. Basel, Karger, 2012, vol 22, pp 181–193

Hyperandrogenism in Adolescent Girls

Sophie Catteau-Jonard · Christine Cortet-Rudelli · Chloé Richard-Proust · Didier Dewailly

Department of Endocrine Gynecology and Reproductive Medicine, Hôpital Jeanne de Flandre, University Hospital, Lille, France

Abstract

When the symptoms of hyperandrogenism are mild in an adolescent girl, it is difficult to establish whether they are related to the physiological androgenization of puberty or to an incipient disease. The most frequent etiology is the polycystic ovary syndrome (PCOS). Its diagnosis is defined in adult women by precise criteria which need to be adapted to the particular case of the adolescent girl. Nonclassic adrenal hyperplasia is the main differential diagnosis to PCOS. Although much less frequent, other etiologies of peripubertal hyperandrogenism such as adrenal or ovarian tumors or Cushing's disease must be considered by analyzing the rapidity of installation and intensity of hyperandrogenic symptoms and by a systematic hormonal work-up. In addition to etiologic measures, the treatment consists of administration of an anti-androgen, mainly cyproterone acetate. In the case of PCOS, the patient needs to be educated regarding the metabolic risks.

Mild symptoms of hyperandrogenism, such as acne or hyperseborrhea, are frequent in adolescent girls [1], and are often associated with irregular menstrual cycles. In most instances, these symptoms are transient and only reflect the immaturity of the hypothalamic-pituitary-ovary axis during the first years following menarche. In some subjects, however, these manifestations can persist and even worsen, and hirsutism may appear, thus revealing an adrenal or ovarian disorder whose most common cause is polycystic ovary syndrome (PCOS).

The management of an adolescent hyperandrogenic girl must achieve three main goals: (1) eliminate a severe cause of hyperandrogenism, such as an adrenal or ovarian tumor, or the nonclassic adrenal hyperplasia (NCAH), (2) recognize PCOS early on in order to set up antiandrogen therapy without delay and to initiate the prevention of obesity and insulin resistance, and (3) distinguish the so-called physiological hyperandrogenism of puberty, which will resume within 1–2 years, from a nascent PCOS.

Physiological Hyperandrogenism of Puberty

At the start of puberty, LH pulsatility is only present during sleep. It then extends to the daytime, with amplification of pulse amplitude and acceleration of frequency. This is accompanied by an increase in androgen plasma levels. These changes parallel those in the GH/IGF-1 axis, whose hyperactivity induces a selective insulin resistance. This phenomenon results in a physiological hyperinsulinism which is responsible for the increase in insulin plasma level and decrease in SHBG and IGFBP-1 liver production [2].

The first menstrual cycles in adolescent girls are frequently anovulatory. When compared to ovulatory cycles, they are characterized by higher serum levels of testosterone (T), androstenedione (A) and LH, with the possibility of mild hyperandrogenic symptoms [3]. In most of adolescent girls, these abnormalities will resume spontaneously within 1–2 years along with the regularization of their menstrual cycles. Conversely, in some others, they will worsen, with progressive constitution of PCOS features, such as hirsutism, anovulation, increased plasma T, A and LH levels and ovarian enlargement (see below). At this time, however, it is difficult to distinguish biologically and ultrasonically those adolescents with such an evolution from the ones with 'physiological mini-PCOS' due to the normal maturational process of puberty [4]. Some features, however, are predictive (see below), in particular the association with oligomenorrhea which should not be viewed too quickly as a normal feature of the first gynecological years [5].

Diagnosis of Hyperandrogenism in Female Adolescents

Clinical Assessment

When an adolescent girl is referred for hyperandrogenism, the first visit must include a thorough record of history and a careful physical examination.

Although infrequent, some clinical symptoms must be carefully searched for, since they draw the clinician's attention toward a severe disease: (a) rapidly growing hirsutism, with other signs of virilization such as clitoromegaly, temporal balding, voice deepening, and increasing muscle mass, which are indicative of an adrenal or ovarian tumor, (b) symptoms of hypercorticism (Cushing syndrome), and (c) galactorrhea, indicative of a prolactinoma.

In the other situations, symptoms of hyperandrogenism are mild and consist of: (a) hirsutism, whose degree should be quantified according to the Ferriman-Gallwey score, (b) acne, indicative of hyperandrogenism when it occurs early, is inflammatory, and mainly localized in chin, neck and thorax, and (c) alopecia, indicative of hyperandrogenism when it affects the vertex.

Some clinical features are predictive of PCOS: (a) family history of hyperandrogenism and menstrual disorders, (b) history of precocious adrenarche, (c) history of menstrual disorders, mainly oligomenorrhea, persisting more than 2 years after

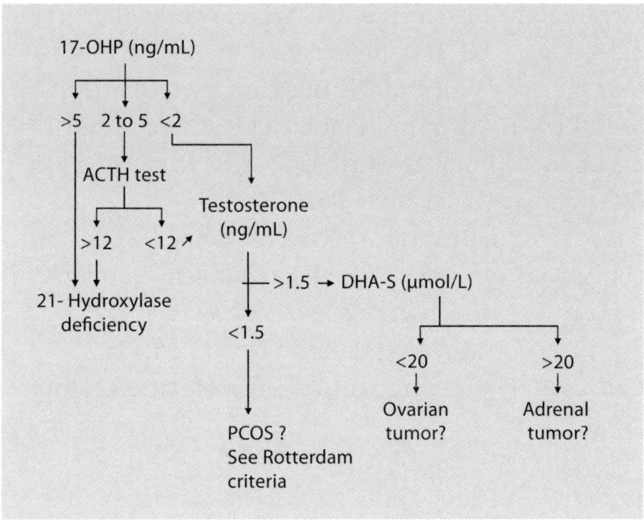

Fig. 1. Flow-chart for the use of hormonal assays in the work-up of hyperandrogenism in adolescent girls.

menarche, (d) obesity (BMI >25) or abdominal adiposity with increased waist/hip ratio (WHR), and (e) presence of acanthosis nigricans.

First Laboratory Assessment

After the first visit, a minimal laboratory screening is mandatory, unless the clinical findings lead to search at once for adrenal or ovarian tumor, or a prolactinoma. Blood sampling must be performed early in the morning, certainly before 10.00 h. This will avoid false negative results due to the circadian decrease in adrenal steroids, mainly 17-hydroxyprogesterone (17-HP) that parallels the one in cortisol and ACTH and occurs later in the day. Second, patients must be investigated in the early follicular phase. This will avoid false positive results due to the steroid production from the corpus luteum. In amenorrheic or oligomenorrheic patients, blood sampling should be performed after a short sequence of progestin treatment.

This laboratory screening must include the assay of total T, DHEAS and 17-HP. Other assays are less useful (e.g. the A assay) or not robust enough (e.g. the free T assay) to fulfill the reliability needed for this first step.

Further Investigations

According to these preliminary results, the diagnostic strategy can follow the flow chart indicated in figure 1:

(a) If an adrenal or ovarian tumor is suspected, adrenal computed tomography or pelvic MRI is indicated, respectively.

(b) If NCAH is suspected (basal 17-HP >2 ng/ml), an ACTH test should be performed. For some authors, the ACTH test is mandatory as soon as the first visit to ascertain the diagnosis of NCAH. However, there is no evidence that its sensitivity in detecting 21-OHD is higher than the one of basal 17-HP determination, providing that the above-mentioned rules are respected [6]. Therefore, the ACTH test is only useful when the morning follicular unsuppressed 17-HP level falls between 2 and 5 ng/ml (6–15 nmol/l), which is the case in approximately 6% of all patients referred for hyperandrogenism (see below).

(c) If the patient is suspected of having PCOS, pelvic ultrasound imaging and metabolic work-up are indicated, in complement to other hormonal assays (see below).

Causes of Hyperandrogenism in Female Adolescents

Polycystic Ovary Syndrome

Pediatric and adult endocrinologists may encounter PCOS as a mildly virilizing state since it is the most frequent cause of hyperandrogenism in female teenagers and in adult women [7].

Pathophysiology: Puberty and PCOS

The intra-ovarian hyperandrogenism is the cardinal feature of PCOS. This disease is programmed but stays quiescent until the puberty because it needs pituitary LH to be expressed. However, LH does not have any more a central role in PCOS and elevated serum LH levels are not constant in patients with PCOS. A second event seems to be necessary to reveal a PCOS. Hyperinsulinism may be the second factor. This metabolic defect may even pre-date the PCOS since it is most likely genetic in nature, although it remains to be proven that this is the case in all patients. An increased body of evidence suggests that it has a role in causing and/or propagating the disease [2]. Hyperinsulinism may interfere early with the pubertal maturation process at the hypothalamic, pituitary, ovarian and adrenal levels, leading to a 'hyperpubertal state'. This may trigger a self-perpetuating process causing the outcome of puberty to be PCOS in genetically susceptible young women.

Nevertheless, in lean and normoinsulinemic women, other still unknown factors, either genetic or environmental, may be basic for the development of PCOS [8].

Abbott et al. [9] hypothesized that the clinical and biochemical features of PCOS can arise as a consequence of genetically determined hypersecretion of androgens by the ovary during in utero life. The resulting hyperandrogenism results in 'programming' of the hypothalamic-pituitary unit to favor excess LH secretion during puberty and encourages preferential abdominal adiposity that predisposes to insulin resistance.

Follicular Abnormalities

In PCOS, the follicular problem is 2-fold [10]: first, early follicular growth is excessive, and second, the selection of one follicle from the increased pool and its further maturation to a dominant follicle does not occur (follicular arrest).

A local excess of androgens secondary to theca-interstitial cell hyperfunction is thought to be involved in the multifollicular aspect of ovaries.

While the excess of small follicles appears as the salient and constant feature of PCO, follicular arrest does not occur constantly in patients with PCOS since some of them do ovulate monthly. Nevertheless, the former influences the latter, as suggested by the strong relationship between the follicle excess and the degree of menstrual disturbances in women with PCOS [11].

Clinical Aspects

Although very variable, the phenotypic features of PCOS can be schematically divided into three components, i.e. hyperandrogenic, anovulatory and dysmetabolic. These three components are not necessarily or fully associated [7].

Hyperandrogenism

Usually, symptoms are moderate and consist of increased male-pattern hair growth, acne, seborrhea or alopecia, which reflect mild androgenic stimulation of the pilosebaceous unit. Hyperandrogenism symptoms frequently commence at the time of puberty. In some cases, hyperandrogenism is expressed before puberty as 'precocious adrenarche' in patients who subsequently develop PCOS, indicating early adrenal involvement [12].

Anovulation

This component of PCOS accounts for oligomenorrhea (i.e. menstrual cycle length ≥3 months) and secondary amenorrhea, which are the most typical features of the anovulatory PCOS. They very often date back to menarche. Primary amenorrhea is uncommon, but PCOS is still found in about 20% of girls referred for this symptom [13]. These patients have no pubertal delay and are frequently overweight. The amenorrhea is quite reversible under short sequences of progestin treatment, without having to add estrogens. This qualifies this amenorrhea as 'normoestrogenic' or 'type 2 anovulation' in the World Health Organization (WHO) classification. About 20% of adolescent and adult patients with PCOS report normal menses. However, this does not mean necessarily that they ovulate each cycle. In one study, 20% of them were in fact anovulatory.

Metabolic Syndrome

Obesity (BMI >25) is observed in 30–50% of adolescent and adult women with PCOS. Most women with PCOS become overweight just before or during puberty and several lines of evidence suggest that the onset of obesity in this period of life could represent a specific risk factor for the subsequent development of PCOS [2]. Obesity of women with PCOS is frequently characterized by a distribution of fat that favors the upper body segment (increased WHR). This type of fat distribution is detected even in adolescent girls with normal BMI [14] and is associated with greater insulin resistance than if fat is located predominantly in the lower body segment. Papular hypertrophic pigmented skin on the nape of the neck, the axillae, chest and vulva is detected in 5–50% of women with PCOS. This dermal manifestation, acanthosis nigricans, is now recognized as a non-specific marker of moderate to severe insulin resistance.

Diagnosis

With the new Rotterdam definition [15], at least 2 of the following 3 criteria are required to define PCOS: (1) oligo and/or anovulation (OA); (2) clinical and/or biochemical signs of hyperandrogenism (HA), and (3) polycystic ovaries (PCO). Most importantly, other etiologies have to be excluded before applying these criteria, in particular congenital adrenal hyperplasia, androgen-secreting tumors, Cushing's syndrome, hypothalamic anovulation and prolactinoma (see below).

Hormonal Markers for PCOS

It is not useful to search an elevated serum LH level and/or an exaggerated LH response to the GnRH test and/or an elevated LH/FSH ratio. Indeed, the sensitivity as well as the specificity of a high LH level in the diagnostic of PCOS are low and not recommended by the Rotterdam consensus.

The research of a biological hyperandrogenism is primordial in order to avoid serious causes of hyperandrogenism (see above; fig. 1). In most cases of PCOS, A and T serum levels are modestly and inconstantly elevated.

Ultrasound Definition of PCO and Anti-Müllerian Hormone

Defining PCO at U/S is an evolving issue, along with technical improvements such as the use of high-frequency probes through vaginal route and image enhancing software. To define PCO, the proposal from the Rotterdam consensus conference [16] is 'either 12 or more follicles measuring 2–9 mm in diameter in the whole ovary and/or increased ovarian volume (>10 cm^3)' (fig. 2). The priority has to be given to the ovarian volume and to the follicle number because both have the advantage to be physical entities that can be measured in real-time conditions and because both are considered as the key and consistent features of PCO. For instance, a close relationship between serum androgen levels and follicle number has been reported, as well as with anti-Müllerian hormone (AMH) [17]. In difficult situations, other ultrasound criteria for PCO may be used, although all have not been fully validated. In adolescent girls, the follicle criterion is difficult to use because it is much less reliable by abdominal than by vaginal route, the latter being most often impossible. Only the volume criterion should be used. In such situations, the assay of serum AMH offers an interesting surrogate to the follicle count [18].

Screening for Metabolic Syndrome

This should include clinical parameters (family history, BMI, WC, blood pressure, search for acanthosis nigricans) and biological parameters (glycemia, insulinemia,

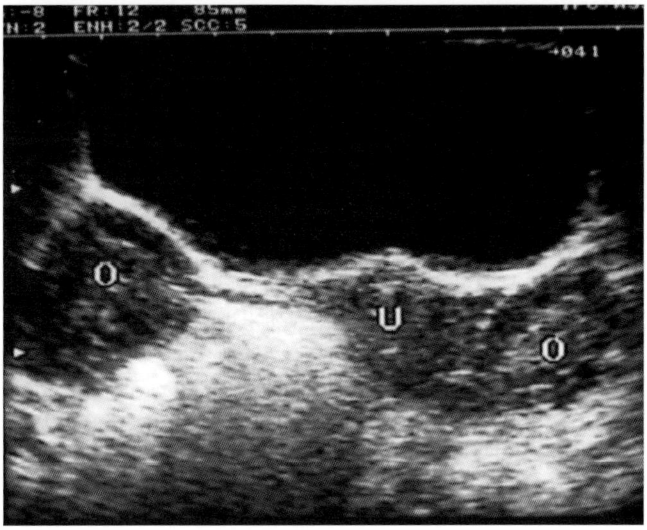

Fig. 2. Sonogram by abdominal route depicting the polycystic appearance of the ovaries in an adolescent girl with PCOS. Note that both ovarian sections are greater than the uterine section. In this representative case, the increased number of subcapsular follicles and the stromal hyperplasia are easily seen.

HDL-cholesterolemia, triglycerides). In addition, obese women with PCOS should be screened for glucose intolerance with an oral glucose tolerance test. No tests for insulin resistance are necessary to make the diagnosis of PCOS nor are they needed to select treatments [15]. In our experience, increased WC and decreased HDL-C were the most frequent metabolic abnormalities found in young (16–20 years) patients with PCOS [19]. It must be emphasized, however, that the adult threshold for a decreased HDL-C (<0.50 g/l in women) seems not appropriate in patients aged less than 20 years. Lowering this threshold to 0.4 g/l, as for children, would seem more judicious but this awaits confirmation [19]. In addition, the use of a metabolic score ≥3 to retain the diagnosis of metabolic syndrome does not seem appropriate for adolescents [19].

The PCOS Phenotypes

The new definition of Rotterdam recognizes 4 PCOS phenotypes: HA+OA+PCO (full-blown syndrome), HA+OA, HA+PCO (so-called ovulatory PCOS) and OA+PCO ('nonhyperandrogenic PCOS').

There is for the moment good agreement that women with asymptomatic PCO should not be considered as having PCOS and conversely that ovulatory women with HA and PCO do have PCOS. On the other hand, phenotype OA+PCO is not widely accepted and other definitions of PCOS still exclude this phenotype [20] although data are accumulating to certify that it is a true PCOS phenotype [21].

Non-Classic Adrenal Hyperplasia

NCAH is encountered with relatively high frequency (1–6%) among adolescent and adult patients with hyperandrogenism. This incidence may vary from one geographic area to another, as reported for classical 21-OHD, because of ethnic and racial clusters.

Pathophysiology

The 21-hydroxylase deficiency is responsible for an oversecretion of 17-HP and other steroids that are upstream this enzymatic step. Gene mutations of cytochrome P450 C21, resulting in NCAH, reduce the activity of 21-hydroxylase to 20–50%. This is not sufficient to impair the physiologically needed cortisol production, providing that the amount of precursor required is much greater than normal, thus compensating for the lower enzyme efficiency. The alteration in the enzyme kinetic is therefore sufficient to explain the excessive accumulation of 21-OH precursors, mainly progesterone and 17-HP, in the presence of a normal stimulation by ACTH. This excess is partly converted to androgens, resulting in adrenal hyperandrogenism. Therefore, NCAH is essentially a hyperandrogenic disorder, without overt abnormality in the gluco- and mineralocorticosteroid pathways.

Cytochrome P450 C21 gene is localized on chromosome 6. In NCAH, the most frequent mutation is V281L. Patients are homozygote or compound heterozygote with another mutation sometimes severe on the other allele. Considering the high frequency of heterozygote in the general population, it is essential to genotype the partner of the patient and to offer genetic counseling if he bears one severe mutation [22].

To understand why NCAH expresses itself only during or after puberty, it must be recalled that the steroidogenic changes accompanying adrenarche result in an increased 17,20-lyase and a decreased 3β-hydroxysteroid dehydrogenase-isomerase activity, thus increasing the adrenal output of Δ5 androgens. Such a phenomenon acting while 21-hydroxylase is partly deficient could be the physiological trigger of hyperandrogenism in NCAH.

Clinical Aspects

Before the age of 7–8 years, NCAH may mimic an idiopathic premature pubarche or, more rarely, a virilizing ovarian or adrenal tumor, especially when there are symptoms of precocious pseudo-puberty, such as accelerated height velocity and clitoromegaly. In the first series, the prevalence of NCAH compared to the other causes of premature pubarche was debated, varying from 0% to more than 20%, mainly because of differences in diagnostic criteria. More recently, it has been estimated at 6–8%, justifying the measurement of the 17-HP morning level in this situation.

Numerous studies have shown that adolescent or adult women with NCAH are seldom more virilized than other women with ovarian causes of hyperandrogenism and that no symptom of hyperandrogenism is specific for NCAH. Furthermore, NCAH may also be detected in individuals having mild symptoms such as acne [23]. Therefore, the clinical presentation cannot be used for the diagnosis of NCAH. Clitoromegaly, male habitus and temporal baldness are infrequent findings, unless the patient suffers from undiagnosed simple virilizing CAH. It has been suggested from a multicenter study including 220 patients that NCAH is a progressive disorder since the prevalence of hirsutism increases with the patient's age [24].

Diagnosis

The diagnosis of NCAH should be considered in those patients selected from a basal 17-HP >2 ng/ml (see above) and in whom the poststimulation 17-HP level exceeds 12 ng/ml (36.4 nmol/l). Between this threshold and the upper normal limit, which is about 3 ng/ml in most studies, there is the range of heterozygotes who are unaffected carriers and that of patients with functional ovarian and/or adrenal hyperandrogenism. The former may have a poststimulation 17-HP level as high as 15 ng/ml, but in any case their basal 17-HP level exceeds 2 ng/ml.

Once the biochemical diagnosis has been obtained, genotypes from adolescent patients with NCAH should be obtained as early as possible in order to be ready for genetic counseling when they desire a pregnancy.

Other Causes

Adrenal and Ovarian Tumors

These causes of hyperandrogenism are rare. The clinical presentation is often suggestive (see above, 'Diagnosis of hyperandrogenism in female adolescents'). The laboratory investigations will rapidly confirm the clinical suspicion and imaging techniques will localize the tumor (see same section above). Some extreme forms of PCOS, such as hyperthecosis, may also present with similar clinical and hormonal features. However, they are very infrequent in adolescents, unless the patient has an extreme insulin resistance (HAIR-AN syndrome), either genetic or secondary to a congenital or acquired portosystemic shunt [25].

Cushing Syndrome

Some adrenal tumors may secrete high amounts of androgens and cortisol. Therefore, the clinical presentation might be dominated by symptoms of glucocorticoid excess. Conversely, these symptoms may be mild in a hyperandrogenic adolescent patient with a pituitary Cushing disease. Therefore, it is wise to check the 24-hour urinary free cortisol level in any doubtful situation, especially in obese patients with full-blown PCOS.

Hyperprolactinemia

PRL excess stimulates the secretion of adrenal androgens, mainly DHEAS. Therefore, a mild hyperandrogenism frequently accompanies the clinical expression of a prolactinoma, but it is seldom the main complaint. Conversely, mild hyperprolactinemia frequently occurs in PCOS, but it has no specific expression and often disappears

Table 1. Serum tumor markers

Marker	Associated tumor
CA 125; CA 19.9	epithelial tumors (especially serous) immature teratoma (rare)
α-Fetoprotein	endodermal sinus tumors embryonal carcinomas mixed germ cell tumors immature teratoma, polyembryoma (rare)
Human chorionic gonadotropin	choriocarcinoma embryonal carcinomas mixed germ cell tumors polyembryoma, dysgerminoma (rare)
Carcinoembryonic antigen	serous tumors, mucinous tumors
Lactate dehydrogenase	dysgerminoma, mixed germ cell tumors
Estradiol	thecomas adult granulosa cell tumors
Testosterone	Sertoli cell tumors Leydig (hilus) cell tumors
F9 embryoglycan	embryonal carcinoma, yolk sac tumor choriocarcinoma, immature teratoma
Inhibin	granulosa-theca cell tumor
Müllerian inhibiting substance	granulosa-theca cell tumor

Hormonal Investigations

Endocrine signs and symptoms are due to abnormal steroid secretion by the tumor: estrogens, androgens or both. Hormonal investigation is rarely indicated and will be oriented by the clinical signs. It should include baseline gonadotrophins (LH, FSH), estradiol, AMH, and androgens. Elevated plasma levels of estrogens and/or androgens (testosterone >150 ng/dl) with low gonadotrophin levels suggest a peripheral gonadal or adrenal tumor. Inhibin B and anti-Müllerain hormone (AMH) are glycoproteins secreted by the granulosa cells of the ovary. They are specific markers of granulosa cell tumors and Sertoli cell tumors [6, 7].

Serum Tumor Markers

The measurement of tumor markers contributes to the diagnosis of certain malignant tumors and indicates postoperative tumor recurrence (table 1). These markers are not specific for ovarian origin but are specific of tissue [8]. α-Fetoprotein is a marker for endodermal sinus tumors (yolk sac tumors), mixed germ cell tumors, and sometimes immature teratomas. Beta-human chorionic gonadotropins (βHCG) are secreted by the cells of choriocarcinomas and occasionally by embryonal carcinomas. Carcinoembryonic antigen has low specificity because it is secreted by the cells of epithelial tumors (intestinal, ovarian, etc.) and germ cell tumors. Elevated serum cancer antigen (CA) 125 and CA 19.9 are typically associated with a malignant epithelial tumor of the ovary [9, 10], but these markers lack specificity. The study of the cancer predisposing genes, P53 and BRCA1 and BRCA2, is not currently part of the management of ovarian tumor in the child.

Management

Management of an ovarian mass is often surgical, which allows for definitive diagnosis by histopathological study. The clinician is generally confronted by one of two situations: either an ovarian mass or a pain syndrome that requires complementary investigations or acute abdominal pain that requires emergency surgery.

In the Emergency Situation: Adnexal Torsion or Rupture

Emergency surgery is performed only in complicated presentations when adnexal torsion or rupture is suspected. Torsion is the most frequent complication of ovarian masses, with an incidence ranging from 3 to 33%. Thus, pain development in the context of an ovarian mass should first raise the suspicion of adnexal torsion. According to several reports, the incidence of adnexal torsion in association with ovarian tumors ranges from 30 to 84%, with most of these tumors being benign. One explanation for this observation is that malignant tumor growth gives rise to peritumoral inflammation at the origin of adhesions [11].

The clinical signs and symptoms of torsion are generally vague: acute subumbilical abdominal pain with vomiting. Pelvic ultrasonography, as the first examination, will show a heterogeneous mass without visualization of the homolateral ovary. A lack of blood flow on Doppler suggests arterial obstruction. Complementary biological testing (tumor markers) is useful before surgery, but no test should delay surgical management because conservation of the adnexae depends on rapid intervention [3, 4].

Laparoscopy rather than laparotomy is the most reliable means of diagnosis because it reveals details of the torsion (number of twists in the adnexa, ovarian cyanosis) and is the means by which detorsion is performed [12]. No report has yet reported a thromboembolic event in the gonadal veins of young girls during detorsion [13]. Evaluating the viability of the ovary remains difficult but several works report the overall re-vascularization of the ovary and recovery of function after detorsion. The surgical approach should be as conservative as possible in order to preserve future fertility; thus, detorsion by laparoscopy or conventional surgery can be performed with puncture of a benign appearing cyst or cystectomy of a dermoid cyst [14–16].

Excision of a more suspicious tumoral mass during the same intervention is probably inadvisable. Ovarian fixation (ovariopexy) is planned by some and debated by others because it may provoke adhesions or modify the relationship between the ovary and fallopian tube, thereby altering future fertility. Moreover, it does not prevent the risk of future torsion [17].

In the Nonemergency Situation

The initial clinical, biological and radiological investigations confirm the presence of an ovarian mass and eliminate other diagnoses like fecalomas, pregnancy, urinary tract disorder, or ascites. The mass is localized to within the intervesico-rectal space by excluding tumors of other spaces. Its fluid, solid or mixed structure is determined. Diagnosis of a complex mass may be difficult, in which case MRI is indicated as it will give more specific information of the various components and will be helpful in determining local or distant tumor extension. The investigations are completed by measurement of tumor markers and steroid hormones.

The recent literature indicates a trend toward laparoscopy in pediatric practice, although conventional surgery still holds a considerable place [18, 19]. The most adapted approach often combines video-assisted surgery, as the two techniques are complementary. First, laparoscopy with an 'open' technique is performed to avoid the risk of pneumoperitoneum caused by a blind technique. This also permits full exploration of the peritoneal cavity and evaluation of the ovarian mass (size, surface, connection between ovarian parenchyma and tumor). Excision of a functional and benign small mass can be performed. Tumor excision can be performed either in the abdominal cavity under laparoscopy or after externalization of the adnexae by a small incision at the level of the iliac fossa. In other cases, ovarian surgery is performed by a broader pelvic approach (Pfannenstiel) following the established practices of oncologic surgery. In a recent study of 45 ovarian torsions, Vaysse's group suggested that laparotomy is preferable when the mass measures more than 75 mm in diameter [20].

Etiologies of Ovarian Masses

Nontumoral Functional Masses

Simple Functional Cysts

Simple ovarian cysts are a frequent development in adolescence. These cysts can be considered a variant of a physiological process, especially in puberty: functional cysts develop when a follicle (follicular cyst) or the corpus luteum (luteinized cyst) fails to involute, and they disappear during the next cycle. They are the most frequent cause of the ovarian masses detected in adolescence. The mean age at appearance is 13.5 years and the cysts are most frequently seen in the first 2 years of reproductive functioning. They are revealed by pain or menstrual disturbance but it is assumed that the true incidence is very much underestimated by a lack of recognition of the asymptomatic forms. The characteristic ultrasonographic image shows a unilocular cyst of 3–8 cm in diameter, with clearly defined borders, thin walls, and strictly fluid contents. The natural course is usually regression within a few days to a few weeks. During monitoring, the adolescent and her family need to be informed of the risk of torsion and advised to consult immediately in the case of acute pain. Management depends on the clinical signs and the cyst size. Monthly ultrasonographic monitoring is recommended for the first 3 months, as well as progestin or estrogen-progestin treatment in some cases [21]. Persistence of the cyst beyond three months or an increase in its volume during monitoring raises the suspicion of an organic cyst (dermoid cyst, purely fluid cystadenoma, or paraovarian cyst), which will require surgical excision. Some authors plan needle aspiration under ultrasonographic control, or laparoscopy if the diameter of the cyst is greater than 5 cm. Certain factors predispose toward ovarian cysts in adolescents: early menarche and long and irregular cycles.

Hemorrhagic Cysts and Endometriomas

The ultrasonogram may indicate intracystic bleeding. It is important to differentiate between slight occult bleeding causing intracystic debris, which should be closely monitored for the development of an intracystic stone, and avascular, apulsatile contents on Doppler examination, which may require cystectomy. Some serous or mucinous tumors can show similar songraphic images and their persistence should prompt intervention. Only histological and cytological analyses will permit definitive diagnosis.

Endometriosis is characterized by severe dymenorrhea that is resistant to the habitual treatment. It is rare in puberty. The retrovaginal wall is a frequent location, with palpation causing pain during rectal examination. Ultrasonography and MRI during menstruation will reveal endometrial nodules on the fallopian tube or ovary. Laparoscopy is a key element in diagnosis. Excision of localized endometriomas may be necessary. Endometriosis is rare in adolescence and will require suppression of ovarian activity by continuous estrogen-progestin or progestin treatment or GnRH analog.

Cysts and Impuberism: Aromatase or 17β-Hydroxylase Deficiency

Rare enzyme abnormalities can cause the recurrence of hemorrhaging ovarian cysts [22]. Certain clinical and hormonal elements will point toward this type of enzyme disorder: the cysts arise in a context of impuberism (absence of breast development and immature uterus) and insufficient ovarian secretion (LH and FSH are elevated and estradiol is undetectable). Aromatase is implicated in the conversion of testosterone into estrogens. The clinical picture of aromatase deficiency associates impuberism, marked virilization, and bleeding ovarian cysts. Estrogen treatment induces feminization, the regression of virilization, menarche, and the disappearance of the ovarian cysts. In the case of 17β-hydroxylase deficiency, hydrocortisone treatment is needed to limit the production of adrenal steroids.

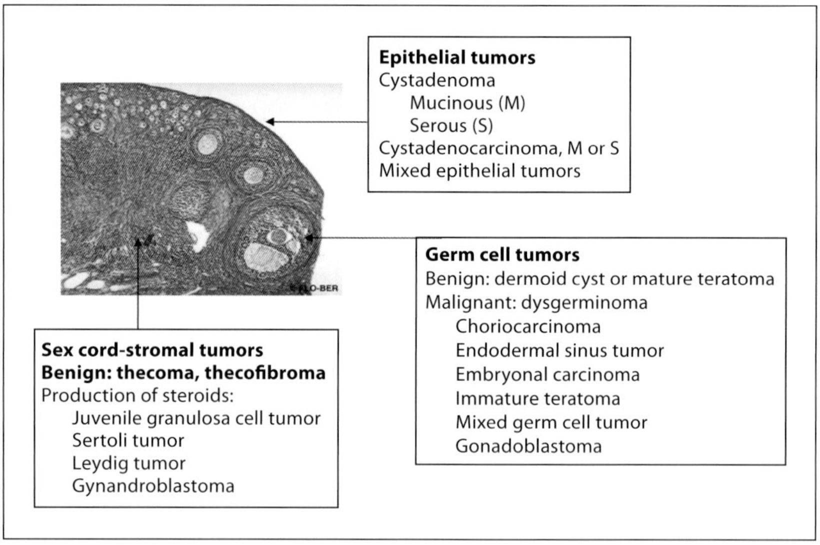

Fig. 1. Ovarians tumors. International classification of the World Health Organization [4].

Benign or Malignant Ovarian Tumors

The World Health Organization (WHO) has classified ovarian tumors on the basis of histological cell type and benign or malignant status [2] (fig. 1). This classification takes into account tumors of germ cell, epithelial, and sex cord-stromal origins. The tumor stage is defined according to the International Federation of Gynecology and Obstetrics (FIGO) and includes local, regional and distant tumor spread [23] (table 2). Depending on the series, ovarian tumors account for 2–25% of all ovarian masses.

Epithelial ovarian neoplasms are rare in patients under the age of 20 years. Epithelial tumors develop on the coelomic epithelium and cysts on the surface of the ovary. The two most frequent histomorphic types are the serous and mucinous forms. In adolescent girls the histoprognostic types are often benign, sometimes borderline (or low malignant potential) but rarely invasive. Germ cell tumors are the most frequent group, they develop from germ cells and are divided into two categories: teratomas (multiple tissue and single tissue) and nonteratomous tumors. Sex cord-stromal tumors represent 5–8% of all ovarian tumors. They can be divided into two groups: tumors developing from the gonadal stroma: fibromas, thecomas, sclerosing stromal tumors, and tumors developing from the sex cord: granulosa cell tumors, Sertoli-Leydig tumors.

Germ Cell Tumors: Dermoid Cysts, Dysgerminomas

The TGM derived from the transformation of primordial germ cells, totipotent cells can remain ‘undifferentiated’ (seminoma), ‘poorly differentiated (embryonal carcinoma) or become differentiated embryonic structures (mature or immature teratoma)

Table 2. Staging ovarian carcinomas according to the International Federation of Gynecology and Obstetrics (FIGO) [23]

Stage I:	Tumor limited to the ovaries
IA:	Tumor limited to one ovary; no ascites present containing malignant cells; no tumor on the external surface; capsule intact
IB:	Tumor limited to both ovaries; no ascites present containing malignant cells; no tumor on the external surfaces; capsules intact
IC:	Tumor classified as either stage IA or IB but with tumor on the surface of one or both ovaries; or ruptured capsule(s); or with ascites containing malignant cells present; or with positive peritoneal washings
Stage II:	Tumor involving one or both ovaries, with pelvic extension
IIA:	Tumor extension and/or metastases to the uterus and/or tubes
IIB:	Tumor extension to other pelvic tissues
IIC:	Tumor either stage IIA or IIB but with tumor on the surface of one or both ovaries; or with capsule(s) ruptured; or with ascites containing malignant cells present; or with positive peritoneal washings
Stage III:	Tumor involving one or both ovaries with peritoneal implants beyond the pelvis and/or retroperitoneal or inguinal lymph node involvement; superficial liver metastasis; tumor is limited to the true pelvis but with histologically proven malignant extension to small bowel or omentum
IIIA:	Tumor grossly limited to the true pelvis with negative nodes but with histologically confirmed microscopic seeding of abdominal peritoneal surfaces
IIIB:	Tumor of one or both ovaries with histologically confirmed implants of abdominal peritoneal surfaces, none >2 cm in diameter; nodes are negative
IIIC:	Abdominal implants >2 cm in diameter and/or positive retroperitoneal or inguinal nodes
Stage IV:	Tumor in one or both ovaries with distant metastases, pleural metastases (histologically +), parenchymal liver metastasis

and extraembryonic (yolk sac tumor secreting the α-fetoprotein and/or secreting choriocarcinoma hCG).

Benign cystic teratomas or dermoid cyst is the only benign germ cell tumor and it represents 95% of germ cell tumors. It occurs in young women (an average of 30 years old), is unilateral in 90% of cases and slow growing [24]. Mature dermoid cysts are generally voluminous (3–30 cm), heterogeneous with multiple components (fat, teeth, hair and bone), and are most often asymptomatic. The sonograms and pelvic X-rays are often characteristic, showing a cystic mass with solid component and calcifications. Diagnosis is based on MRI: the presence of fat in an ovarian tumor is pathognomonic of a mature teratoma, the fatty component results in a high-intensity signal on T_1-weighted images which disappears during fat saturation. This tumor associates multiples tissues: ectodermic (pilo-sebaceous parts, teeth), mesodermic (fat, osteocartilagenous tissue) and endodermic (thyroid tissue) debris. In 10–20% of the cases, both ovaries are affected. Macroscopic examination of the controlateral ovary is thus always indicated (though biopsy is not considered further informative). The treatment is cystectomy with preservation of the healthy ovarian tissue. In all cases, ultrasonographic monitoring is needed for several years to ensure that new cyst development is not missed. Classically, the teratoma is well differentiated, mature and benign, but histological examination is always imperative to detect a malignant component: this would indicate an immature malignant teratoma. The mature teratoma may be associated with another germ cell tumor resulting in a combined tumor with different histological components which have all developed from the same stem cell. Immature multiple tissue teratomas are rare malignant tumors in young women (in their 20s). They are fast growing, with frequent capsular rupture.

Dysgerminomas are nonteratomous tumors. They are one of the most frequently seen malignant tumors in young women. Tumor growth is rapid with frequent capsular rupture, and the solid component is predominant. Fluid tumors of this type are extremely rare. These tumors secrete tumor markers. The pure seminomas are seen especially after 15 years. An abnormal secretion of α-fetoprotein reflects the presence of yolk material, even if the quota is not found histologically, it is the same for hCG that shows the presence of cells syncitiotrophoblastic cells. These very specific markers can make a positive diagnosis of malignant germ cell tumors and monitor tumor progression (remission, relapse). At FIGO stage IA, the prognosis is good. Treatment is surgical by salpingo-ovariectomy. Bilateral tumors are seen in 20% of the cases. Prognosis is more reserved for widespread forms that will require adjuvant chemotherapy. Other malignant tumors (carcinomas, embryonic teratomas, choriocarcinomas) are treated by surgery limited to the affected ovary followed by chemotherapy, depending on the stage and progression. The overall prognosis is good, with cure and preservation of fertility.

Recent data seem to indicate that surgical management must take into account the tumor size and the marker levels. For a tumor with a diameter greater than 75 mm or positive markers, laparotomy is the preferred surgical choice.

Tumors of the Epithelium: Cystadenomas

Epithelial tumors increase in frequency during the second decade of life, from 16% at 14 years of age to 28% at 17 years. They are rarely malignant before 20 years. They develop on the celomic epithelium and cysts on the surface of the ovary There are two types of cystadenoma: serous and mucinous. Serous cystadenomas are more common (fig. 2). It is cystic tumor which is often bilateral, uni- or bifocal with a thin wall, homogenous signal intensity on MRI with no solid component. Mucinous cystadenomas are multi-lobed with thick and irregular walls and mucoid contents but no solid component. Their development is often rapid. The incidence of borderline tumors rises with age and are characterized by the presence of vegetations or endocystic or exocystic papillary excrescences covering the surface of the ovary [25]. A malignant component (cystadenocarcinoma) is nevertheless found in 7–30% of the cases. In 2009, a French study of 42 cystadenomas in girls younger than 16 years found that the mean age at diagnosis was 11.5 years and that 22% of

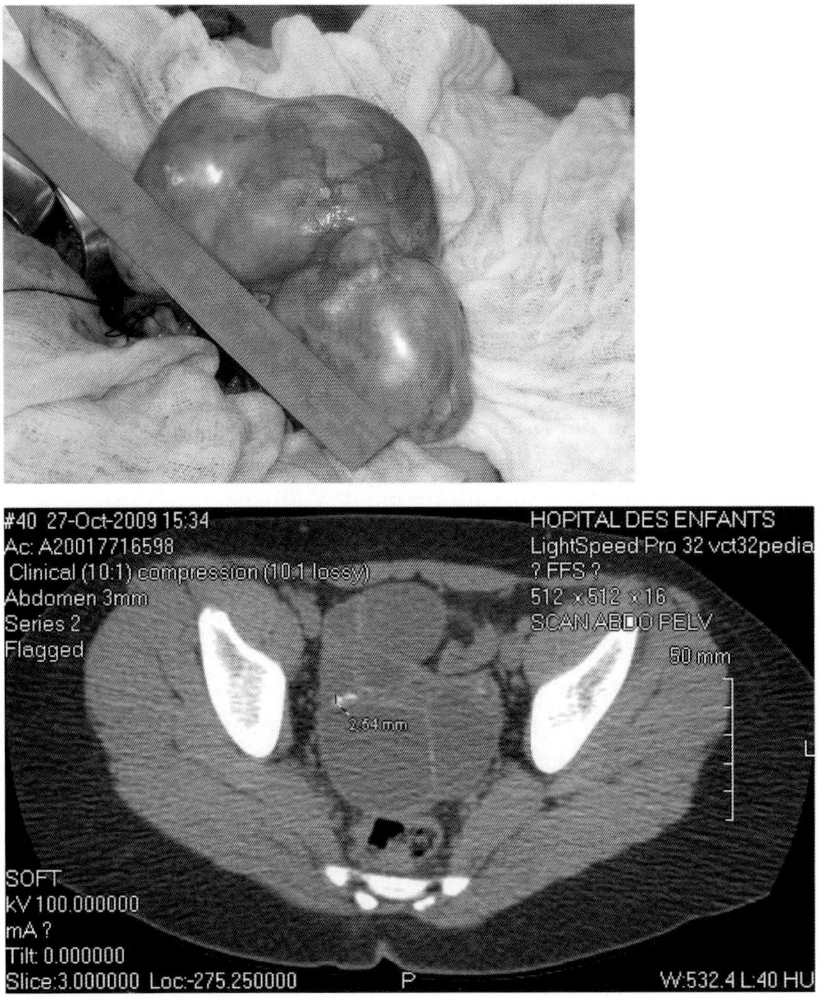

Fig. 2. Voluminous serous cystadenoma in a 10-year-old girl (peroperative photo and scan).

the tumors were bilateral [26]. Cystectomy should be performed with total removal of the cyst wall and preservation of the healthy ovary. Regular monitoring for several years is needed because of the risk of recurrence. This risk is higher for mucinous cystadenomas.

Sex Cord-Stromal Tumors

This group of tumors has the particularity of being associated with hormonal activity such as the production of estrogens or androgens. Most of these tumors are benign (fibrothecoma, sclerosing stromal tumor) or limited to the ovary at diagnosis.

Sex cord-stromal tumors include granulosa cell and Leydig-Sertoli cell tumors, as well as stromal tumors. All have endocrine activity and secrete estrogens, androgens and specific hormone markers (inhibin B and AMH) [6, 7]. Granulosa cell tumors cause precocious pseudo puberty in the prepubertal girl and metrorrhagia or amenorrhea with virilization in the young pubertal girl [27]. The mean age of appearance is 7–9 years. The juvenile form has a low risk of malignancy, as opposed to the adult form. On MRI, the solid component is often seen as a low intensity signal on T_1-weighted images and a clearly low-intensity signal on T_2-weighted images because of the fibrous stroma. These tumors show little local spread and the capsule is generally conserved. They are classed as FIGO stage IA. Treatment is strictly surgical: ovariectomy or tumorectomy. Ultrasonographic monitoring and marker level testing is needed for several years. Other prognostic factors include FOXL2 gene expression. FOXL2 is implicated in ovarian development and function and its expression is found to be diminished in granulosa tumors [28].

Other types of tumor are extremely rare, like gonadoblastomas, which develop in 7–10% of the cases of gonadal dysgenesis with fragment Y (Turner syndrome).

Conclusions

Ovarian tumors are mostly benign and their frequency increases with age. Most cysts are functional and adnexal torsion is the main complication. Ultrasonography is the diagnostic tool of choice; MRI is an essential complement to imaging of tumors with heterogeneous solid components. If there is a surgical indication, the surgery must conform to oncologic standards and must be as conservative as possible to preserve future fertility.

References

1 Pfeifer SM, Gosman GG: Evaluation of adnexal masses in adolescents. Pediatr Clin N Am 1999;46: 573–592.

2 Serov SF, Scully RE, Sobin LH: Histological typing of ovarian tumours. International Histological Classification of Tumours, No 9. Geneva, World Health Organization, 1973, pp 37–55.

3 Dane B, Dane C, Kiray M, Cetin A: Sonographic findings in adnexal torsion: a report of 34 cases. Arch Gynecol Obstet 2009;279:841–844.

4 Shadinger LL, Andreotti RF, Kurian RL: Preoperative sonographic and clinical characteristics as predictors of ovarian torsion. J Ultrasound Med 2008;27:7–13.

5 Chiou SY, Lev-Toaff AS, Masuda E, Feld RI, Bergin D: Adnexal torsion: new clinical and imaging observations by sonography, computed tomography, and magnetic resonance imaging. J Ultrasound Med. 2007;26:1289–1301.

6 Lappohn RE, Burger HG, Bourna J: Inhibin is a marker of granulosa cell tumor. Acta Obstet Gynecol Scand 1992;155–161.

7 Gustafson ML, Lee MM, Scully RE, Moncure AC, Hirakawa T, Goodman A, Muntz HG, Donahoe PK, McLaughlin DT, Fuller AF: Müllerian inhibiting substance as a marker for ovarian sex-cord tumor. N Engl J Med 1992;326:466–471.

8 Schwartz PE: Ovarian masses: serologic markers. Clin Obstetric Gynecol 1991;34:423.

9 Skates SJ, Horick N, Yu Y, Xu FJ, Berchuck A, Havrilesky LJ, De Bruijn HW, Van der Zee AG, Woolas RP, Jacobs IJ, Zhang Z, Bast RC Jr: Preoperative sensitivity and specificity for early stage ovarian cancer when combining cancer antigen CA 125II, CA 15-3, CA 72-4, and macrophage colony stimulating factor using mixtures of multivariate normal distributions. J Clin Oncol 2004;22: 4059–4066.

10 Zhang Z, Yu Y, Xu F, Berchuck A, Van Haaften Day C, Havrilesky LJ, De Bruijn HW, Van Der Zee AG, Woolas RP, Jacobs IJ, Skates S, Chan DW, Bast RC Jr: Combining multiple serum tumor markers improves detection of stage I epithelial ovarian cancer. Gynecol Oncol. 2007;107:526–531.
11 Templeman C, Fallat ME, Blinchevsky A, Hertweck P: Noninflammatory ovarian masses in girls and young women. Obstet Gynecol 2000;96:229–233.
12 Rousseau V, Massicot R, Darwish AA, Sauvat F, Emond S, Thibaud E, Nihoul-Fekété C: Emergency management and conservative surgery of ovarian torsion in children: a report of 40 cases. J Pediatr Adolesc Gynecol 2008;21:201–206.
13 Templeman C, Hertweck SP, Fallat ME: The clinical course of unresected ovarian torsion. J Pediatr Surg 2000;35:1385–1387.
14 Broach AN, Mansuria SM, Sanfilippo JS: Pediatric and adolescent gynecologic laparoscopy. Clin Obstet Gynecol 2009;52:380–389.
15 Oltmann SC, Fischer A, Barber R, Huang R, Hicks B, Garcia N: Cannot exclude torsion – a 15-year review. J Pediatr Surg 2009;44:1212–1216.
16 Lo Lm, Chang SD, Horng SG, Yan TY, Lee CL, Liang CC: Laparoscopy versus laparotomy for surgical intervention of ovarian torsion. J Obstet Gynaecol Res 2008;34:1020–1025.
17 Ares M, Sarihan H: Oophoropexy in children with ovarian torsion. Eur J Pediatr Surg 2004;14:168–171.
18 Piippo S, Mustaniemi L, Lenko H, Aine R, Maenpaa J: Surgery for ovarian masses during childhood and adolescence: report of 79 cases. J Pediatr Adolesc Gynecol 1999;12:223–227.
19 Karpelowsky JS, Hei ER, Matthews K: Laparoscopic resection of benign ovarian tumours in children with gonadal preservation. Pediatr Surg Int 2009;25: 251–254.
20 Galinier P, Carfagna L, Delsol M, Ballouhey Q, Lemasson F, Lemandat A, Moscovici J, Guitard J, Pienkowski C, Vaysse P: Ovarian torsion: management and ovarian prognosis: a report of 45 cases. J Pediatr Surg 2009;44:1759–1765.
21 Kanizsai B, Orley J, Szigetvari I, Doszpod J: Ovarian cyst in children adolescents: their occurrence, behavior, and management. J Pediatr Adolesc Gynecol 1998;11:85–88.
22 Conte FA, Grumbach MM, Fisher CR, Simpson ER: A syndrome of female pseudohermaphrodism, hypergonadotrophic hypogonadism and multicystic ovaries associated with missence mutations in the gene encoding aromatase (p450arom). J Clin Endocrinol Metab 1994;78:1287.
23 International Federation of Gynecology and Obstetrics (FIGO) Cancer Committee: Staging announcement. Gynecol Oncol 1986;25:303–306.
24 Valteau-Couanet D, Dubrel M, Dufour C, Couanet D, Hartmann O, Patte C: Malignant ovarian tumors in childhood. Arch Pediatr 2008;15:781–782.
25 Tsai JY, Saigo PE, Brown C, La Quaglia MP: Diagnosis, pathology, staging, treatment and outcome of epithelial ovarian neoplasm in patients age <21 years. Cancer 2001;91:2065–2070.
26 Massicot R, Rousseau V, Darwish A, Sauvat F, Jaubert F, Nihoul Fekete C: Serous and seromucinous infantile ovarian cystadenomas: a study of 42 cases. Eur J Obstet Gynecol Reprod Biol 2009;142: 64–67.
27 Kalfa N, Patte C, Orbach D, Lecointre C, Philippe F, Brauner R, Pienkowski C, Rubie H, Guedj AM, Paris F, Lumbroso S, Sultan C: Delayed recognition of endocrine disorders worsens the prognosis for granulosa cell tumors in pre or post pubertal girls. Horm Res 2004;62(suppl 2):38.
28 Kalfa N, Philibert P, Patte C, Tibhaud E, Pienkowski C, Ecochard A, Boizet-Bonhoure B, Fellous M, Sultan C: Juvenile granulosa cell tumor: clinical and molecular expression. Gynecol Obstet Fertil 2009; 37:33–44.

Audrey Cartault
Unité d'Endocrinologie, Génétique et Gynécologie Médicale, Hôpital des Enfants
330, avenue de Grande-Bretagne
FR–31026 Toulouse Cédex (France)
Tel. +33 33 534 558 556, E-Mail cartault.a@chu-toulouse.fr

Breast Asymmetry
A small asymmetry is frequent, but sometimes the asymmetry is very marked and very detrimental aesthetically [12]. Differential diagnosis is unilateral hypertrophy. The palpation of this too voluminous breast reveals a normal supple tissue without any nodule. If the morphological aspect of the breast is at stage S5, normalization of the two breasts with the same volume is not possible. The only treatment is surgical.

A Becker nevus is frequently associated with a unilateral mammary hypoplasia achieving an asymmetry [13]. This hamartoma appears more often at puberty. Its clinical characteristics are characterized by a clear brown stain sometimes with coats. At the physiopathologic level, an increased number of androgen receptors are present and may be responsible of this underlying mammary hypoplasia.

Abnormality of Form
The breast must be different from the harmonious standard breast. Tuberous breast is a small breast with a tight implantation base associated with a very large nipple. The mammary gland makes a hernia through the nipple [14]. The treatment is surgical.

Aberrations or Diseases Linked with Stromal Tissue Development

The new classification ANDI is well suited for mammary hypertrophy. From the normal volume of the breast to the simple hypertrophy or major hypertrophy like gigantomastia, all the stages from normal development to pathological disease can be described.

Mammary Hypertrophy: Aberration of Development
Mammary hypertrophy, which is a simple exaggeration of normal volume of the breast, can be embarrassing leading to a physical discomfort, creating disturbances of vertebral static and psychological trouble. Clinically, the mammary gland is voluminous but supple. Medical treatment with 19-nortestosterone derivatives has been proposed 16 (10–25th) to 10 (10–25th) days per cycle with good results [15]. Progestogens (pregnane or norpregnane derivatives) have also been used in this context, but these therapeutics remain to be evaluated. The decision for surgical treatment can be made without any age limits.

Gigantomastia: Disease
Gigantomastia represents a pathological situation whose suddenness of apparition and speed of evolution makes it an emergency. It is a sudden increase of mammary volume occurring early in reproductive life. Sometimes, the gigantomastia can be asymmetric. The breasts are firm, painfully strained with inflammatory signs on the breast skin.

Reported for the first time by Durston in 1669, no aetiology can clearly explain this phenomenon. Classically, a hypersensitiveness to estrogens has been evocated, but no estrogen receptors are present and plasma estradiol levels are normal [16]. A dysimmunitary process has been evocated (especially in the presence of inflammatory signs) because hypertrophy may occur in women with autoimmune diseases like rheumatoid polyarthritis, Hashimoto's thyroiditis and myasthenia [17].

Reduction surgical treatment is often necessary to relieve these young women. The ideal time for this surgical treatment is after stabilization of the disease.

After the surgery, a follow-up is desirable because recurrences have been described, leading, if major, to mastectomy with mammary prosthesis.

Aberrations or Diseases of Ductal Development

Ductal Ectasia: Anatomophysiologic Variation

Ductal ectasia is more frequent in middle-aged women. At adolescence, ectasia has been described as an exaggeration of sinus ductal whose epithelium disposed in 'accordion' pleats allows the dilatation and stagnation of secretions.

At the initial stage of ductal ectasia, a variant of the normality, a pathologic step can occur such as an abscess, where the secretion stagnation leads to epithelium ulceration with secretions avoiding secondary ductal inflammation.

Clinically, ductal ectasia appears as a retro-areolar tumor of 1–3 cm in size, sensitive, discreetly blue and sometimes associated with brownish even bloody nipple discharge, either spontaneous or provoked by a discrete palpation of the nipple. Its development is rapid and takes place early in reproductive life before or after the menarche. Ultrasound confirms a hydroid lesion. The spontaneous evolution is mostly favorable with regression of the tumefaction and disappearance of nipple discharge. In the follow-up, the risk is nipple infection because of the vulnerability of the nipple. Several steps can occur in the same or the contralateral breast, or both.

If the evolution is long or if nipple discharge persists, surgical treatment can be decided on. The histological lesion is ductal ectasia. It is a distension of one ductal duct associated with an inflammatory reaction, conjunctive fibrosis and sometimes benign epithelial hyperplasia.

The nipple discharge reported during the evolution of ductal ectasia must be distinguished from a sebaceous gland juxta-areolar discharge set on the areola (Montgomery tubercle). Cure is spontaneous without treatment [18].

Breast Abscess: Disease

Classically described postpartum, breast abscess has been reported at adolescence. Retro-areolar abscess is the most frequent. It is the consequence of the ductal ectasia infection with rupture of ductal duct in surrounding tissue and abscess formation. According to the stage at discovery, the nodule is at various sizes, with or without inflammatory signs often with fever. Early medical treatment can lead to cessation of the symptoms. This treatment associates local anti-inflammatory dressings and systemic antibiotherapy. The frequency of recurrences necessitates a long duration of antibiotherapy even after the disappearance of clinical symptoms. For some authors, the umbilical nipple is a risk factor of these recurrent abscesses. If the medical treatment is ineffective, surgery can be proposed. Recurrence is frequent after a simple incision and drain. A global resection of the concerned duct is therefore advised [19].

Aberrations or Diseases of Lobular Development

Before the perimenarcheal period, the mammary gland consists of a few ducts only. During the perimenarcheal development, the principal changes are ducts sprouting and addition of lobular structures. Estrogenes induce connective tissue and vascular growth which is required for the new ducts development. The lobules develop particularly during the early reproductive life at 15–25 years of age. Different types of lobules have been described by Russo and coworkers [20, 21]. Each period of reproductive life (like pregnancy, breastfeeding or menopause) is associated with more and more differentiated lobules. This explains the frequency of fibroadenoma during early reproductive life. Indeed, fibroadenoma is an exaggeration of the development of various structures of the lobules. Although fibroadenomas are classified as benign diseases, they can almost be considered as aberrations of normal development [22].

Fibroadenoma: Aberration of Normal Development

The lobular origin explains many features of fibroadenoma, for instance his frequency during the menarcheal period at the time of maximal lobular development. Fibroadenoma is the most common breast tumor of adolescence. Indeed, its discovery is certainly less frequent by clinical examination than by ultrasound which usually detects deeper fibroadenomas. The characteristics of adolescent fibroadenoma are accurate enough to be diagnosed certainly after only clinical examination. Often, the tumor is noticed accidentally by the adolescent herself. It is a firm, smooth, round or bosselated, painless and very mobile tumor. His encapsulation explains this mobility [23].

The size of fibroadenoma is usually 1–3 cm. During the growth phase, the tumor doubles in size in 6–12 months and is then likely to remain static for the rest of the patient's life or gradually decreases in size or disappears. In a study, Dent et al. [24] followed 99 young women with a clinical and cytological diagnosis of single or multiple fibroadenoma. They found that 107 lumps disappeared on the 279 tumors followed over 7–9 years. There is no relationship between the probability of either disappearance, initial size or multiple features in a same woman, but with young age less 20 years [24, 25]. Development of the fibroadenoma is hormone dependent [26–29]. This hormone dependence diminishes rapidly with the evolution of the lesion and the apparition of the fibrosis without hormonal receptors, a further possible explanation for the plateauing in the growth curve [26]. Ultrasound confirms the evident clinical diagnosis. The ultrasonic features of fibroadenoma are a round or oval sharp contour, weak internal echoes in a uniform distribution and intermediate attenuation, more evident if the tumor is young.

The histological features of fibroadenoma are an exaggeration of normal lobular development. The proliferation of stromal element and epithelial element is regular, maintaining a normal relationship as in a normal lobule. Then, there is a progressive sclerosis of the stromal element and the epithelial element disappears.

For some authors [27–29], fibroadenoma occurs in women with estrogen-progesterone imbalance leading to an 'unopposed estrogen effect'. Progesterone appeared to oppose the estrogen effects on the breast epithelial cells. Based on this rationale, some clinicians, at least in our country, propose progestin treatment for various benign breast disorders, e.g. fibroadenoma. 19-Nor-testosterone derivatives, used 16–20 days per cycle, have been proposed with good clinical and ultrasound results [15]. Pregnane or norpregnane derivatives have also been proposed but remain to be evaluated.

Removal of all fibroadenomas is a classical position, but for an adolescent, a few reasons can explain a more flexible approach.

- A recurrence after surgery at the site of previous removal or near it in the same breast or in the controlateral one is possible [30].
- Fibroadenomas are often multiple. A repeating surgery is not recommended for an adolescent in an aesthetic approach [31, 32].
- Furthermore, lumps can become smaller or disappear.
- Medical treatment with progestins provides good results.
- The risk of malignancy is negligible for women less than 20 years. It allows a conservative approach without fear.

The conservative attitude can be decided if clinical and ultrasound examination show unequivocally benign characteristics. Fine-needle aspiration can confirm if clinical or ultrasound features are not entirely typical. After the triple assessment (clinical, ultrasound and cytology), the diagnosis is confirmed and sure, but sometimes the cytological feature can be florid if the fibroadenoma is young.

Patients can be discharged after 6 months if the lesion remains stable or regressed. A classical clinical surveillance only is necessary. The conservative policy should be reconsidered if the tumor increases in size.

If there is a doubt regarding the nature of the presumed fibroadenoma or if the patient wishes to be rid of it, surgery is decided [33]. The surgical approach must be as aesthetic as possible. A periareolar excision is better from this point of view.

Giant Fibroadenoma: Disease

If fibroadenoma simplex can be considered as an aberration of normal lobule development, a giant fibroadenoma is a disease.

It is a large tumor greater than 5 cm at onset or soon after menarche. This encapsulated breast mass with rapid enlargement compresses the adjacent breast tissue with the development of skin ulcers and prominent veins. This sudden growth is opposite to the hypothesis that giant fibroadenoma arises from the continued progression of small fibroadenoma. It is possible that giant fibroadenoma is a separate condition de novo. The clinical feature is a large well-demarcated breast mass, firmer than the rest of the breast, opposite to breast asymmetry or unilateral hypertrophy.

A giant fibroadenoma in this age group may be associated with multiple smaller fibroadenomas in the same breast or in the opposite.

Giant fibroadenoma has been described as being more common in the black population [34].

On the basis of clinical diagnosis, surgery can be recommended as the size imposes surgery and a cosmetic approach is recommended [35]. Tumor fragmentation is possible.

The histological features are the same as for fibroadenoma simplex, with a normal relationship between epithelial and stromal elements. The florid feature of this proliferation can lead to considerable confusion with cytosarcoma phyllodes being very rare under the age of 20. The phyllode tumor is distinct from the giant fibroadenoma both macroscopically and histologically, the diagnosis is a histological one.

To diagnose the phyllode tumor, both epithelial and fibrous stromal elements must be present, with the stroma showing cellularity, irregularity, hyperchromatism and significant mitosis [36]. The stroma is notably more cellular than in fibroadenoma and is dominant in relation to the epithelial component. Under the age of 20, they almost invariably behave in a benign manner. All should be treated by enucleation. This tumor shows no recurrence locally, if completely excised. Many diagnoses of phyllode tumor are certainly made in excess.

Multiple Fibroadenomas

Fibroadenomas are often multiple, occurring concurrently or successively in both breasts. Haagensen [37] shows an incidence of 16% in his experience. Sometimes the development of multiple fibroadenomas, among which a size upper than 5 cm can be reported, is brutal with a breast invaded by the fibroadenomatous disease. It is, as for giant fibroadenoma, a real disease. The treatment of these multiple fibroadenomas is not surgical due to the risk of aesthetic damages. Medical treatment can be discussed. The use of progestin 19-nortestosterone derivatives, if early, has shown a diminution of the fibroadenoma size and sometimes disappearance of some tumors.

Aberrations or Disease Associated with Cyclical Variations of Breast Tissue

In the adolescent, the aberrations associated with cyclical variations of mammary gland have very little clinical presentations. Indeed, in the early pubertal period, cyclical mastalgia is exceptional. But, the longer time since the first menstruations raises the higher probability to observe rises in cyclical hormonal mastalgia. Cyclical mastalgia must be defined with strict clinical criteria; appearance before the menstruations during more than 4 days, disappearance some days after the menstruations, and bilaterality.

Cancer

Breast cancer constitutes only about 1% of childhood cancers and <0.1% of all breast cancers occur in this age group [38–42]. Three clinical presentations are identified:

1 Primary malignancy of the breast; carcinoma (juvenile secretory carcinoma), sarcoma or lymphoma.
2 Metastasis disease: rhabdomyosarcoma or leukaemia [43]; non-Hodgkin's lymphoma.
3 Secondary malignancy: postradiation therapy (mantle irradiation).

Mammography is not helpful in the diagnosis of breast cancer. It is less sensitive in detecting malignancies in younger patients than in older ones. An accurate strategy is essential to discover the rare malignancy. Physical examination is essential to perform surgical biopsy:

(a) if eccentric subareolar mass is not centralized beneath the areola in a child before puberty, and

(b) since in adolescents with malignancy (current or former), metastasis lesions are more common than primary lesions.

Conclusion

Breast diseases at adolescence show their own characteristics linked to the development process and physiology of the mammary gland. The distinction between aberration (divergence of normal development) and disease, as proposed by the ANDI classification applies to the adolescence context particularly well. Moreover, the absence of malignancy pathology at this age makes possible reassurance of women early at the first consultation. The diagnoses are more often performed only clinically. Sometimes, resorting to complementary investigation is necessary and ultrasound is the best investigation. Indeed, mammography is not contributory at this age.

References

1 Hughes LE, Mansel RE, Webster DJTW: Aberrations of normal development and involution (ANDI): a new perspective on pathogenesis and nomenclature of benign breast disorders. Lancet 1987;ii:1316–1319.

2 Hughes LE, Mansel RE: Aberrations of normal development and involution (ANDI): a concept of benign breast disorders based on pathogenesis; in Hughes LE, Mansel RE, Webster DJT (eds): Benign Disorders and Diseases of the Breast, ed 2. Philadelphia, Saunders, 2000, pp 21–34.

3 Hughes LE, Mansel RE: Breast anatomy and physiology; in Hughes LE, Mansel RE, Webster DJT (eds): Benign Disorders and Diseases of the Breast, ed 2. Philadelphia, Saunders, 2000, pp 7–20.

4 De Silva NK, Brandt ML: Disorders of the breast in children and adolescents. 1. Disorders of growth and infections of the breast. J Pediatr Adolesc Gynecol 2006;19:345–349.
5 Marshall WA, Tanner JM: Variations in pattern of pubertal changes in girls. Arch Dis Child 1969;44: 291–303.
6 Wellings SR, Jense HM, Mascum MG: An atlas of subgross pathology of the human breast with reference to possible precancerous lesions. J Nat Cancer Inst 1975;55:231–273.
7 Herman-Giddens ME, Slora EJ, Wasserman RC: Secondary sexual characteristics and menses in young girls seen in office practice; a study from the pediatric research in office settings networks. Pediatrics 1997;99:505–512.
8 Greydanus DE, Matyytsina L, Gains M: Breast disorders in children and adolescents. Prim Care Clin Office Pract 2006;33:455–502.
9 Dehner LP, Hill DA, Deschryver K: Pathology of the breast in children, adolescents, and young adults. Semin Diagn Pathol 1999;16:235–47.
10 Lewis EJ, Crutchfield CE 3rd, Prawer SE: Accessory nipple and associated conditions. Pediatr Dermatol 1997;14:333–334.
11 Fokin AA, Robicsek F: Poland's syndrome revisited. Ann Thorac Surg 2002;74:2218–2225.
12 Netscher D, Mosharrafa A, Laucirica R: Massive asymmetric virginal breast hypertrophy. South Med J 1996;89:434–437.
13 Friedel J, Heid E, Dallara JM, Grosshans E: Naevus pharmacologiques ou fonctionnels. Ann Dermatol Venerol 1991;118:645–654.
14 Ribeiro L, Canzi W, Buss A: Tuberous breast: a new approach. Plast Reconst Surg 1998;101:42–52.
15 Mauvais-Jarvis P, Kuttenn F: Benign breast disease; in Bardin CW (ed): Current Therapy in Endocrinology and Metabolism, part 3. Philadelphia, BC Decker Press, 1994, pp 364–370.
16 Jabs AD, Frantz AG, Smith-Vanitz A: Mammary hypertrophy is not associated with increase estrogen receptors. Plast Reconstr Surg 1990;86:64–66.
17 Touraine P, Youssef N, Alyanakian MA, et al: Breast inflammatory gigantomastia in a context of immune-mediated diseases. J Clin Endocrinol Metab 2005;90:5287–5294.
18 Markins F, Giacomontions M, Salisbury S: Nipple discharge and breast lump related to Montgomerry's tubercle in adolescents females. J Pediatr Surg 1988; 23:718–720.
19 De Silva NK, Brandt ML: Disorders of the breast in children and adolescents. 2. Breast masses. J Pediatr Adolesc Gynecol 2006;19:415–418.
20 Russo J, Calaf G, Roi L, Russo IH: Influence of gland age and topography on cell kinetics of normal breast tissue. J Natl Cancer Inst 1987;78:413–418.
21 Russo J, Russo IH: Toward a physiological approach to breast cancer prevention. Cancer Epidemiol Biomark Prev 1994;3:353–364.
22 Dixon JM, Mansel RE: Congenital problems and aberrations of normal breast development and involution Br Med J 1994;309:797–800.
23 Simmons JY: Fibroadenomas in adolescence. Curr Opin Obstet Gynecol 2009;21:402–406.
24 Cant PJ, Maden MV, Close PM, et al: Case for conservative management of selected fibroadenomas of the breast. Br J Surgery 1987;74:857–859.
25 Dent DM, Cant PJ: Fibroadenoma. World J Surg 1989;13:706–710.
26 Martin PM, Kuttenn F, Serment H, Mauvais-Jarvis P: Progesterone receptors in breast fibroadenomas. J Steroid Biochem 1979;11:1295–1298.
27 Kuttenn F, Fournier S, Durand JC, Mauvais-Jarvis P: Estradiol and progesterone receptors in breast fibroadenomas. J Clin Endocrinol Metab 1981;52: 1225–1229.
28 Mauvais-Jarvis P, Kuttenn F, Gompel A: Antiestrogen action of progesterone in breast tissue. Breast Cancer Res Treatment 1986;8:179–187.
29 Korenman SG: The endocrinology of breast cancer. Cancer 1980;46:874–878.
30 Dobie V, Walsh J, Lamb J, Dixon JM: Natural history of fibroadenoma of the breast; in Mansel RE (ed): Recent Developments in the Study of Benign Breast Disease. London, Parthenon Publishing, 1994, pp 75–81.
31 Neinstein LS: Breast disease in adolescents and young women. Pediatr Clin North Am 1999;46:607–629.
32 Hindle W, Alonzo L: Conservative management of breast fibroadenomas. Am J Obstet Gynecol 1991; 164:1647–1649.
33 West K, Rescorta F, Scherrer LR, Grosfeld J: Diagnosis and treatment of symptomatic breast masses in the pediatric population. J Pediatr Surg 1995;30:182–187.
34 Naidu AG, Thomson SR, Nirmul D: Giant fibroadenoma in black and Indian adolescents. S Afr J Surg 1989;27:171–172.
35 Chang DS, McGrath MH: Management of benign tumors of the adolescent breast. Plast Reconstr Surg 2007;120:13e–19e.
36 Rajan PB, Cranor ML, Rosen PP: Cystosarcoma phyllodes in adolescent girls and young women: a study of 45 patients. Am J Surg Pathol 1998;22:64–69.
37 Haagensen CD: Diseases of the Breast. Philadelphia, Saunders, 1986.

38 Tea MK, Asseryanis E, Kroiss R, Kubista E, Wagner T: Surgical breast lesions in adolescent females. Pediatr Surg Int 2009;25:73–75.
39 Altman AJ, Schwartz SD: Malignant Diseases of Infancy, Childhood and Adolescence, ed 2. Philadelphia, Saunders, 1983, pp 1–505.
40 Corpon CA, Black CT, Singletary SE, Andrassy EJ: Breast cancer in adolescent females. J Pediatr Surg 1995;30:322–324.
41 Shannon C, Smith IE: Breast cancer in adolescents and young women. Eur J Cancer 2003;39:2632–2642.
42 Rogers DA, Lobe TE, Rao N: Breast malignacy in children. J Pediatr Surg 1994;29:48–51.
43 Hays DM, Donaldson SS, Shimada H, et al: Primary and metastatic rhabdomyosarcoma in the breast: neoplasms of adolescent females, a report from the Intergroup Rhabdomyosarcoma Study. Med Pediatr Oncol 1997;29:181–189.

Dr. C. Duflos
Service Endocrinologie-Médecine de la Reproduction, Hôpital Pitié-Salpêtrière
10, rue Marguerite
FR–75017 Paris (France)
Tel. +33 1 4766 2421, E-Mail catherineduflos@hotmail.fr

Sultan C (ed): Pediatric and Adolescent Gynecology. Evidence-Based Clinical Practice. 2nd, revised and extended edition. Endocr Dev. Basel, Karger, 2012, vol 22, pp 222–229

Cervical Cancer Prevention – Current Perspectives

J. Monsonego

Institute of the Cervix, Paris, France

Abstract

This report addresses several areas including the progress made toward global implementation of currently licensed human papillomavirus (HPV) vaccines, and monitoring impact of HPV vaccination programs that can be implemented within developed and less-developed countries. For the sake of completeness, a short update on the evolution of HPV testing in primary screening programs at present and after HPV vaccine introduction has also been included.

Human Papillomavirus Vaccine Efficacy and Safety Profile

The human papillomavirus (HPV) bivalent vaccine (16–18) and the HPV quadrivalent vaccine (6–11–16–18) are generally safe and extremely effective in preventing HPV16 and HPV18 infections and HPV16/18-related precancerous cervical lesions [1–5]. In clinical trials, the quadrivalent vaccine was also shown to prevent HPV6/11/16/18-related precancerous vulvar or vaginal lesions, and genital warts [4, 6]. Administration of vaccine before sexual debut most likely provides maximal benefit and currently, 10- to 13-year-old females are the focus of HPV immunizations programs in many countries. Although there are limited follow-up data on vaccinated cohorts, demonstration of durable protection throughout the course of the trials, and of immune memory with antigen challenge 4.5 years after the completion of the initial vaccine series, supports long-term protection [7]. Only time will tell if the protection is sufficiently durable to eliminate the need for routine boosting years after the initial vaccine series is completed. Several additional questions concerning the use of these vaccines in boys, older adults, and populations with a high burden of HIV are being addressed in ongoing trials. Other issues related to implementation of immunization programs, feasibility of 2 vs. 3 doses of vaccine, herd immunity, and cost are being evaluated in demonstration projects and mathematical models. Whether prophylactic administration of HPV vaccine will prevent oro-pharyngeal HPV16 or HPV18 infections and the associated cancers remains to be determined but there is no reason to suspect that it will not.

The EUROGIN statement on cervical cancer prevention was produced soon after the publication of decisive trials of quadrivalent and bivalent virus-like particle (VLP) human papillomavirus (HPV) vaccines (against HPV16, HPV18, HPV6 and HPV11, and HPV16 and HPV18, respectively). These included efficacy trials involving virological and precancerous cervical disease endpoints among women aged 15–26 years, and immunologic bridging trials with endpoints of safety and VLP serum antibody levels in female and male adolescents (reviewed in Schiller et al. [8]; data updated recently [9]). For vaccines, efficacy against all considered endpoints associated with HPV vaccine types, including cervical intraepithelial neoplasia grade 2 or worse (CIN2+), among young women not yet infected at the time of vaccination was greater than 95%.

As expected, more limited protection was noted for both vaccines among women infected with HPV vaccine types before vaccination and against endpoints associated with any HPV type. Neither vaccine was found to clear existing HPV infection or [10] or slow rates of progression from infection to CIN [11]. These trials therefore demonstrated that both HPV vaccines are most effective when given to females naïve to HPV vaccine types.

Important progress was made in 2008 in understanding experience with HPV vaccine introduction in many countries [12] and in the evaluation of the cost-effectiveness of different vaccination strategies [13]. Over 100 world countries approved one or both vaccines, and those implementing mass vaccination programs are rapidly increasing. Developed countries such as the United States, Canada, Australia and New Zealand were the first to make this move [14]. Australia has already reported an encouraging coverage of school-based vaccination in different regions (70% or more) [15]. The decision to introduce HPV vaccines was also unusually rapid among the European Union (EU) Member States [16]. Indeed, a majority of the 27 EU Member States made a recommendation to integrate HPV vaccination into their respective national immunization programs.

The recommended age for routine vaccination was 11–13 years except in France (14–23 years, according to sexual history) and Germany (12–17 years). Temporary catch-up vaccination, up to age 17 or 18, has also been recommended or initiated in a few countries [16, 17]. It is of concern that data on HPV vaccination acceptance in many EU countries are not available, and that market sales data suggest that in some countries (e.g. France and Germany) women at the upper limit of the recommended age group have received more vaccine than younger girls.

In developing countries, where 80% of cervical cancer cases occur, the potential benefits of HPV vaccines are enormous. HPV vaccines are licensed in many low and middle income countries but few such countries have recommended HPV vaccine introduction for national immunization programs due to other programmatic and

Together these data provide another major confirmation of the value of HPV testing as a primary screening test (followed by cytological triage of HPV-positive women) and further support for a screening algorithm. When a highly sensitive test is used, there is no justification for performing any screening among women under the age of 25 years, among whom over treatment and possible consequences (e.g. premature delivery) [32, 33] suggest that more harm than good is done. A challenge for this approach is to avoid unnecessary investigation and treatment of HPV-positive/cytology-negative women, for who repeat testing is currently recommended after 6–12 months. This is particularly important for women aged less than 30, or even 35 years, among whom transient HPV infections are more common [34].

New adjunct tests such as HPV type-specific tests may help to determine which of these women need immediate referral and which can be safely monitored at longer intervals. Evidence is mounting that typing for HPV16 is particularly important because of its faster progression time and stronger link with CIN3 or worse [35], whereas HPV types 18 and 45 are more strongly associated with adenocarcinoma [36] and endocervical lesions.

As noted above, the lower specificity of HPV DNA tests compared to cytology remains an issue, especially for younger women in whom much HPV infection is benign and transient. It is desirable to minimize the number of women allocated to short-term repeat testing (e.g. HPV-positive/cytology-negative women) and several approaches are currently under development to try to improve test specificity while retaining high sensitivity, including tests that detect persistent HPV DNA, HPV mRNA tests, tests that assess proliferation and cell cycle markers, and p16 detection by staining of cytology slides as well as through detection by ELISA New data have shown that using mRNA testing as primary screening test is accurate, extremely sensitive for the detection of HG CIN and more specific than HPV DNA testing [37] allowing to reduce unnecessary colposcopies, follow-up and treatment.

Screening of Vaccinated Women

It is unlikely that screening will be modified in older adolescents and young women receiving HPV vaccines under catch-up programs. However, girls vaccinated before age 15 years will not need screening for another 10 years, so the current priority for women over 25 years of age should be to introduce HPV test-based screening [24]. This will also provide the necessary experience to use this test in vaccinated women when they reach screening age. Developing efficient screening algorithms for vaccinated women will require periodic evaluation and modification. For example, cytology-based screening will have a lower positive predictive value for CIN2+ because vaccination with moderate to high coverage is expected to substantially lower the prevalence of high-grade lesions caused by HPV16 and HPV18. There will, however, only be a minimal reduction of false-positive tests due to lower grade cervical abnormalities resulting from reactive changes related to low-risk HPV types and other agents. Abnormal cytology results will be less common, and this is likely to be a problem for cytologists, since maintaining the concentration to spot a few abnormal cells will be more difficult when they are very rare.

HPV testing followed by triage using cytology, as proposed in 2008 [9, 24], may be more appropriate because of the opportunity it creates for cytotechnicians to read only smears that are more likely to contain lesions. It has recently been shown that the accuracy in reading smears from HPV-positive women is increased as compared to blind reading. Automated cytology, especially using p16 staining to identify cells that need careful study, may also be a viable approach for triage of HPV-positive women, although this has not yet been established. New testing approaches using persistent HPV DNA detection, mRNA, proliferation markers and cell cycle proteins may also help to refine screening algorithms and merit formal evaluations. Finally, as more options for HPV detection and triage of HPV-positive findings become available, quality-assurance and standardization of assays is of paramount importance for any test considered for high volume screening programs.

Many different combinations of screening programs and immunization campaigns can be conceived according to the resource levels available in different parts of the world [24]. Immunization programs have shown, within and between countries, a greater potential to reach underprivileged populations than most other medical interventions. If high coverage of adolescents (e.g. through school-based programs) can be achieved, HPV vaccination may especially benefit population subsets who are underserved by screening programs. With 85% coverage, HPV16 and HPV18 vaccination may, for instance, raise the fraction of cancers avoided by a fairly good, though not perfect, screening program from 50 to 82%. On a world scale, this corresponds to lack of HPV vaccination in the populations most likely not to undergo adequate cervical cancer screening in their lifetime.

References

1 FUTURE II Study Group: Quadrivalent vaccine against human papillomavirus to prevent high-grade cervical lesions. N Engl J Med 2007;356:1915–1927.

2 Harper DM, Franco EL, Wheeler CM, Moscicki AB, Romanowski B, Roteli-Martins CM, Jenkins D, Schuind A, Costa Clemens SA, Dubin G, HPV Vaccine Study Group: Sustained efficacy up to 4.5 years of a bivalent L1 virus-like particle vaccine against human papillomavirus types 16 and 18: follow-up from a randomised control trial. Lancet 2006;367:1247–1255.

3 Villa LL, Costa RL, Petta CA, et al: High sustained efficacy of a prophylactic quadrivalent human papillomavirus types 6/11/16/18 L1 virus-like vaccine through 5 years follow-up. Br J Cancer 2006;95:1459–1466.

4 Garland SM, Hernandez-Avila M, Wheeler CM, Perez G, Harper DM, Leodolter S, Tang GW, Ferris DG, Steben M, Bryan J, Taddeo FJ, Railkar R, Esser MT, Sings HL, Nelson M, Boslego J, Sattler C, Barr E, Koutsky LA; Females United to Uniterally Reduce Endo/Ectocervical Disease (FUTURE) I Investigators: Quadrivalent vaccine against human papillomavirus to prevent anogenital diseases. N Engl J Med 2007;356:1928–1943.

5 Paavonen J, Jenkins D, Bosch FX, Naud P, Salmeron J, Wheeler CM, Chow SN, Apter DL, Kitchener HC, Castellsague X, de Carvalho NS, Skinner SR, Harper DM, Hedrick JA, Jaisamrarn U, Limson GA, Dionne M, Quint W, Spiessens B, Peeters P, Struyf F, Wieting SL, Lehtinen MO, Dubin G, HPV PATRICIA Study Group: Efficacy of a prophylactic adjuvanted bivalent L1 virus-like particle vaccine against infection with human papillomavirus types 16 and 18 in young women: an interim analysis of a phase III double-blind, randomised controlled trial. Lancet 2007;369:2161–7210.
6 Giuliano AR, Tortolero-Luna G, Ferrer E, Burchell AN, de Sanjose S, Kjaer SK, Munoz N, Schiffman M, Bosch FX: Epidemiology of human papillomavirus infection in men, cancers other than cervical and benign conditions. Vaccine 2008;26(Suppl 10: K17–K28.
7 Olsson SE, Villa LL, Costa RL, Petta CA, Andrade RP, Malm C, Iversen OE, Hoye J, Steinwall M, Riis-Johannessen G, Andersson-Ellstrom A, Elfgren K, von Krogh G, Lehtinen M, Paavonen J, Tamms GM, Giacoletti K, Lupinacci L, Esser MT, Vuocolo SC, Saah AJ, Barr E: Induction of immune memory following administration of a prophylactic quadrivalent human papillomavirus (HPV) types 6/11/16/18 L1 virus like particle (VLP) vaccine. Vaccine 2007; 25:4931–4939.
8 Schiller JT, Castellsagué X, Villa LL, Hildesheim A: An update of prophylactic human papillomavirus L1 virus-like particle vaccine clinical trial results. Vaccine 2008;26(suppl 10):K53–K61.
9 Franceschi S, Cuzick J, Herrero R, Dillner J, Wheeler CM: EUROGIN 2008 roadmap on cervical cancer prevention. Int J Cancer 2009;125:2246–2255.
10 Hildesheim A, Herrero R, Wacholder S, Rodriguez AC, Solomon D, Bratti MC , Schiller JT, Gonzalez P, Dubin G, Porras C, Jimenez SE, Lowy DR, Costa Rican HPV Vaccine Trial Group: Effect of human papillomavirus 16/18 L1 virus like particle vaccine among young women with preexisting infection: a randomized trial. JAMA 2007;298:743–753.
11 The FUTURE II Study Group: Effect of prophylactic human papillomavirus L1 virus-like-particle vaccine on risk of cervical intraepithelial neoplasia grade 2, grade 3, and adenocarcinoma in situ: a combined analysis of four randomised clinical trials. Lancet 2007;369:1861–1868.
12 WHO Strategic Advisory Group of Experts (SAGE): Meeting of the immunization Strategic Advisory Group of Experts, November 2008 – conclusions and recommendations. Wkly Epidemiol Rec 2009; 84:1–16.
13 Kim JJ, Goldie SJ: Health and economic implications of HPV vaccination in the United States. N Engl J Med 2008;359:821–832.
14 Barr E, Sings HL: Prophylactic HPV vaccines: New interventions for cancer control. Vaccine 2008;26: 6244–6257.
15 Brotherton JML, Deeks SL, Campbell-Lloyd S, Misrachi A, Passaris I, Peterson K, Pitcher H, Scully M, Watson M, Webby R: Interim estimates of human papillomavirus vaccination coverage in the school-based program in Australia. Commun Dis Intell 2008;32:457–461.
16 King LA, Levy-Bruhl D, O'Flanagan D, Bacci S, Lopalco PL, Kudjawu Y, et al: Introduction of human papillomavirus (HPV) vaccination into national immunisation schedules in Europe: results of the VENICE 2007 survey. Euro Surveill 2008;13: pii:18954.
17 Koulova A, Tsui J, Irwin K, Van DP, Biellik R, Aguado MT: Country recommendations on the inclusion of HPV vaccines in national immunization programmes among high-income countries, June 2006–January 2008. Vaccine 2008;26:6529–6541.
18 Goldie SJ, Diaz M, Kim SY, Levin CE, Van MH, Kim JJ: Mathematical models of cervical cancer prevention in the Asia Pacific region. Vaccine 2008;26(suppl 12):M17–M29.
19 Wright TC Jr, Bosch FX: Is viral status needed before vaccination? Vaccine 2008;26(suppl 1):A12–A15.
20 Sycuro LK, Xi LF, Hughes JP, Feng Q, Winer RL, Lee SK, O'Reilly S, Kiviat NB, Koutsky LA: Persistence of genital human papillomavirus infection in a long-term follow-up study of female university students. J Infect Dis 2008;198:971–978.
21 Muñoz N, for the Future II Steering Committee: The efficacy of quadrivalent HPV (types 6/11/16/18) L1 virus-like particle (VLP) vaccine against HPV6 /11/16/18-related cervical and external genital disease in women aged 24 to 45. EUROGIN 2008, Nice, 2008, abstr SS19–SS13.
22 Brown DR, Kjaer SK, Sigurdsson K, et al: The impact of quadrivalent human papillomavirus (HPV; types 6, 11, 16, and 18) L1 virus-like particle vaccine on infection and disease due to oncogenic nonvaccine HPV types in generally HPV-naive women aged 16–26 years. J Infect Dis 2009;199: 926–935.
23 Wheeler CM, Kjaer SK, Sigurdsson K, et al: The impact of quadrivalent human papillomavirus (HPV; types 6, 11, 16, and 18) L1 virus-like particle vaccine on infection and disease due to oncogenic nonvaccine HPV types in sexually active women aged 16–26 years. J Infect Dis 2009;199:936–944.

24 Franco EL, Cuzick J: Cervical cancer screening following prophylactic human papillomavirus vaccination. Vaccine 2008;26(suppl 1):A16–A23.
25 Cuzick J, Clavel C, Petry KU, Meijer CJ, Hoyer H, Ratnam S, Szarewski A, Birembaut P, Kulasingam S, Sasieni P, Iftner T: Overview of the European and North American studies on HPV testing in primary cervical cancer screening. Int J Cancer 2006;119:1095–1101.
26 Mayrand MH, Duarte-Franco E, Rodrigues I, Walter SD, Hanley J, Ferenczy A, Ratnam S, Coutlée F, Franco EL, Canadian Cervical Cancer Screening Trial Study Group: Human papillomavirus DNA versus Papanicolaou screening tests for cervical cancer. N Engl J Med 2007;357:1579–1588.
27 Ronco G, Segnan N, Giorgi-Rossi P, Zappa M, Casadei GP, Carozzi F, et al: Human papillomavirus testing and liquid-based cytology: results at recruitment from the new technologies for cervical cancer randomized controlled trial. J Natl Cancer Inst 2006;98:765–774.
28 Cuzick J, Szarewski A, Mesher D, Cadman L, Austin J, Perryman K, Dalla Palma P, Del Mistro A, Folicaldi S, Gillio-Tos A, Nardo G, Naldoni C, Schincaglia P, Zorzi M, Confortini M, Cuzick J, New Technologies for Cervical Cancer Working Group: Long-term follow-up of cervical abnormalities among women screened by HPV testing and cytology: results from the Hammersmith study. Int J Cancer 2008;122:2294–2300.
29 Bulkmans N, Berkhof J, Rozendaal L, van Kemenade FJ, Boeke A, Bulk S, Voorhorst FJ, Verheijen RH, van Groningen K, Boon ME, Ruitinga W, van Ballegooijen M, Snijders PJ, Meijer CJ: Human papillomavirus DNA testing for the detection of cervical intraepithelial neoplasia grade 3 and cancer: 5-year follow-up of a randomised controlled implementation trial. Lancet 2007;370:1764–1772.
30 Naucler P, Ryd W, Tornberg S, Strand A, Wadell G, Elfgren K, Rådberg T, Strander B, Johansson B, Forslund O, Hansson BG, Rylander E, Dillner J: Human papillomavirus and Papanicolaou tests to screen for cervical cancer. N Engl J Med 2007;357:1589–1597.
31 Dillner J, Rebolj M, Birembaut P, Petry KU, Szarewski A, Munk C, de Sanjose S, Naucler P, Lloveras B, Kjaer S, Cuzick J, van Ballegooijen M, Clavel C, Iftner T, Joint European Cohort Study: Long term predictive values of cytology and human papillomavirus testing in cervical cancer screening: joint European cohort study. BMJ 2008;337:a1754.
32 Sadler L, Saftlas A, Wang W, Exeter M, Whittaker J, McCowan L: Treatment for cervical intraepithelial neoplasia and risk of preterm delivery. JAMA 2004;291:2100–2106.
33 Arbyn M, Kyrgiou M, Simoens C, Raifu AO, Koliopoulos G, Martin-Hirsch P, Prendiville W, Paraskevaidis E: Perinatal mortality and other severe adverse pregnancy outcomes associated with treatment of cervical intraepithelial neoplasia: meta-analysis. BMJ 2008;337:a1284.
34 Ronco G, Giorgi-Rossi P, Carozzi F, Confortini M, Dalla Palma P, Del Mistro A, Gillio-Tos A, Minucci D, Naldoni C, Rizzolo R, Schincaglia P, Volante R, Zappa M, Zorzi M, Cuzick J, Segnan N, New Technologies for Cervical Cancer Screening Working Group: Results at recruitment from a randomized controlled trial comparing human papillomavirus testing alone with conventional cytology as the primary cervical cancer screening test. J Natl Cancer Inst 2008;100:492–501.
35 Franceschi S, Clifford GM: A study of the impact of adding HPV types to cervical cancer screening and triage tests. J Natl Cancer Inst 2005;97:938–939.
36 Smith JS, Lindsay L, Hoots B, Keys J, Franceschi S, Winer R, Clifford GM: Human papillomavirus type distribution in invasive cervical cancer and high-grade cervical lesions: a meta-analysis update. Int J Cancer 2007;121:621–632.
37 Monsonego J: Clinical value of HPV mRNA testing in primary screening. IPV Conference, Malmö, 2009.

J. Monsonego, MD
Institute of the Cervix
174, rue de Courcelles
FR–75017 Paris (France)
Tel. +33 1 47 66 05 29, Fax +33 1 47 66 74 70, E-Mail jmonsonego@wanadoo.fr

Sultan C (ed): Pediatric and Adolescent Gynecology. Evidence-Based Clinical Practice. 2nd, revised and extended edition. Endocr Dev. Basel, Karger, 2012, vol 22, pp 230–250

Chronic Pelvic Pain in the Adolescent

Caitlin W. Hicks · Ellen S. Rome

Section of Adolescent Medicine, Cleveland Clinic Children's Hospital, Cleveland Clinic Lerner College of Medicine at Case, Cleveland, Ohio, USA

Abstract

Chronic pelvic pain occurs commonly in the adolescent and can be a diagnostic and therapeutic challenge for the clinician, the adolescent, and her family. Defined as lower quadrant or lower abdominal pain lasting 3–6 months or longer, chronic pelvic pain can lead to missed school and activities, decreased functioning, and decreased quality of life in the adolescent. Both the primary care clinician and the pediatric gynecologist need to be aware of the most common causes of chronic pelvic pain in the adolescent, including surgical and nonsurgical, gynecologic versus other pathology including the psychosomatic, and the role of the mind in control of somatic pain in the adolescent. Adding to this complexity is the standard adolescent sense of invulnerability; a knowledge of adolescent development remains essential to the delivery of appropriate gynecologic care for this age group. Education and communication with both the adolescent and her family requires sensitivity, especially in cultures where adolescent sexuality is taboo or discouraged. This chapter will discuss the developmental stages of adolescence and how that impacts care of the patient with chronic pelvic pain at the varying ages, the issue of confidentiality when obtaining a sexual history on the adolescent, and etiologies of chronic pelvic pain specific to the adolescent, including gynecologic and nongynecologic causes. Diagnostic and treatment considerations for chronic pelvic pain in the adolescent will also be addressed.

Special Challenges in the Adolescent Population: Stages of Adolescence and Confidentiality

Approximately 3–5% of all visits by adolescents aged 11–21 years to a primary care provider involve a chief complaint of chronic abdominal pain [1]. Recent estimates suggest that as much as USD 166 million is spent annually on treatment of chronic pelvic pain in the United States alone, making this a significant medical problem in both pediatric and adult medical practices [2].

Early adolescence (11–14 years) is characterized by the onset of puberty, with changes in the body resulting in thelarche, adrenarche, and menarche [3]. In early adolescence, the teen functions much like Alice in Wonderland: does she have enough of this, or too much of that, and is she normal? In middle adolescence (15–17 years), the focus shifts from self to peers, with the dominant question moving from 'Am I normal'? to 'Am I liked'? Peers become more important than parents, and fitting in may involve risk-taking on multiple fronts, including sexually. The ability to foresee consequences requires abstract thought, which develops late in adolescence (if at all!). For a teen, 'long-term relationship' may mean 3 weeks, and waiting to initiate sexual activity may mean 3 months. Given this mindset of invulnerability, negotiating condom use every time with every partner can be difficult, as is knowing that mild lower abdominal pain may be related to last weekend or last month's sexual activity with the development of pelvic inflammatory disease. Long-term consequences have a very different meaning to the teen than to her parent. A mother may be highly concerned about future fertility, but the adolescent may not be able to envision life much beyond the current season or school year. Therefore, the evaluation and management of pelvic pain within this population requires not only knowledge of the various etiologies, but also insight into the stages of adolescent development.

Adding to the complexity is the nature of the adolescent visit, with 2 patients: the adolescent and her mother. Families of adolescents with chronic pelvic pain may have sought multiple opinions 'unsuccessfully', with insufficient management of the pain and little or no return of functionality. Fear of cancer, endometriosis, or another condition may drive the medicine-seeking behavior. Communication is essential, and the medical history requires sensitivity, or knowing which questions should be asked with a parent present, plus confidentiality, or knowing which questions should be saved for when the parent is out of the room. Adolescents may not wish their parents to see them as sexual beings, and may withhold key pieces of a history out of shame or embarrassment, or merely a desire for privacy. The successful medical interview creates a positive tone for all future interactions, builds trust among teen and clinician, and among parent and clinician, with the astute clinician also serving as a bridge to open the lines of communication between the two. A good history will illuminate the hidden agenda of each, ideally early in the visit rather than in the classic pattern of 'Oh By the Way' as the clinician is reaching the door to leave the room. The classic mnemonic for the confidential adolescent medicine history is the HEADS examination, as depicted in table 1. After the clinician has asked standard questions about the nature of the pain, and wishes to ask questions of a more sensitive nature, confidentiality must be established. One way to do this is to ask the patient if she prefers the parent in the room for the examination, or if she prefers her mother to politely exit until after the examination. The clinician can then ask if she wants to have private time during the examination, before, or after, and also whether she wants alone time first or whether she wants her mother to have private time first. While she is deciding, the clinician can state, 'Everything we talk about alone without your parent is confidential, meaning that I will not share your private concerns with your parent, unless you tell me something life-threatening or dangerous. In the same way, everything I talk about with your

Table 1. The HEADS Questions, Useful in the Adolescent History

Home: who lives at home? What happens when there is an argument in the home? (ex. 'It's fine except when dad drinks'. 'Really, what happens then?' 'Well, he hits me in the stomach and beats up mom').
Education: current grade level in school, and current academic achievement. Is the child age appropriate in school? Academic underachievement can be a red flag for underlying psychosocial pathology, and a cause of chronic abdominal pain.
Activities: How does the teen fill their time? Are they in a gang? Do they carry a gun? And can they not carry it to your office next time?
Drugs, cigarettes, alcohol? Do their friends smoke? Do they smoke? How much, how often, have they tried to quit, when and how? How long does a pack last? For drugs, which kinds and how often? For alcohol, how much, how often? Have they ever had any blackouts or passouts? Have they ever had sex while under the influence of drugs or alcohol?
D is also for **depression/suicide:** have they ever been seriously depressed? Ever wished they were dead? If yes, how often? Ever thought about killing themselves? Have they had a plan? Have they actually tried? If so, which ways?
Sex: have they engaged in oral sex, anal sex, vaginal sex? How many lifetime partners? Any prior sexually transmitted diseases or pregnancies? Do they use condoms? Sometimes, most of the time, or all the time? What do they use for their second method of contraception? Are they attracted to guys, girls, or both? Has anyone ever tried to make them do something sexually that made them uncomfortable?

parent is private, meaning I will not share your parent's private concerns with you without their permission unless they tell me something life-threatening or dangerous to you.' In establishing confidentiality and its limits, the clinician is more likely to create a safe environment in which the teen and her parent can share their private concerns. A mother may ask that her daughter be given 'the virginity test', fearing that pelvic pain may represent a sexually transmitted infection (STI) but afraid to know the answer. An adolescent may have myths or misperceptions about how her body works. Having the chance to ascertain these hidden agendas can shape the visit and provide windows of opportunity to educate both parties and prevent disease.

Another barrier to the adolescent visit is the pediatricians' reluctance to check below the waist in this population, despite the fact that lower abdominal pain in young women is usually attributed to gynecologic disorders. Primary care and emergency room physicians are often reluctant to obtain gynecologic histories and perform pelvic examinations in these patients [3]. Many teenagers have their pain dismissed as 'all in their heads' without proper evaluation; all adolescents with chronic pelvic pain deserve to be taken seriously, especially since a significant percentage will have underlying pathology [4]. Evaluation of an adolescent patient with pelvic pain should be fairly aggressive, as adequate diagnosis and early therapy is essential in order to improve the quality of life and preserve the reproductive prognosis in these young women [5].

Other Aspects of the History and Physical Examination

Establishing a good rapport with an adolescent patient can facilitate a thorough history and physical and provide a good deal of information to determine the etiology of the pain without the use of extensive diagnostic studies [3]. Given the vast array of possible causes of pelvic pain, it is essential that the clinician obtain a thorough and complete history from the patient upon initial evaluation. The clinician should begin with a history of present illness that describes the location, frequency, and duration of the pain, as well as exacerbating and relieving factors, relationship and timing of the pain to menses, vaginal discharge or itching, dysuria or urinary frequency/urgency, food intake, bowel symptoms and patterns, and associated nausea and/or vomiting [6]. Does the pain wake her from sleep? A positive answer suggests organic rather than functional pathology. Children and adolescents can also rate the pain on a scale of 1–10, with developmentally challenged patients using the scale with smiling to frowning faces to correspond to the numbers. Such a scale also helps the teen and care provider track severity of pain over time. The impact of pain on the patient's school performance, extracurricular and social activity, sleep, mood, and family interactions should also be explored with the parent in the room as a 'reality check'. Does she miss school but not weekend activities? Are there other stressors in her life? Parental divorce, relationship challenges, 'girl drama' or stress from peers, can all add to or exacerbate abdominal pain. Has she tried any medicines? Prescription or over the counter? Which ones, how much, and how often? Any complimentary medicines tried?

Following the pain-specific history, information regarding significant past medical and surgical history should be obtained. Family history should include any history of endometriosis, inflammatory bowel disease and irritable bowel syndrome, celiac disease, depression, interstitial cystitis, lupus, and cancer [3]. In addition, a menstrual history including age at menarche, menstrual pattern, onset and character of menstrual cramps and other menstruation associated symptoms, and response to analgesic medication is pertinent. Does the pain start before menses? Does she get midcycle pain? Finally, as mentioned above in the HEADS examination, a carefully collected sexual history including past and present sexual activity, dyspareunia, pregnancy, sexual or physical abuse, and alcohol or drug use must be obtained, all asked with the parent out of the room; otherwise, the teenager may feel unable to disclose issues of sexuality, abuse, or other events [5]. All questions should be asked nonjudgmentally, with open body language. Good eye contact with the teen is essential, conveying a message of caring and respect for what she has to say. This trust is essential to being able to intervene effectively and engage the teen in a partnership to enhance her physical well-being.

Upon completion of the medical interview, a complete physical examination including musculoskeletal assessment, abdominal palpation, pelvic examination in the nonvirginal adolescent, and rectoabdominal examination at a minimum in the virginal patient [5]. The abdomen should be examined for any scars, hernias, masses, or trigger points, and the back should be inspected for scoliosis and palpated for costovertebral angle tenderness [3]. Special attention should be paid to the abdomen and pelvis to localize the pain, check for referred pain, rebound and guarding, identify any masses, and assess for peritoneal signs and for organomegaly [6]. During the pelvic examination, the external genitalia, urethra, and hymen should be examined for any congenital abnormalities, and any lesions, point tenderness, or discharge should be noted [3]. The bimanual examination should assess uterine size, shape, and symmetry, the presence of adnexal and/or cervical motion tenderness, and be able to identify any adnexal mass or thickening. In addition, the posterior cul-de-sac should be assessed for pain and nodularity [6]. With proper education and a sensitive style, most adolescents can successfully undergo a pelvic examination, even those who have not yet been sexually active. Use of a Huffman speculum in this scenario is preferred, with the Pederson (next size up) speculum reserved for those girls who have already had sexual intercourse. For the obese young lady, a Graves speculum or a Pederson with a surgical glove finger with the tip cut off can be used, to keep vaginal wall folds from obstructing visibility. Rectoabdominal examination can be used in those girls who cannot tolerate a pelvic examination, and should help exclude adnexal tenderness or masses. A saline moistened Q tip can help determine length of vaginal canal, with gentle probing helping to find some vaginal septums. Ultrasonography (US) can clarify anatomy further, especially in the hands of a skilled adolescent-sensitive radiologist. In some centers, MRI is used to determine pelvic anatomy when a Müllerian anomaly is suspected. CT serves an important role in patients with nonlocalizing symptoms, an indeterminate US evaluation, or in patients who require a wider search beyond the field of view available with US. In addition, the widespread availability of and familiarity with CT have helped to expand its role in the emergency evaluation of the female patient with acute pelvic pain.

Laboratory Studies

Laboratory evaluation for the adolescent patient with pelvic pain should typically include a complete blood count with differential; an erythrocyte sedimentation rate and/or C-reactive protein; a urinalysis and, as indicated, a urine culture; stool Guiaic testing for occult blood; a pregnancy test, and nucleic acid amplification tests

(NAATs) for *Neisseria gonorrhoeae* and *Chlamydia trachomatis* if sexually active. Tests for trichomonas and bacterial vaginosis (wet prep or vaginal swab) can also be useful. Lubricant should not be used for any speculum examination or digital vaginal examination unless cervical specimens have already been obtained [7]. With the new guidelines from the American College of Obstetricians and Gynecologists [8], a Pap smear is recommended starting at age 21 years, but not specifically as part of the evaluation for chronic pelvic pain.

The Role of Laparoscopy

Diagnostic laparoscopy tends to be reserved for those adolescent girls whose pain has not been adequately managed with simple stepwise treatment as outlined below. The early use of diagnostic laparoscopy in more refractory cases of chronic pelvic pain can often lead to a more precise diagnosis when less invasive methods fail [9]. Laparoscopy can diagnose endometriosis or other specific pelvic pathology. Negative laparoscopy findings are also useful, as they provide reassurance to patients and their parents that pelvic structures are normal, and often lead to symptomatic improvement in adolescent females with pelvic pain; a landmark study published by Goldstein [10] in 1989 reported that 74% of patients with intractable pelvic pain were symptomatically improved after a negative laparoscopy. Laparoscopy entails surgical risk, added costs, and requires specific skill geared towards recognition of disease in the adolescent, which may vary from disease processes found in the adult. The goal is to avoid laparoscopy in those girls who truly have normal pelvises and no disease, using other modalities effectively to manage the pain.

In a study of 46 adolescent girls ages 13–21 years with chronic pelvic pain lasting over 3 months despite nonsteroidal anti-inflammatory drugs (NSAIDs) and continuous hormone therapy, Laufer et al. [7] found that 70% had endometriosis on laparoscopy. Laparoscopic findings of all girls are found in table 2. Anecdotally, adhesions of unknown origin in a young girl without prior surgery resulted in fairly specific, localized tenderness in the mid right quadrant. Laparoscopic lysing of the adhesions resulted in a full return to functionality, pain free, with happy patient and happy family over long-term follow-up. When in doubt of the diagnosis, the carefully selected patient without a high risk of secondary gain in surgery can have great benefit from both negative and positive laparoscopic findings.

Causes of Chronic Pelvic Pain in the Adolescent

Classically, the causes of pelvic pain are divided into acute versus chronic and gynecologic versus nongynecologic [4]. Acute pelvic pain starts over a short time (anywhere from a few minutes to a few days), whereas chronic pelvic pain is defined as

Table 2. Laparoscopic findings in adolescent girls with chronic pelvic pain nonresponsive to NSAIDS and continuous hormone therapy

Laparoscopic findings	Number (%)
Visible endometriosis	31/46 (67.4)
Adhesions	11/46 (23.9)
Prior surgery	8
Endometriosis found	3
Endometriosis not present	5
No prior surgery	3
Endometriosis found	3
Endometriosis not present	0
Grossly normal pelvis	5/46 (10.9)
Functional cysts	4/46 (8.7)
Paratubal cysts	4/46 (8.7)
Müllerian anomalies	3/46 (6.5)
With endometriosis	1
Without endometriosis	2

From Laufer et al. [92].

cyclic or acyclic pelvic pain that persists for at least 3–6 months, requires medical or surgical evaluation and intervention, and can cause functional disability [11]. While both gynecologic and nongynecologic diagnoses should be considered in the etiology of pelvic pain, the more common causes of pelvic pain in the adolescent include pelvic inflammatory disease, undertreated dysmenorrhea, hemorrhaghic corpus luteum cysts, endometriosis and pelvic adhesions [4].

Specific Etiologies, Diagnosis and Treatment

Acute Pelvic Pain

Ectopic Pregnancy

Despite recent declines, the current adolescent birth rate continues to be much higher in the United States than in most other developed countries, averaging 54.4 per 1,000 adolescents aged 15–19 years of age [12]. With nearly 36% of high-school students admitting to being sexually active on our annual Youth Risk Behavior Survey [13], a high index of suspicion for pregnancy in the adolescent remains warranted when she presents with acute or chronic pelvic pain.

Several disease processes, either specific to pregnancy or with an increased incidence in pregnant patients, can cause pelvic pain [14]. In a normal intrauterine pregnancy, women may experience pain due to round ligament strain, 'morning sickness' with the associated nausea and abdominal pain, or as a result of a urinary tract infection, which occurs with greater frequency during pregnancy. More serious causes of pelvic pain during pregnancy include threatened or incomplete miscarriage, rupture of corpus luteum cyst, ectopic pregnancy, septic miscarriage with peritonitis and acute urinary retention due to a retroverted gravid uterus or an impacted ovarian cyst in the pelvis [15]. Transvaginal US, combined with quantitative β-human chorionic gonadotropin (β-HCG) analysis, is an excellent tool for identifying various pregnancy entities in the pregnant patient with pelvic pain [14]. In normal pregnancies, quantitative HCG performed in the same lab at initial presentation and at 48 hours should reveal an increase of at least 66%, at 72 hours, it should increase by 114%. Rates of increase lower than those numbers suggest an ectopic pregnancy, which constitutes a medical and/or surgical emergency. With a high index of suspicion, ectopic pregnancies can be diagnosed early, thereby allowing medical or minimally invasive surgical treatment and decreasing the risk of interfering with a women's reproductive potential [4].

Ovarian Torsion: A Surgical Emergency

Ovarian torsion involves partial or complete rotation of the ovarian pedicle on its axis, which results initially in impaired lymphatic and venous drainage and eventual loss of arterial perfusion [16]. While torsion in adults is often associated with an ovarian cyst or benign neoplasm, torsion in adolescents more often occurs in the absence of an associated adnexal mass and is felt to be due to increased mobility of the vascular pedicle [17]. The pain associated with ovarian torsion occurs suddenly, may be acute enough to wake the teen from sleep or keep them from falling asleep, and persists if the ovary remains torsed. Occasionally, the ovary may intermittently twist, resulting in intense pain that then resolves completely between episodes; this acute pain may occur during sexual intercourse, with change of position, or other movement, with chronicity associated with intermittent torsion.

The pain of torsion can be quite severe and occurs more commonly on the right side [18, 19]. Torsion can be difficult to diagnose clinically because the presenting symptoms, including pain, nausea, and vomiting, are nonspecific and similar to many causes of acute abdomen [20]. Delay in treatment can lead to ovarian necrosis [5]; if ovarian torsion is suspected, US with duplex Doppler imaging is the study of choice [21].

Traditionally, treatment approach to ovarian torsion in adolescents is oophorectomy [22–25]. Recent data suggests that when the size of the abdominopelvic mass is less than 75 mm, laparoscopy allowing detorsion, aspiration of a benign-appearing cyst, and upholding of the ovary in the abdominal cavity, is safe and effective in children and adolescents [26]. Therefore, a more conservative approach after detorsion of ovaries remains preferable to surgical removal, unless the torsed structure is clearly necrosed and not viable [26].

series reported an incidence of IC of 39% among adolescent females with pelvic pain, dysmenorrhea, dyspareunia, and urinary symptoms [84], which is consistent with findings from previous studies involving adult women [85, 86]. As a result, health care providers should question young women presenting with chronic pelvic pain about urinary symptoms and dyspareunia, and should consider simultaneous evaluation of the bladder by cystoscopy and hydrodistension if and when they choose to order a diagnostic laparoscopy [84].

Nongynecologic Causes of Chronic Pelvic Pain
Irritable bowel syndrome (IBS) is the most common cause of nongynecologic chronic pelvic pain among adolescents, occurring in approximately 15–20% of patients [87]. IBS is defined as chronic abdominal pain (usually in the lower segment) associated with a change in the consistency or frequency of stools that is relieved by defecation. Patients may also complain of the passage of mucus or abdominal bloating. According to diagnostic criteria developed for the pediatric population, these symptoms should be present for at least 12 weeks and not necessarily consecutively for the past 12 months [88]. The disorder has no structural, biochemical, or physiologic diagnostic markers, and is therefore a diagnosis of exclusion medical management of IBS is directed at alleviating the most predominant symptoms. Antispasmodics are the most frequently used medication, along with fiber bulking agents, anti-diarrheals, and psychological and behavioral interventions including cognitive-behavioral therapy, psychotherapy, hypnosis, relaxation training, and family or group therapy [3].

Finally, psychosocial causes may also account for some cases of chronic pelvic pain in the adolescent patient. After medical causes have been precluded by a detailed history and physical examination plus judicious use of any necessary laboratory and imaging tests, clinicians should consider psychosocial causes in their differential diagnosis. Sexual abuse can result in somatic symptoms including headaches and abdominal and/or pelvic pain. Parental stress or recent divorce can be manifested in a teenager as chronic pelvic pain and, in this case, the patient and parent must understand that the pain is real and is being physiologically experienced by the patient [5]. Past studies have repeatedly demonstrated an association between negative emotions such as anxiety and depression and pelvic pain [89–91]. The use of techniques including biofeedback, relaxation training, or ongoing counseling may be useful to help train the affected teenager to ameliorate or control his/her pain completely, using mind over body [5]. Some patients with pelvic pain of psychosocial cause may improve with adjunctive psychological therapy or with the evaluation and treatment offered by intensive pain programs [4].

Conclusions

Chronic pelvic pain remains a significant cause of absenteeism from school and decreased participation in school-related functions [47–50]. Such absences diminish opportunities for successful educational, psychosocial, and cognitive development during the critical period of adolescent growth. The early diagnosis and appropriate management of adolescent pelvic pain can improve daily functioning and improve future reproductive health outcomes in this population, and thus must be approached aggressively [3]. The clinician must use his/her knowledge of adolescent development and skills as an artful historian to weave together accurate facts in a sensitive manner to reach a timely diagnosis.

Determining the cause of pelvic pain in the adolescent patient is often a clinical challenge. When evaluating a patient with pelvic pain, the physician not only needs to differentiate acute versus chronic, gynecologic versus nongynecologic, surgical emergency versus a longer term problem. This differential must include pregnancy and pregnancy-related complications, even in the girl who states that she is not sexually active; STIs and PID; primary dysmenorrhea; endometriosis; reproductive tract anomalies; ovarian cysts; pelvic adhesions; adnexal torsion; appendicitis; interstitial cystitis; IBD, and psychosocial etiologies. Radiologic imaging, including US, CT and MRI can be invaluable in making a diagnosis [21], and laparoscopy is an important adjunct in the evaluation and treatment of pelvic pain [62].

Above all, negotiation of a trusting relationship between clinician and patient, clinician and the mother, with the clinician helping to facilitate communication between the parent and child, can ensure compliance with needed therapies, adequate follow up to prevent sequelae, and improve outcomes.

References

1 Smith MS, Tyler DC, Womack WM, et al: Assessment and management of recurrent pain in adolescence. Pediatrician 1989;16:85–93.

2 Rein DB, Kassler WJ, Irwin KL, et al: Direct medical cost of pelvic inflammatory disease and its sequelae: decreasing, but still substantial. Obstet Gynecol 2000; 95:397–402.

3 Song AH, Advincula AP: Adolescent chronic pelvic pain. J Pediatr Adolesc Gynecol 2005;18:371–377.

4 Goldfarb AF: Clinical Problems in Pediatric and Adolescent Gynecology. New York, Chapman & Hall, 1996.

5 Steege JF, Metzger DA, Levy BS: Chronic Pelvic Pain: An Integrated Approach. Philadelphia, Saunders, 1998.

6 Holland-Hall CM, Brown RT: Evaluation of the adolescent with chronic abdominal or pelvic pain. J Pediatr Adolesc Gynecol. 2004;17:23–27.

7 Emans SJH, Laufer MR, Goldstein DP, et al: Pediatric and Adolescent Gynecology, ed 5. Philadelphia, Lippincott Williams & Wilkins, 2005.

8 ACOG Practice Bulletin No 109: Cervical cytology screening. Obstet Gynecol 2009;114:1409–1420.

9 Frates MC, Laing FC: Sonographic evaluation of ectopic pregnancy: an update. AJR Am J Roentgenol 1995;165:251–259.

10 Goldstein DP: Acute and chronic pelvic pain. Pediatr Clin North Am 1989;36:573–580.

11 ACOG Committee on Practice Bulletins – Gynecology: ACOG practice bulletin No 51: chronic pelvic pain. Obstet Gynecol 2004;103:589–605.

12 Singh S, Darroch JE: Adolescent pregnancy and childbearing: levels and trends in developed countries. Fam Plann Perspect 2000;32:14–23.

13 Eaton DK, Kann L, Kinchen S, et al: Youth risk behavior surveillance–united states, 2007. MMWR Surveill Summ 2008;57:1–131.

14 Webb EM, Green GE, Scoutt LM: Adnexal mass with pelvic pain. Radiol Clin North Am 2004;42: 329–348.

15 Kilpatrick CC, Orejuela FJ: Management of the acute abdomen in pregnancy: a review. Curr Opin Obstet Gynecol 2008;20:534–953.

16 Lee EJ, Kwon HC, Joo HJ, et al: Diagnosis of ovarian torsion with color Doppler sonography: depiction of twisted vascular pedicle. J Ultrasound Med 1998;17:83–89.
17 Rha SE, Byun JY, Jung SE, et al: CT and MR imaging features of adnexal torsion. Radiographics 2002;22:283–294.
18 Schultz LR, Newton WA Jr, Clatworthy HW Jr: Torsion of previously normal tube and ovary in children. N Engl J Med 1963;268:343–346.
19 Servaes S, Zurakowski D, Laufer MR, et al: Sonographic findings of ovarian torsion in children. Pediatr Radiol 2007;37:446–451.
20 Houry D, Abbott JT: Ovarian torsion: a fifteen-year review. Ann Emerg Med 2001;38:156–159.
21 Vandermeer FQ, Wong-You-Cheong JJ: Imaging of acute pelvic pain. Clin Obstet Gynecol 2009;52:2–20.
22 Spigland N, Ducharme JC, Yazbeck S: Adnexal torsion in children. J Pediatr Surg 1989;24:974–976.
23 Kokoska ER, Keller MS, Weber TR: Acute ovarian torsion in children. Am J Surg 2000;180:462–465.
24 Cass DL, Hawkins E, Brandt ML, et al: Surgery for ovarian masses in infants, children, and adolescents: 102 consecutive patients treated in a 15-year period. J Pediatr Surg 2001;36:693–699.
25 Beaunoyer M, Chapdelaine J, Bouchard S, et al: Asynchronous bilateral ovarian torsion. J Pediatr Surg 2004;39:746–749.
26 Galinier P, Carfagna L, Delsol M, et al: Ovarian torsion: management and ovarian prognosis – a report of 45 cases. J Pediatr Surg 2009;44:1759–1765.
27 Bau A, Atri M: Acute female pelvic pain: ultrasound evaluation. Semin Ultrasound CT MR 2000;21:78–93.
28 Flum DR, Morris A, Koepsell T, et al: Has misdiagnosis of appendicitis decreased over time? A population-based analysis. JAMA 2001;286:1748–1753.
29 Balthazar EJ, Birnbaum BA, Yee J, et al: Acute appendicitis: CT and US correlation in 100 patients. Radiology 1994;190:31–35.
30 Malik AA, Bari SU: Conservative management of acute appendicitis. J Gastrointest Surg 2009;13:966–970.
31 Centers for Disease Control: Sexually Transmitted Diseases Surveillance, 2007.
32 Allsworth JE, Lewis VA, Peipert JF: Viral sexually transmitted infections and bacterial vaginosis: 2001–2004 national health and nutrition examination survey data. Sex Transm Dis 2008;35:791–796.
33 Forhan SE, Gottlieb SL, Sternberg MR, et al: Prevalence of sexually transmitted infections among female adolescents aged 14 to 19 in the united states. Pediatrics 2009;124:1505–1512.
34 Westrom L, Joesoef R, Reynolds G, et al: Pelvic inflammatory disease and fertility. A cohort study of 1,844 women with laparoscopically verified disease and 657 control women with normal laparoscopic results. Sex Transm Dis 1992;19:185–192.
35 Murphy P, Kirkman A, Hale RW: A national survey of women's attitudes toward oral contraception and other forms of birth control. Womens Health Issues 1995;5:94–99.
36 Rome ES: Pelvic inflammatory disease: the importance of aggressive treatment in adolescents. Cleve Clin J Med 1998;65:369–376.
37 Ho MK, Lo JY, Lo AC, et al: Evaluation of replacing the existing diagnostic strategy for *Neisseria gonorrhoeae* and *Chlamydia trachomatis* infections with sole molecular testing of urine specimens in a sexually transmitted infection clinic setting. Sex Transm Infect 2009;85:322–325.
38 Centers for Disease Control and Prevention, Workowski KA, Berman SM: Sexually transmitted diseases treatment guidelines, 2006. MMWR Recomm Rep 2006;55(RR-11):1–94.
39 Sam JW, Jacobs JE, Birnbaum BA: Spectrum of CT findings in acute pyogenic pelvic inflammatory disease. Radiographics 2002;22:1327–1334.
40 Beigi RH, Wiesenfeld HC: Pelvic inflammatory disease: new diagnostic criteria and treatment. Obstet Gynecol Clin North Am 2003;30:777–793.
41 Jossens MO, Eskenazi B, Schachter J, et al: Risk factors for pelvic inflammatory disease: a case control study. Sex Transm Dis 1996;23:239–247.
42 Westrom L: Incidence, prevalence, and trends of acute pelvic inflammatory disease and its consequences in industrialized countries. Am J Obstet Gynecol 1980;138:880–892.
43 Lareau SM, Beigi RH: Pelvic inflammatory disease and tubo-ovarian abscess. Infect Dis Clin North Am 2008;22:693,708, vii.
44 Rome ES: Pelvic inflammatory disease in the adolescent. Curr Opin Pediatr 1994;6:383–387.
45 Lidegaard O, Helm P: Pelvic inflammatory disease: The influence of contraceptive, sexual, and social life events. Contraception 1990;41:475–483.
46 Andersch B, Milsom I: An epidemiologic study of young women with dysmenorrhea. Am J Obstet Gynecol 1982;144:655–660.
47 Klein JR, Litt IF: Epidemiology of adolescent dysmenorrhea. Pediatrics 1981;68:661–664.
48 Svanberg L, Ulmsten U: The incidence of primary dysmenorrhea in teenagers. Arch Gynecol 1981;230:173–177.
49 Harlow SD, Park M: A longitudinal study of risk factors for the occurrence, duration and severity of menstrual cramps in a cohort of college women. Br J Obstet Gynaecol 1996;103:1134–1142.

50 Schroeder B, Sanfilippo JS: Dysmenorrhea and pelvic pain in adolescents. Pediatr Clin North Am 1999;46:555–571.
51 Alvin PE, Litt IF: Current status of the etiology and management of dysmenorrhea in adolescence. Pediatrics 1982;70:516–525.
52 Harel Z: Dysmenorrhea in adolescents and young adults: etiology and management. J Pediatr Adolesc Gynecol 2006;19:363–371.
53 Smith SK, Kelly RW: Effect of platelet-activating factor on the release of PGF-2 alpha and PGE-2 by separated cells of human endometrium. J Reprod Fertil 1988;82:271–276.
54 Nigam S, Benedetto C, Zonca M, et al: Increased concentrations of eicosanoids and platelet-activating factor in menstrual blood from women with primary dysmenorrhea. Eicosanoids 1991;4:137–141.
55 Harel Z, Lilly C, Riggs S, et al: Urinary leukotriene (LT) E(4) in adolescents with dysmenorrhea: a pilot study. J Adolesc Health 2000;27:151–154.
56 Marjoribanks J, Proctor ML, Farquhar C. Nonsteroidal anti-inflammatory drugs for primary dysmenorrhoea. Cochrane Database Syst Rev 2003;4:CD001751.
57 Owen PR: Prostaglandin synthetase inhibitors in the treatment of primary dysmenorrhea: outcome trials reviewed. Am J Obstet Gynecol 1984;148:96–103.
58 Dawood MY: Nonsteroidal anti-inflammatory drugs and changing attitudes toward dysmenorrhea. Am J Med 1988;84(5A):23–9.
59 Karnaky KJ: Development of the oral contraceptives. Am J Obstet Gynecol 1975;123:771–772.
60 Chan WY, Dawood MY: Prostaglandin levels in menstrual fluid of nondysmenorrheic and of dysmenorrheic subjects with and without oral contraceptive or ibuprofen therapy. Adv Prostaglandin Thromboxane Res 1980;8:1443–1447.
61 Creatsas G, Deligeoroglou E, Zachari A, et al: Prostaglandins: PGF2 alpha, PGE2, 6-keto-PGF1 alpha and TXB2 serum levels in dysmenorrheic adolescents before, during and after treatment with oral contraceptives. Eur J Obstet Gynecol Reprod Biol 1990;36:292–298.
62 Goldstein DP, deCholnoky C, Emans SJ, et al: Laparoscopy in the diagnosis and management of pelvic pain in adolescents. J Reprod Med 1980;24: 251–256.
63 Reese KA, Reddy S, Rock JA: Endometriosis in an adolescent population: the Emory experience. J Pediatr Adolesc Gynecol 1996;9:125–128.
64 Laufer MR, Goitein L, Bush M, et al: Prevalence of endometriosis in adolescent girls with chronic pelvic pain not responding to conventional therapy. J Pediatr Adolesc Gynecol 1997;10:199–202.
65 Clement PB: History of gynecological pathology. IX. Dr. John Albertson Sampson. 1921. Int J Gynecol Pathol 2001;20:86–101.
66 Ailawadi RK, Jobanputra S, Kataria M, et al: Treatment of endometriosis and chronic pelvic pain with letrozole and norethindrone acetate: a pilot study. Fertil Steril 2004;81:290–296.
67 Amsterdam LL, Gentry W, Jobanputra S, et al: Anastrazole and oral contraceptives: A novel treatment for endometriosis. Fertil Steril 2005;84:300–304.
68 Chwalisz K, Perez MC, Demanno D, et al: Selective progesterone receptor modulator development and use in the treatment of leiomyomata and endometriosis. Endocr Rev 2005;26:423–438.
69 Porcu E, Venturoli S, Dal Prato L, et al: Frequency and treatment of ovarian cysts in adolescence. Arch Gynecol Obstet 1994;255:69–72.
70 Steinkampf MP, Hammond KR, Blackwell RE: Hormonal treatment of functional ovarian cysts: a randomized, prospective study. Fertil Steril 1990;54: 775–777.
71 Spanos WJ: Preoperative hormonal therapy of cystic adnexal masses. Am J Obstet Gynecol 1973;116: 551–556.
72 Alexander-Williams J: Do adhesions cause pain? Br Med J (Clin Res Ed) 1987;294:659–660.
73 Duffy DM, diZerega GS: Adhesion controversies: pelvic pain as a cause of adhesions, crystalloids in preventing them. J Reprod Med 1996;41:19–26.
74 Cheong Y, William Stones R: Chronic pelvic pain: aetiology and therapy. Best Pract Res Clin Obstet Gynaecol 2006;20:695–711.
75 Economy KE, Laufer MR: Pelvic pain. Adolesc Med 1999;10:291–304.
76 Goldstein DP, deCholnoky C, Leventhal JM, et al: New insights into the old problem of chronic pelvic pain. J Pediatr Surg 1979;14:675–680.
77 Peters AA, van Dorst E, Jellis B, et al: A randomized clinical trial to compare two different approaches in women with chronic pelvic pain. Obstet Gynecol 1991;77:740–744.
78 Swank DJ, Swank-Bordewijk SC, Hop WC, et al: Laparoscopic adhesiolysis in patients with chronic abdominal pain: a blinded randomised controlled multi-centre trial. Lancet 2003;361:1247–1251.
79 Sant GR, Hanno PM: Interstitial cystitis: current issues and controversies in diagnosis. Urology 2001;57(6 suppl 1):82–88.
80 Rosamilia A, Dwyer PL: Interstitial cystitis and the gynecologist. Obstet Gynecol Surv 1998;53:309–319.

81 Hanno PM, Landis JR, Matthews-Cook Y, et al: The diagnosis of interstitial cystitis revisited: Lessons learned from the national institutes of health interstitial cystitis database study. J Urol 1999;161:553–557.
82 Curhan GC, Speizer FE, Hunter DJ, et al: Epidemiology of interstitial cystitis: a population based study. J Urol 1999;161:549–552.
83 Mattox TF: Interstitial cystitis in adolescents and children: a review. J Pediatr Adolesc Gynecol 2004; 17:7–11.
84 Rackow BW, Novi JM, Arya LA, et al: Interstitial cystitis is an etiology of chronic pelvic pain in young women. J Pediatr Adolesc Gynecol 2009;22:181–185.
85 Propert KJ, Schaeffer AJ, Brensinger CM, et al: A prospective study of interstitial cystitis: results of longitudinal follow-up of the interstitial cystitis data base cohort. the interstitial cystitis data base study group. J Urol 2000;163:1434–1439.
86 Chai TC: Diagnosis of the painful bladder syndrome: current approaches to diagnosis. Clin Obstet Gynecol 2002;45:250–258.
87 Hyams JS, Burke G, Davis PM, et al: Abdominal pain and irritable bowel syndrome in adolescents: a community-based study. J Pediatr 1996;129:220–226.
88 Rasquin-Weber A, Hyman PE, Cucchiara S, et al: Childhood functional gastrointestinal disorders. Gut 1999;45(suppl 2):II60–II68.
89 Sigmon ST, Dorhofer DM, Rohan KJ, et al: The impact of anxiety sensitivity, bodily expectations, and cultural beliefs on menstrual symptom reporting: a test of the menstrual reactivity hypothesis. J Anxiety Disord 2000;14:615–633.
90 Harlow BL, Cohen LS, Otto MW, et al: Early life menstrual characteristics and pregnancy experiences among women with and without major depression: the Harvard study of moods and cycles. J Affect Disord 2004;79:167–176.
91 Strine TW, Chapman DP, Ahluwalia IB: Menstrual-related problems and psychological distress among women in the United States. J Womens Health (Larchmt) 2005;14:316–323.
92 Laufer MR, Goitein L, Bush M, et al: Prevalence of endometriosis in adolescent girls with chronic pelvic pain not responding to conventional therapy. J Pediatr Adolesc Gynecol 1997;10:199–202.

Ellen S. Rome, MD, MPH
Section of Adolescent Medicine, Cleveland Clinic Children's Hospital
Cleveland Clinic Lerner College of Medicine at Case
9500 Euclid Avenue, A120
Cleveland, OH 44195 (USA)
Tel. +1 216 444 3566, E-Mail romee@ccf.org

Sultan C (ed): Pediatric and Adolescent Gynecology. Evidence-Based Clinical Practice. 2nd, revised and extended edition. Endocr Dev. Basel, Karger, 2012, vol 22, pp 251–270

Congenital Developmental Defects of Derivates of Müllerian Ducts

Jan Hořejší

Department of Obstetrics and Gynecology, Charles University Prague, 2nd Medical Faculty and Teaching Hospital Praha-Motol, Prague, Czech Republic

Abstract

Congenital developmental defects of Müllerian derivates, understandable with the knowledge of embryological development of Wolffian and Müllerian ducts, are defects of canalisation (= gynatresias), defects in fusing, combined defects and uterovaginal agenesis. Gynatresias should be suspected in the newborn, but distinguished in puberty, on the basis of menstrual blood retention, as hymeneal atresia (haematocolpos), aplasia partis distalis vaginae (haematocolpos partialis), transversal vagina septum and aplasia of vagina and uterine cervix (isolated haematometra). Particular operations are described. Defects in the fusing of Müllerian ducts from the point of view of surgery could be single-coated or double-coated. Incomplete reduplication with unilateral renal aplasia syndrome could present as hemihaematocolpos, hemihaematometra and haematometra in rudimental horn. For diagnosis of these disorders menstrual blood retention is necessary. Surgical treatment in the first two types includes resection of the common wall and haematometra in rudimental horn needs metroplasty or hemihysterectomy. Congenital absence of uterus and vagina (Rokitanski Küster) appears in genetically, endocrinologically and psychosexually normal females. Diagnosis is based on clinical examination and ultrasonography. Initial examination should be nonsurgical (dilatation method). All surgical corrections create a place for the future vagina and reach its epithelization. Different procedures are criticised. The author recommends and describes Vecchietti's laparoscopic surgery

The development of the genitals is complicated not only by the genetically contingent formation of gonads, but also by the origination, development and disappearance of mesonephric (Wolffian) ducts, and the origination, development, fusing and canalisation of the paramesonephric (Müllerian) ducts and their opening into the urogenital sinus.

Congenital developmental defects of the derivatives of Müllerian ducts occur in a wide spectrum of variations; their clinical presentation varies according to anatomical configuration from the simplest (e.g. hymenal atresia) to defects that are very complicated. Nevertheless, their incidence is not high (estimated 1:10,000–20,000 girls born). That is why the literature often cites only the causality of individual cases or their small groups. But even authors that often diagnose and operate on these defects have dissimilar experience and their classification is rather various. The principles of 'evidence-based medicine' in this matter are therefore difficult to assert. In this chapter, for the description and division of developmental defects of the derivatives of Müllerian ducts, we start from the embryological development of genitals, presupposing that this knowledge enables the correct understanding, diagnosis and operation of these defects. We emphasize that the basic principle of the surgical therapy of Müllerian developmental defects is and must be respect for the free outflow of menstrual blood, the possibility of normal female intercourse and, of course, chiefly the opportunity to get pregnant. Some defects and their resolution lay the foundations for future indisputable indication of ending the pregnancy with an elective caesarean section; on the other hand, in other cases, nothing stands in the way of delivery per vias naturales. Where this imperative does not exist, it depends on the management of the delivery and on both the concrete obstetric situation and experience of the obstetrician. From the aforementioned it follows that in the diagnosis and resolution of less frequent and complicated congenital defects in derivatives of Müllerian ducts, focus should be on centres that have experience with this and those to which just such focus brings, deepens and hones the necessary experience.

Some developmental defects (namely those of the external genitals) are so conspicuous that they can already be detected and diagnosed in newborns; others only appear during examination for growth disorders or other somatic anomalies (e.g. Turner syndrome); others express themselves as late as puberty (delayed puberty, difficulties caused by the retention of menstrual blood during atresia). Some manifest themselves as primary amenorrhea and should be accordingly revealed at 15 years of age, others not until somatosexual maturity when they cause difficulties during intercourse or render it impossible and, finally, some are not revealed until the investigation of fertility disorders in adult women. Even treatment is similarly (including surgery of congenital developmental defects) performed during various stages of a woman's life.

To correctly understand congenital defects of the internal genitals or so-called female genital ducts in women, it is necessary to realize basic facts from embryological development (fig. 1): Wolffian mesonephric ducts originate in embryos that are 25–30 days old and represent ducts draining the mesonephros (ductus mesonephrici). From these the ureteric bud grows out which, in the upward direction, reaches the metanephrogenic blastema and induces there the development of the kidneys, and itself changes into the ureter. The ureteric bud is at this time separating from the Wolffian duct and already opens independently into the urogenital sinus. At 42 days of embryonal development, Müllerian ducts start to develop. They run along Wolffian mesonephric ducts and therefore are called paramesonephric ducts.

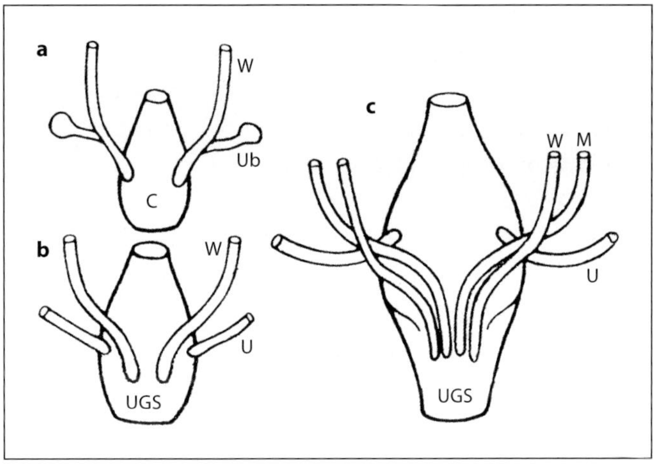

Fig. 1. Schema of embryonal development of deferent urogenital tract. (**a**) Embryo 25–30 days; (**b**) embryo 35–38 days; (**c**) embryo 42–48 days. C = Cloaca; UGs = urogenital sinus; W = ductus mesonefricus Wolfi; M = ductus paramesonefricus Mülleri; Ub = ureteral bud; U = ureter.

Wolffian ducts represent a guiding structure for them which corresponds to their sufficient coming together so that they may fuse and form the so-called uterovaginal canal, and are even responsible for coalescence of both uterovaginal canals together and its emptying into the urogenital sinus in the place of the so-called Müllerian eminence. The aforesaid implies that the development of the urinary and female genital organs is very closely related in early stages. That is why even developmental defects of the female genital ducts are often associated with developmental defects of the uropoetic system and during diagnosis of one there should always be consideration of the other and a search for them. Genital glands do not affect the development of the female genital ducts with one exception: Sertoli cells of embryonic testes (and even dysgenic testes) in an embryo about 48 days old secrete a substance that inhibits the development of Müllerian ducts, the so-called MIF – Müllerian inhibiting factor. This substance is secreted in the area of the gubernaculum testis where it crosses the base of the paramesonephric Müller ducts and destroys the homolateral Müllerian duct. If both testes are developed, then derivatives of Müllerian ducts are missing entirely. If only one testicle is present (even dysgenetical), then derivatives of Müllerian ducts cannot be found on the side where it is developed, the uterus is thus unicornuate and, as a rule, hypoplastic and, of course, has one Fallopian tube.

Defects in the Development of Paramesonephric (Müllerian) Ducts and Their Derivatives

These are divided into 'horizontal' defects = defects of canalisation, and further, 'vertical' defects = defects in fusing, and combined defects. Congenital absence of uterus and vagina belongs to Müllerian anomalies as well (table 1).

Table 1. Classification of congenital defects of derivates of Müllerian ducts

Defects of canalisation-gynatresias
Hymenal atresia
Retrohymenal atresia
Aplasia partis distalis vaginae
Transversal vaginal septum
Atresia cervicis uteri
Vaginal aplasia
Defects in the fusing of Müllerian ducts
Single-coated defects
Uterus subseptus
Uterus septus
Double-coated defects
Uterus arcuatus
Uterus bicornis
Uterus bicorporeus unicolis
Uterus duplex (uterus bicorporeus bicolis)
• Uterus duplex cum vagina subsepta septa
• Uterus duplex cum vagina duplice (uterus didelphys)
Combined defects in the development of Müllerian ducts (syndrome of incomplete duplication in the internal genitals)
Aplasia of the uterus and vagina

Defects of Canalisation – Gynatresias

Defects of canalisation, i.e. gynatresias (fig. 2), originate either in defects of drainage of the uterovaginal funiculus in any of its parts or a failure to connect the uterovaginal canal to the cloaca and thus into the urogenital sinus. Gynatresia may also be the result of partial failure to form derivatives of Müllerian ducts (e.g. partial aplasia of the vagina). The first suspicion of gynatresia should be mentioned already during examination of the genitals of the newborn: as an effect of newborn estrogenization, the uterine cervix secretes viscous mucous which flows out of the vagina and hymenal opening outwards, so it may be seen on the vulva. The presence of this mucous on the genitals of a newborn is a marker of correct development of the female genital ducts. On the other hand, the absence of this mucous on the genitals signals some form of gynatresia: this fact should be noted in paediatric documentation in such a way that it may be actively searched for in puberty. Also, we must inform the mother of this and emphasize that, at the time of the beginning of puberty, she must proactively seek out a gynaecologist so that the defect may be ruled out in time or correctly diagnosed and surgically corrected at the right time. During the period of genital maturation, at first mucous accumulates above the imperforated hymen, as a rule asymptotically,

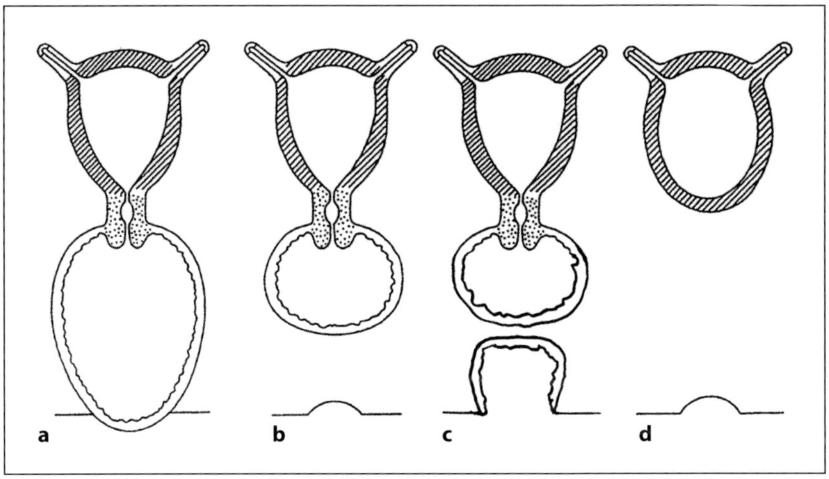

Fig. 2. Different types of gynatresias. **a** Hymenal atresia (haematocolpos). **b** Partial vaginal aplasia (haematocolpos partial). **c** Transversal vaginal septum (haematocolpos partial). **d** Cervical and vaginal aplasia (isolated haematometra).

and later menstrual blood. The origination of the menstrual blood retention is an absolutely basic condition for it to be possible to differentially-diagnostically discern between three basic types of gynatresia. This is not possible earlier.

Hymenal Atresia

The most common gynatresia is hymenal atresia – imperforate hymen (fig. 2a). The natural hymenal opening is missing and therefore mucous cannot flow out of the genitals (at puberty mucocolpos develops) and after menarche, menstrual blood creates haematocolpos.

Clinical Presentation

A patient with normal and sufficient development of secondary sex characteristics has yet to menstruate; on the other hand, she experiences repeated pain in the underbelly in roughly monthly intervals which increase in intensity month after month. In further progression, the retention of menstrual blood fills the uterus (haematometra) and Fallopian tubes (haematosalpinges). The vagina and uterus, unfastened by retained blood, bulge the underbelly and lower part of the abdomen. The pulling upward of the urinary bladder and pressure on the urethra may induce acute urine retention. Only quite rarely do signs of peritoneal irritation caused by retrograde outflow of menstrual blood into the peritoneal cavity appear during hymenal atresia. A unique complication is also rupture of haematometra with an emptying out of the retained blood into the peritoneal cavity with the development of sudden abdominal incidence. Spontaneous bursting of the athletic hymen (which is essentially 'self-healing' of this defect) is likewise rare as well. During examination we may see the region of the hymen without an opening, lividly coloured and bulging. There is more bulging with increased intraabdominal pressure (e.g. coughing). With rectal examination we may palpate ovoid cystically-tense swelling which begins immediately at the level of the perineum (or anal opening), entirely fills the small pelvis and reaches various upward heights, many times to the navel or even higher. If the retention is of a greater extent, it is not possible to differentiate between the vagina and uterus. This resolution is aided by ultrasound examination which also eventually uncovers the creation of haematosalpinges. Further examination (CT, MRI or even laparoscopy) is indicated rarely only for rather than being about a type of defect, informs about insufficient experience of the doctor.

Therapy

Therapy is simple – surgical creation of a sufficiently spacious opening in the hymen and ensuring its permanent clearness. A large number of surgical methods have been described (slicing of the hymen with one incision or an X-shaped incision, cutting out a triangular or oval part of the hymen with suturing of the early bleeding edges, etc.). We ourselves perform and recommend a very simple solution: we cut simply through the hymen where it is most protruded and introduce large Péan forceps into the opening and with their forcible opening tear the hymen until the opening is sufficiently large. This method has the advantage that the tissue of the hymen tears where it is thinnest and therefore does not bleed. Permanent and sufficient clearness of the created opening is ensured by inserting a hollow dilatory phantom (best made of a 10- or 20-ml syringe) for a week to 10 days. The operation is of course performed under general anaesthesia and requires fastidious asepsis, because the contents of hematometra are an ideal environment for the breeding of bacteria and the origination of an acute inflammation which is especially dangerous where haematosalpinges have already been created. Therefore the operation should be performed fundamentally during hospitalization. The described solution is definitive, patients are able to freely menstruate following it, they don't have problems during their first intercourse or in their further sexual lives, and they can give birth per vias naturales.

Retrohymenal Atresia

Retrohymenal atresia originates as a defect in the connection of the 'Müllerian' parts of the vagina to the cloaca. Their clinical presentment and treatment does not vary significantly from hymenal atresia.

Aplasia partis distalis vaginae – partial aplasia of the vagina – present itself through the creation of haematocolpos partialis (fig. 2b).

Clinical Presentation

The clinical presentation is the same as for hymenal atresia, but the external genitals are not bulged or livid. During rectal palpation, we feel cystic resistance up to a number of centimetres above the level of the anus. For correct diagnosis, ultrasound examination is very important.

Therapy

Therapy is colpostomy: after splitting the mucosa of the external genitals with a dull preparation in the urorectal space, we proceed upward all the way to the bottom of the haematocolpos partialis. There we establish fixation stitches, open the cavity between them and suction out the old menstrual blood retention. Although the vagina was created using only its part (usually about half), as its wall has been stretched by retention, there is enough of it to pull it down to the level of the external genitals and fixate it there with a suture. This not only removes the retention, but the defect is perfectly covered by the vaginal mucosa. After healing of the sutures, the vaginal entrance is both visually and palpably anatomically normal, and does not have a tendency to secondary closure and, as a rule, there is no need for any further surgery, neither immediately nor after to enable sexual life. Also, delivery is possible per vias naturals, and the colpostomy itself does not indicate an elective caesarian section. An unpleasant situation is presented by the condition where, during partial aplasia only a very small part of the vagina developed. That is why even a small amount of 'material' to bridge the distance where the vagina is not formed. Colpostomy is difficult to perform and we must be prepared for complications (stenosis, synechias) that require re-canalisations and dilatations. Not even the usual finding of haematocolpos partialis nor in the described complicated cases have we ever been forced to perform a hysterectomy; we always managed to preserve the function of the uterus and to create a functional vagina.

Transversal Vaginal Septum

Transversal vaginal septum (fig. 2c) is usually localised between the middle and upper part of the vaginal length. It could be complete or incomplete.

Clinical Presentation

In complete transversal vaginal septum, the clinical presentation is the same as in the haematocolpos partialis with missing distal part of the vagina, but on examination we reveal the distal part of the vagina formed normally. The vagina appears shorter and ends at the transversal septum. Incomplete transversal vaginal septum is a stenosis, which gives the vagina a shape of a sand-glass clock. Menstrual blood flows through the stenosis and does not create retention. The defect causes dyspareunia, not only for shortness of the lower vaginal segment, but also the attempt to overpower the stenosis during intercourse could be painful.

Therapy

Transversal vaginal septum should be solved surgically by excision of stenotic part with a circular suture 'end-to-end'. In cases of complete transverse vaginal septum surgery should be acutely performed acutely due to the obstruction and retention of menstrual blood – haematocolpos partialis forms. In cases of the incomplete transversal septum surgery could be postponed till the start of sexual activity. Operated vagina will be patent enough for sexual intercourse, but scars surrounding the former stenosis are not elastic enough to allow vaginal delivery without serious injuries.

Atresia Cervicis Uteri

Atresia cervicis uteri is a rare defect whereby the uterine cervix is solid and does not have a cavity which is the cause of the creation of isolated hematometra in a normal vagina. This defect is corrected by surgical creation or clearing, i.e. canalisation of the canal of the uterine cervix as a rule by combined abdomino-vaginal procedure.

Vaginal Aplasia

Vaginal aplasia – complete absence of the vagina – is, as a rule, associated even with aplasia of the uterine cervix in normal configuration of the uterine corpus (fig. 2d). Isolated hematometra develops in puberty. This congenital defect is fortunately very rare and the literature, as a rule, recommends removal of the haematometra by hysterectomy. We do not agree with this, and always try to preserve a functional uterus and even the possibility of fertilization.

Clinical Presentation

The clinical presentation is the same as for gynatresia, but difficulties – the pain which repeats itself monthly – rapidly escalate. Palpation per rectum we can feel the bottom of tension-cystic retention very high; diagnosis is specified by proficient ultrasonographic examination and MRI could be very helpful. Surgical therapy is possible, even if demanding; the surgeon must be well-versed in malformations of the internal genitals and must be able to choose a more or less individual approach for each patient.

Therapy

It is necessary to create a canalised neocervix and neovagina at the same time. In principal, it is possible to select a surgical method only 'from below' or combined abdomino-vaginal. The creation of a 'neocervix' and 'neovagina' is not difficult from the perspective of surgical techniques; more difficult and important is maintaining their clearness by establishing a dilatational phantom of the cervix and vagina. These devices must remain in situ until the full epithelization of the neocervix and neovagina which usually takes 8–10 weeks and, of course, requires hospitalization. Even after removal of both devices, it is necessary to mind the clearness of both, sometimes it is perhaps necessary to repeat canalisation and dilatation of the neocervix. This method is not very demanding considering the surgery itself, but on postoperative care. We operate girls at the time of menarche (12–13 years) that are not at this time fully motivated to preserve their menstrual function and fertility, to bear such long-term care with plenty of unpleasant experiences. For this reason psychological

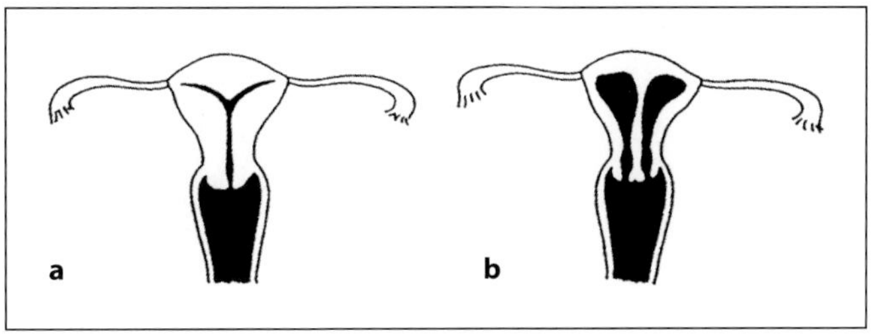

Fig. 3. One-coated uterine duplication. **a** Uterus subseptus. **b** Uterus septus.

support of the patient is very important (clinical psychologist, all nursing personnel and namely the parents). Nonetheless, of our 18 patients, we managed to preserve a functional uterus 16 times and two patients even experienced pregnancy which progressed completely without complications and we helped them deliver 3 healthy children by caesarean section.

Defects in the Fusing of Paramesonephric (Müllerian) Ducts ('Vertical Defects')

Defects is the fusing of paramesonephric (Müllerian) ducts run the gamut of malformations from the simplest, only hinted at, to full duplication of the uterus and vagina. In all types of duplication, there are always found only two Fallopian tubes, in which case each side has its own Fallopian tube (from the upper part of the Müllerian ducts). From a practical perspective, we divide duplicated uterine defects into single- and double-coated defects.

Single-Coated Defects

In single-coated defects (fig. 3), the uterus is monolithic in appearance (using laparoscopy or laparotomy), as a rule wider and only its cavity is partially or wholly duplicated. This includes:

- uterus subseptus (fig. 3a): the cavity is from the fundus downwards not fully separated by the septum which does not reach all the way to the internal cervical os,
- uterus septus (fig. 3b): the cavity is separated by the complete septum all the way to the cervix, sometimes even continuing all the way to the vagina.

Double-Coated Malformations

In double-coated malformations (fig. 4) the partial or full duplication of the uterus is discernable even from the external shape:

- uterus arcuatus (fig. 4a) has concave contours of the uterine fundus instead of the normal convex, the shape of the uterine cavity is usually similar,
- uterus bicornis (fig. 4b) has a body discernibly cleft into two horns, from each withdraws one Fallopian tube,

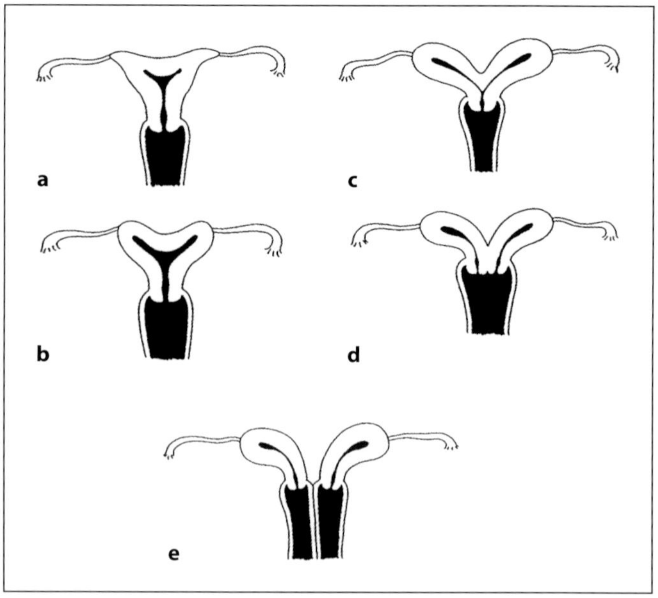

Fig. 4. Double-coated uterine duplication. **a** Uterus arcuatus. **b** Uterus bicornis. **c** Uterus bicorporeus unicolis. **d** Uterus duplex (bicorporeus bicolis). **e** Uterus duplex (bicorporeus bicolis) cum vagina duplilce – 'uterus didelphis'.

– uterus bicorporeus unicolis (fig. 4c) has a duplicated corpus which, however, issues into one cervix;
– uterus duplex (uterus bicorporeus bicolis – fig. 4d) means complete duplication of the uterus. Duplication may continue even to the vagina which is divided only partially – uterus duplex cum vagina subsepta septa, or fully – uterus duplex cum vagina duplice (= uterus didelphys – fig. 4e).

The term 'uterus didelphys' is often used for any duplication of the uterus, but correctly it is used only for uterus duplex cum vagina duplice, because such internal genitals are characteristic of marsupials (dydelphis oposum).

Clinical Presentation

Duplicated malformations of the uterus do not cause menstrual blood retention and therefore do not bring any troubles to girls or adolescent young women. It is usually diagnosed incidentally or at maturity with fertility disorders when a woman repeatedly miscarries or cannot become pregnant. During pregnancy, these defects underlie irregular positioning of the foetus in the uterus (e.g. transverse positioning or breach presentation). This is not always the case, namely full duplication of the internal genitals does not preclude a normally progressing pregnancy and an uncomplicated spontaneous delivery.

Therapy

If the duplicated defect does not cause the aforementioned fertility disorders, it is not treated. In the opposite case it must be surgically corrected: in single-coated

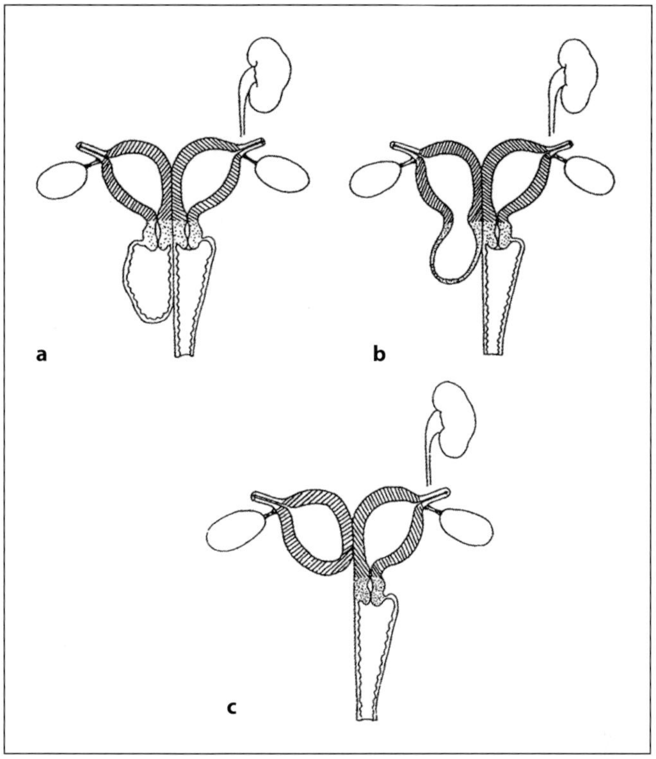

Fig. 5. Internal reduplication syndrome.
a Hemihaematocolpos-.
b Hemihaematometra.
c Haematometra in rudimental horn.

duplication a hysteroscopic resection is done, double-coated defects are corrected using metroplasty per laparotomiam.

Vagina Duplex
Vagina septa (= vagina duplex) or vagina subsepta can cause troubles during intercourse (dyspareunia) or even make intercourse impossible at all, which is resolved by resection of the septum (= common, pressed together parts of the walls of both vaginas). Even if asymmetrical duplication of the vagina need not cause a woman troubles, the septum should be surgically removed before a woman plans her pregnancy so the delivery may be conducted per vias naturales.

Combined Defects in the Development of Müllerian Ducts

Combined defects in the development of Müllerian ducts (syndrome of incomplete duplication of the internal genitals – fig. 5) are caused by the fact that they have not fused and, in addition, one of them has not descended all the way to the paramesonephric Müllerian eminence during embryonic development and has not joined the cloaca. As a result, the derivative of this one Müllerian duct is atretic. Because

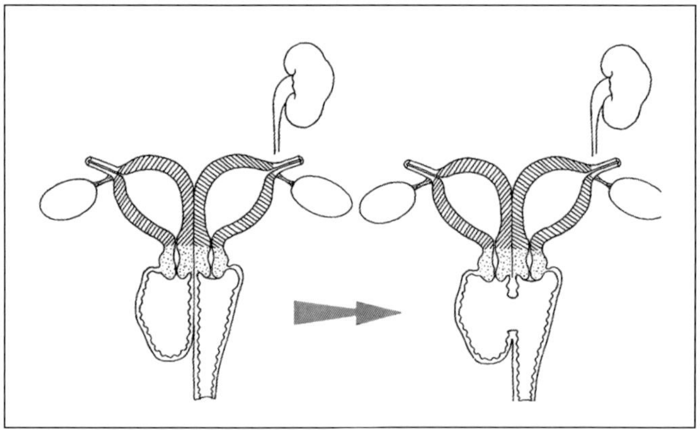

Fig. 6. Surgery in hemihaematocolpos.

the primary cause is a defect in the Wolffian duct, this malformation is associated with aplasia of the kidney and ureter on the side affected by atresia. The absence of the kidney with this defect is absolutely regular. That is why in girls who have been found in childhood to have aplasia of the kidney we must actively search for this defect in puberty. Incomplete duplication manifests itself after menarche: while menstrual blood flows freely from a uterus with a normal vagina, the side affected by atresia retains blood. According to how caudally the development of the Müllerian duct reaches, hemihaematocolpos, hemihaematometra, or haematometra in cornu rudimentario develops.

Clinical Presentation

The clinical presentation is the same as for gynatresia, but the girl menstruates freely from the side not affected by the defect. Examination reveals 'cystic' swelling in the pelvis that, as a rule, encroaches very low above the vaginal entrance. Ultrasonography assists diagnosis as well as the absence of one kidney; MRI is rarely indicated.

Surgical Therapy of Hemihaematocolpos or Hemihaematometra

Surgical therapy of hemihaematocolpos or hemihaematometra consists of the creation of a wide channel of the atretic cavity into the normal vagina (= marsupialization of the atretic cavity) in a way that enables the free outflow of menstrual blood from both parts (fig. 6). Patients do not have any problems with their sex lives in adulthood and may even become pregnant. During pregnancy on the originally patent side, it is possible to try delivery per vias naturales; during gravidity on the originally atretic side of the uterus, a primary caesarean section should be indicated.

In the syndrome of incomplete duplication at the level of hemihaematocolpos, it is possible to sometimes prove the existence of a thin connection between both uterine cervixes. Menstrual blood from the atretic system then flows out in the form of a weak lengthy bleeding or brown discharge several days after menses and sometimes lasting even till the next menses. This type of malformation is referenced in the literature as Herlyn-Verner syndrome or Wunderlich syndrome. Anatomical details could be clarified by the ultrasonography using contrast media. Also this anomaly should be solved using marsupialisation of the atretic cavity into normal vagina.

Haematometra in Cornu Rudimentario
Haematometra in cornu rudimentario (fig. 5c) has the same clinical presentation, but rectal examination palpates resistance very high; ultrasound examination and eventually MRI specifies the diagnosis. This state must be dealt with laparotomically: either, using metroplastics, a rudimentary horn is connected to the other uterus and their cavities are thus joined (the advantage is that the other fallopian tube remains preserved) or both the rudimentary horn and fallopian tube are removed by hemihysterectomy. Pregnancy is possible, but it is, however, considered risky and delivery is conducted per sectionem caesaream.

In general, it is possible to say that the syndrome of incomplete duplication may have an entire range of variations more or less in their details differing from those described as the syndrome of incomplete duplication of the internal genitals, and labelled with the names of the authors who described them. Therefore orientation in the literature is difficult and thus, here, we hold to description on the basis of the embryological explanation of the source of this defect. The difficulties are certainly the correct diagnosis and correct tactics of surgical correction which require good knowledge of the problems and experience with resolving these malformations. The complexity and relatively low incidence of these defects explains and emphasizes the requirement that patients be sent to centres focused on these problems.

As a consequence of the defective development of Müllerian ducts, namely in gynatresia, there is even a frequent incidence of vaginal adenosis (the finding of endocervical type ectopic islands on the vaginal walls of the mucosa). In a broader sense, this is considered a precancerous carcinoma of the vagina. Accordingly, we should, in the postoperative correction of Müllerian anomalies, conduct a targeted search during the postoperative period and monitor patients. Fortunately, after resolving the atresia, centres of vaginal adenosis usually disappear spontaneously.

Aplasia of the Uterus and Vagina

Aplasia of the uterus and vagina, generally known as Rokitansky-Kuster syndrome (in some cases additionally Mayer-Hauser syndrome), is a serious congenital developmental defect whose incidence is estimated at 1 in 5,000–10,000 female newborns. This defect belongs among disorders of the female genital ducts that originate from the middle and caudal part of the derivatives of the ductus paramesonefricus Mülleri.

The so-called uterovaginal primordium does not form, and consequently neither does the uterus nor vagina. In their place there is only thin tissue in the urorectal space.

Clinical Presentation

A girl with well-developed secondary sex characteristics has not had menses yet, but does not suffer from any pain (as in the case of gynatresia). Sometimes the patient comes to the doctor's office because she cannot have intercourse. The external genitals are normal in appearance; the external meatus of the urethra is positioned normally but often has a fimbriate appearance. There are sometimes depressions parauretrally which, during probing, are only a few millimetres deep and do not lead anywhere. The mucosa of the entrance to the vagina sometimes looks as if it is scarred, but even with probing with a thin probe it is not possible to find any passage deeper. The place where the hymen usually forms the opening of the vagina is sunken and foveolate. This hollow is actually a vestigial cloacal part of the vagina that was not able to connect to the 'Müllerian' part of the vagina. This hollow is very important from the perspective of future surgical and non-surgical correction of this defect as will be presented further. The upper part of the urorectal tissue space reaches all the way to the bottom of the pouch of Douglas. There is diagonal peritoneal duplication in this peritoneal space analogous to the ligamentum latum uteri (plica lata uteri) which is naturally empty or contains only small knotty muscular tissue which is unluminized remains of Müllerian ducts. From these run laterally fallopian tubes that are thin but otherwise normal in appearance with fimbriae supplied with an abdominal orifice. The fallopian tubes are developed completely normally, follicles ripen within them and it is possible to even prove a diphase cycle and ovulation. In contrast to their usual position, the ovaries are located higher and more laterally so that they are often not palpable; rectal examination palpates 'an empty small pelvis'. Also, their localization and the evaluation of their morphology using transabdominal ultrasound examination may be difficult. If sonographic examination is done by an experienced ultrasonographer, the absence of a sonographic picture of the uterus may be considered sufficient evidence of its aplasia, a condition which usually need not be confirmed with either MRI or computer tomography. We reject laparoscopy solely for the purpose of diagnosis as the patient will have to undergo laparoscopy anyway during creation of the vagina using Vecchietti's method by way of laparoscopy. A good and sufficient endocrine function of the ovaries can be confirmed by determination of the circulating gonadotrophic hormones, oestrogen and progesterone, but also is implicit from well-developed secondary sex characteristics: Afflicted girls are often attractive in appearance with wholly feminine phenotype and female contours of their figure (female pelvis type, Jayle index is less than 1, i.e. wider hips than shoulders). In contrast to the androgen insensitivity syndrome, pubic hair of the feminine type is well-developed, axillary pubescence is likewise normal. Girls usually have nice tresses. The syndrome is often associated with malformations of the uropoetic tract (e.g. dystopia of the kidney in the small pelvis) and with disorders of the skeleton and middle ear.

Psychosexual feelings of these patients are always clearly feminine; they seek heterosexual contact and long for intercourse. Of course afflicted girls will never menstruate and likewise pregnancy with aplasia of the uterus is ruled out. Because they do not have a vagina, they could not have normal intercourse in the female manner. The absence of menstruation and impossibility of getting pregnant, carrying to term and delivery of their own child is for patients a frustrating and definitive discovery that, during completion of the diagnosis, we must inform them of, but we may at least create or help create a substitute for the vagina in such a way that she may have intercourse that is satisfying both for her and her partner. With these patients it is possible to discuss the option of a surrogate mother, i.e. the possibility that the ova of the afflicted woman will be fertilized in vitro, carried to term and delivered by another healthy woman in the IVF system program. From the standpoint of medical expertise in today's IVF techniques, this does not pose any difficulties; it is however a complicated legal problem and for that reason is unlawful in most European countries. Because the number of women afflicted in this manner and longing to have families in vain is relatively large, it would be very desirable to resolve the legal side of this procedure in a way that women without a uterus and vagina would be able to have a child using their own genetic material without having to circumvent the law of that country or have to undergo IVF in another country.

Therapy

As I have already specified, it is possible to create or help create a neovagina for women afflicted in such a manner. For this purpose there have been worked out a large number of procedures and modifications. The principle of creating a neovagina is the same for all methods: create a cavity in the urorectal space – a space for the creation of a vagina and ensure that this cavity is covered with epithelium. This space in the urorectal space is easily created for it is made up of only thin tissue which it is possible to tunnel well with a sharp or (better) dull preparation all the way to the normal size of a female vagina. The diverse surgical procedures differ mainly in how they attain coverage of the mucosa.

Discussion

The simplest method of creating a neovagina is the dilatation method (Franck). The vagina is created by gradual pushing in of the entrance to the vaginal mucosa to greater depth. The tissue of the urorectal space cleaves during dilatation and the vaginal mucosa entrance continually covers it; the neovagina is therefore instantly covered by a tiled, layered epithelium during dilatation. Dilatation is first carried out by the patient who pushes the mucosa hollow in the dead-end entrance to the vagina into greater depth with her own finger. Later she uses a dilatation phantom that she either holds herself and pushes into the urorectal space or a phantom fixed to a bicycle seat (Ingram); eventually the dilatation phantom may be extended using a screw mechanism until the desired depth and spaciousness of the neovagina is achieved (Uzel). The creation of a neovagina using dilatation may even be achieved with a vibrator; some women have even created it with repeated intercourse or attempts at intercourse. The method of dilatation therapy and its result are favourably affected by local application of preparations containing estriol on the vaginal mucosa entrance. Contraindication of the creation of a vagina using dilatation is too small a distance between the opening of the urethra and the place from which it is necessary to dilatate. In this case an attempt at dilatation could expand and damage the external meatus of the urethra and lead to intercourse in the urinary blad der. Provided there is no such contraindication, the dilatation method should be the method of first choice.

The arguments for non-surgical dilatation methods are, according to Heinz, the following:

- vaginal dilatation is the least invasive treatment used to manage vaginal aplasia,
- long term vaginal dilatation is eventually needed post surgery mainly in cases where the patient has no sexual partner yet,
- to avoid surgery and pain in afflicted patients.

A girl can carry out the first steps towards dilatation even at a young age (perhaps at the age of 10–12 years). As presented by Heinz, aside from her own dilatation therapy, the afflicted better and more naturally familiarizes herself with her sexual organs, and future dilatation and future sex life will then be more natural and successful for her. If dilatation therapy is contraindicated or its result is unsatisfactory, it is necessary to select a surgical method of correction for this defect.

During this surgical method, to cover the neovagina, the following are used:

– A discretionary dermoepidermal graft (McIndoe Bannister) from the buttocks or thigh, sutured to the dilatation phantom, is submerged into the prepared space in the spatium urorectale and is set there until the graft heals. This takes about 3 weeks but even then the dilatation phantom must be established permanently for minimally 2 months, and even after the patient must use a dilator daily for a long time. If these conditions are not fulfilled, the neovagina wrinkles and shrinks; on the other hand, if they are respected, the neovagina is perfectly created and has the appearance of a normal vagina after hysterectomy. The patient retains scar tissue in the place of the taking of the graft, sometimes with a healing keloid. This method is very demanding of the patient and is not routinely performed today.

– A peg made of foam rubber or another phantom is introduced into the prepared space by which the neovagina epithelializes from the edge of the mucosa of the external genitals (Gambarov). It takes a very long time, the effect is very insufficient, and after achieving epithelialization requires long-term dilatation.

– A peg made of foam rubber and covered with amnionic membranes is introduced into the space. These support epithelialization of the edges – that is the external genitals. The moulage with amnionic membranes must be changed regularly, epithelialization is lengthy and the effect is far from perfect. This method is no longer used due to the risk of HIV and other infections of the amnionic membranes.

– The peritoneum of the pouch of Douglas is mobilized, pulled down and stitched to the external genitals; at the height of the 'vaginal arch' it is separated by a suture (Davidov). Also, this peritoneum serves to quicken the epithelialization of the neovagina from the edges of the mucosa of the entrance to the vagina.

– An excluded part of the bowel (sigmoid bowel – Capraro, large intestine – Galego, cecum – Morton and Dewhurst, or even the ileum-Wilfingfseder) is used to cover the neovagina. This method is still sometimes used by surgeons. It is demanding with respect to operational technique (resection of the intestines, pulling down caudally the excluded parts of the intestine even with its mesentery). The resulting effect is sufficiently spacious, but the neovagina is covered with epithelium of the intestinal type which may be traumatized by intercourse; additionally the intestine retains its secretory activity so that viscous secretions constantly flow from the genitals. This method is in harsh conflict with the principle that the vagina is and should be covered with mucosa with multilayer squamous epithelium and, as such, actually imitates anal sex instead. Gynaecologists consider this method of surgical correction obsolete and staunchly reject it.

– William's method (with Creatsas´modifiction) creates the vagina from the mucosa of the external genitals from which, after a curved incision, creates a horned pouch. Skin is stitched across it as in suturing medial episiotomy. A woman may have intercourse soon after the operation, but, in the beginning, the vagina is directed parallel to the perineum; only gradually is the created covering of the vagina submerged into the correct position. In accordance with the degree of pubescence of the external genitals, hair may then grow even in the vagina; if the border of the incision is led too far to the front, the external meatus of the urethra may get all the way to the beginning of the neovagina and, during micturition, urine may run into it. The method may be improved by preparing a space in the urorectal space for submerging the created neovagina and the 'neovagina' is placed in it already during the operation. The operation is very sparing; the surgical procedure is quick and has a good postoperative effect. It is possible, among others, to use it in cases where, due to internal risk, in the finding of a dystopic kidney in the small pelvis or for other risks (including lengthier anaesthesia necessary for laparoscopic procedures), it is necessary to operate briefly and it is even possible to use an epidural or only local infiltrated anesthesia.

Most of the described surgical methods of creating a neovagina obscure the witty method of Vecchietti. The vagina is created by gradual, relatively quick submersion of a dilatation phantom into the urorectal space with simultaneous pulling of the mucosa of the entrance to the vagina in such a way that the neovagina is continuously covered by mucosa with squamous epithelium. The vagina is therefore created similarly to the dilatation method, but the phantom is not pushed into the urorectal space 'from beneath', but is pulled in there with traction wires. Vecchietti described

24 Vecchietti G: Neovagina nella sindrome di Rokitansky-Kuster-Hauser. Attual Ostet Ginecol 1965;11:131–147.
25 Fedele L, Busacca M, Candiani M, Vignali M: Laparoscopic creation of a neovagina in Mayer-Rokitansky-Kuster-Hauser syndrome by modification of Vecchietti's operation. Am J Obstet Gynecol 1994;171:268–269.
26 Major T, Borsos A, Bacsko G: Application of mini-invasive surgery in Mayer-Rokitansky-Kuster-Hauser syndrome. Acta Chir Hung 1997;36:219–220.
27 Bruna JL, Belleanne G, Grafeillec N, Asland A-F, Brund GH: Long-term results after neovagina creation in Mayer-Rokitanski-Kuster-Hauser syndrome by Vecchietti's operation. Eur J Obstet Gynecol Reprod Endocrinol 2002;103:168–172.

Prof. Jan Hořejší, MD, DrSc
Department of Obstetrics and Gynecology, Charles University Prague
2nd Medical Faculty and Teaching Hospital Praha-Motol
CZ–150 06 Praha 5 – Motol (Czech Republic)
Tel. +420 22443 8200, E-Mail jan.horejsi@lfmotol.cuni.cz

Sultan C (ed): Pediatric and Adolescent Gynecology. Evidence-Based Clinical Practice. 2nd, revised and extended edition. Endocr Dev. Basel, Karger, 2012, vol 22, pp 271–286

Eating Disorders throughout Female Adolescence

F. Dominé · C. Dadoumont · J.-P. Bourguignon

Service de Pédiatrie, CHU de Liège, Chênée, Belgium

Abstract

Eating disorders (EDs) are conditions which are becoming more and more widespread among adolescents and they often lead them to seek the opinion of a professional health caregiver, including gynecologists and pediatricians. EDs, and particularly anorexia nervosa (AN), are usually classified as psychological or psychiatric disorders, but they may have major somatic implications and complications as osteoporosis, nutritional deficiencies, cerebral atrophy, cardiac and metabolic disorders. A key issue in the management is prevention or reduction of both the serious somatic consequences and the important mental health consequences (e.g. depression, psychosocial withdrawal, phobia and suicide), integrating different perspectives (psychological or psychiatric – individual and familial –, genetic, nutritional, pediatric, gynecological). Adolescence is a critical period for the onset of EDs though they may also involve younger children. In this case, the consequences on the development (height, weight, puberty) can also be significant. In this review, we will focus on eating disorders in adolescent girls with an emphasis on AN. We describe variations in ED characteristics and their management depending on age at occurrence. A possible ED should be considered by pediatricians consulted about delayed female growth and puberty as well as gynecologists in patients with primary or secondary amenorrhea or infertility.

Eating disorders (EDs) represent, beyond asthma and obesity, conditions leading more and more adolescents to seek the opinion of a professional health caregiver, including gynecologists and pediatricians [1]. Though it is commonly agreed that EDs are much more frequent in girls, a recent study based on a self-administered and anonymous questionnaire showed that 50% of boys aged 16–20 years expressed concern about their weight and body image and almost 20% were involved in some disturbed eating behaviors [2]. While EDs, particularly anorexia nervosa (AN) are usually classified as psychological or psychiatric disorders, they may have major somatic implications on account of several reasons. The weight changes (loss or gain) due to impaired energy balance, the deficits in specific dietary components and the weight control methods set up by those young people, such as purgative behaviors, may compromise health. In addition, AN involves alterations of homeostatic processes that may have somatic consequences independent of weight or nutritional changes. A key issue in the management is prevention or reduction of both the disastrous mental health consequences of EDs (e.g. depression, psychosocial withdrawal, phobia and suicide) and the serious somatic consequences (e.g. osteoporosis, obesity or nutritional deficiencies, cerebral atrophy, cardiac and metabolic disorders).

Because EDs result from a complex and still elusive pathogenesis and are more or less resistant to management strategies irrespective of the discipline, they are challenging the patients, the families and beyond them the clinicians and the scientists, despite efforts reflected in the abundant literature about this topic. Consistent with this, the management of EDs requires integration of different perspectives (psychological or psychiatric – individual and familial –, genetic, nutritional, pediatric, gynecological) in an attempt to maximize support to the patient and the family.

Adolescence is a critical period for the onset of eating disorders. Puberty involves profound endocrine and physical changes together with psychic and cognitive remodeling and underlying CNS structural modifications [3]. Understandably, the profound physical and mental changes challenging normal adolescents together with social models idealizing thinness in young people can account for increased susceptibility to develop body shape concerns and EDs at the time of adolescence. In the USA, two thirds of adolescent girls were found to worry about remaining/becoming thin [4]. More recently, it appeared that, among adolescent girls, above 55% were involved in unhealthy weight control methods such as laxative abuse, self-induced vomiting, severe food restriction, fasting, draconian diet [5].

In this review, we will focus on eating disorders in adolescent girls with an emphasis on AN. This condition is of particular interest for pediatricians who may be consulted about disorders of growth and puberty as well as gynecologist who see those patients because of primary or secondary amenorrhea or infertility. Importantly, however, a variety of health care providers including dieticians and psychologists may be first consulted by patients with EDs and have each to introduce the patient to interdisciplinary management as a crucial issue.

Definition and Diagnostic Criteria: Eating Disorders versus Disordered Eating

The conditions classically evoked as EDs are AN and bulimia nervosa (BN). These two major disorders, also called 'full ED' meet diagnostic criteria that are listed in DSM-IV manual of the American Psychiatric Association [5] and summarized in table 1. Diagnostic criteria stated slightly differently were proposed in the International Classification of Diseases (ICD) established by the WHO [7]. For comparison purposes, they are also listed in table 1. Though AN and BN might be seen as opposing conditions, they share common characteristics including pursuit of thinness, fear of weight gain, and cognitive overinvestment of everything that

Table 1. Criteria of eating disorders according to DSM IV-R* and IDC of WHO**

Anorexia nervosa	Bulimia nervosa	EDNOS
Voluntary food intake limitation.* Weight loss self-induced by avoidance of 'fattening foods' and one or more of the following: self-induced vomiting; self-induced purging; excessive exercise; use of appetite suppressants and/or diuretics.** Refusal to maintain body weight at or above a minimally normal weight for age and height (e.g. weight loss leading to maintenance of body weight less than 85% of that expected; or failure to make expected weight gain during period of growth, leading to body weight less than 85% of that expected).*, ** BMI 17.5 or less.** Intense fear of gaining weight or becoming fat, even though underweight.* Disturbance in the way in which one's body weight or shape is experienced, undue influence of body shape on self-evaluation, or denial of the seriousness of the current low body weight.* Body-image distortion in the form of a specific psychopathology whereby a dread of fatness persists as an intrusive, overvalued idea and the patient imposes a low weight threshold on himself or herself.** Amenorrhea: In postmenarcheal females, absence of at least three consecutive menstrual cycles.* Widespread endocrine disorder involving the hypothalamic-pituitary-gonadal axis manifested in women as amenorrhea (without replacement or contraceptive pill) and in men as a loss of sexual interest and potency. Possibly elevated levels of growth hormone and cortisol, changes in the peripheral metabolism of the thyroid hormone, and abnormalities of insulin secretion.** Absence of preexisting psychiatric disease.* Types: restricting vs. binge-eating/purging*	Recurrent episodes of binge eating characterized by both of the following:* Eating, in a discrete period of time (e.g. within any 2-hour period), an amount of food that is definitely larger than most people would eat during a similar period of time and under similar circumstances.* A sense of lack of control over eating during the episode (e.g. a feeling that one cannot stop eating or control what or how much one is eating).* Persistent preoccupation with eating, and an irresistible craving for food.** Recurrent inappropriate compensatory behavior in order to prevent weight gain, such as self-induced vomiting, misuse of laxatives, diuretics, enemas, or other medications; fasting, or excessive exercise.* Other compensatory behaviors: alternating periods of starvation; use of drugs such as appetite suppressants, thyroid preparations.** When bulimia occurs in diabetic patients they may choose to neglect their insulin treatment.** The binge eating and inappropriate compensatory behaviors occur, on average, at least twice a week for 3 months.* Self-evaluation unduly influenced by body shape and weight.* The disturbance does not occur exclusively during episodes of anorexia nervosa.* The psychopathology consists of a morbid dread of fatness and the patient sets herself or himself a sharply defined weight threshold, well below the premorbid weight that constitutes the optimum or healthy weight in the opinion of the physician. There is often, but not always, a history of an earlier episode of anorexia nervosa, the interval between the two disorders ranging from a few months to several years. This earlier episode may have been fully expressed, or may have assumed a minor cryptic form with a moderate loss of weight and/or a transient phase of amenorrhea.** Types: purging vs. nonpurging (exercise and fasting to compensate).	Eating disorders not otherwise specified include disorders of eating that do not meet the criteria for any specific eating disorder (AN or BN).*, ** (1) In female patients, all the criteria for anorexia nervosa met except that menses are regular.* (2) All the criteria for anorexia nervosa met except that, despite significant weight loss, the patient's current weight is in the normal range.* (3) All the criteria for bulimia nervosa met except that the binge eating and inappropriate compensatory mechanisms occur less than twice a week or for less than 3 months.* (4) Normal body weight and regular use of inappropriate compensatory behavior after eating small amounts of food (e.g. self-induced vomiting after consuming two cookies).* (5) Repeatedly chewing and spitting out, but not swallowing, large amounts of food.* Binge eating disorder: recurrent episodes of binge eating in the absence if regular inappropriate compensatory behavior characteristic of bulimia nervosa.*

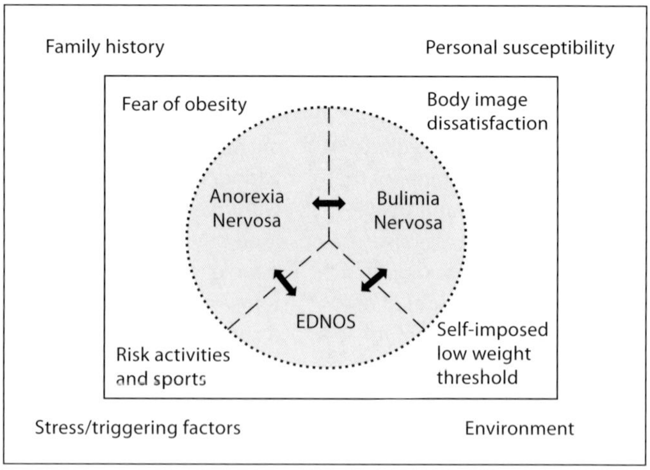

Fig. 1. Schematic representation of the interconnections between the three forms of eating disorders, some predisposing conditions and pathogenetic factors.

refers to food. Quite frequently, anorectic girls fear becoming bulimic and bulimic girls hope for becoming anorectic. Forty to 50% of patients with AN develop BN after months or years [8].

The current concept is to consider, besides AN and BN, the eating disorders not otherwise specified (EDNOS), also called 'partial or atypical ED' (table 1). The EDNOS may be more frequent than AN and BN, clustering the large family of disturbed behaviors in relation with feeding. Obviously, there are no unequivocal criteria defining EDNOS since those disorders include any condition that does not strictly meet the criteria of AN or BN. As illustrated schematically in figure 1, the EDNOS are currently viewed as an intermediate condition between simply dieting and full EDs [1]. Partial EDs are often impermanent and spontaneously resolving but evolution through full ED is possible [9]. The adolescents involved in strict dieting in order to lose weight are more likely to develop a full ED within one to three years [10]. In a study involving 16-year-old girls with a partial ED, 7% developed full ED subsequently [11]. The earlier treatment is initiated, the better is prognosis since the risk of developing a more complicated and persisting disorder is reduced [1]. Therefore, prevention, screening and early management of EDNOS is recommended instead of a 'wait and see' option [12].

In the clinical setting, the diagnosis of AN lies on a triad: anorexia, weight loss and amenorrhea. Anorexia is a self-imposed severe restriction of food intake, hunger being thus effective but controlled. The symptom of anorexia is frequently rationalized by the patient who provides explanations such as dysfunction of digestion or food intolerance. Somatic complaints centered on the abdomen and digestion, are commonly associated. Purgative conducts (self-induced vomiting, laxative abuse, compulsive exercises) can also be associated. A potomania is often present in the daytime.

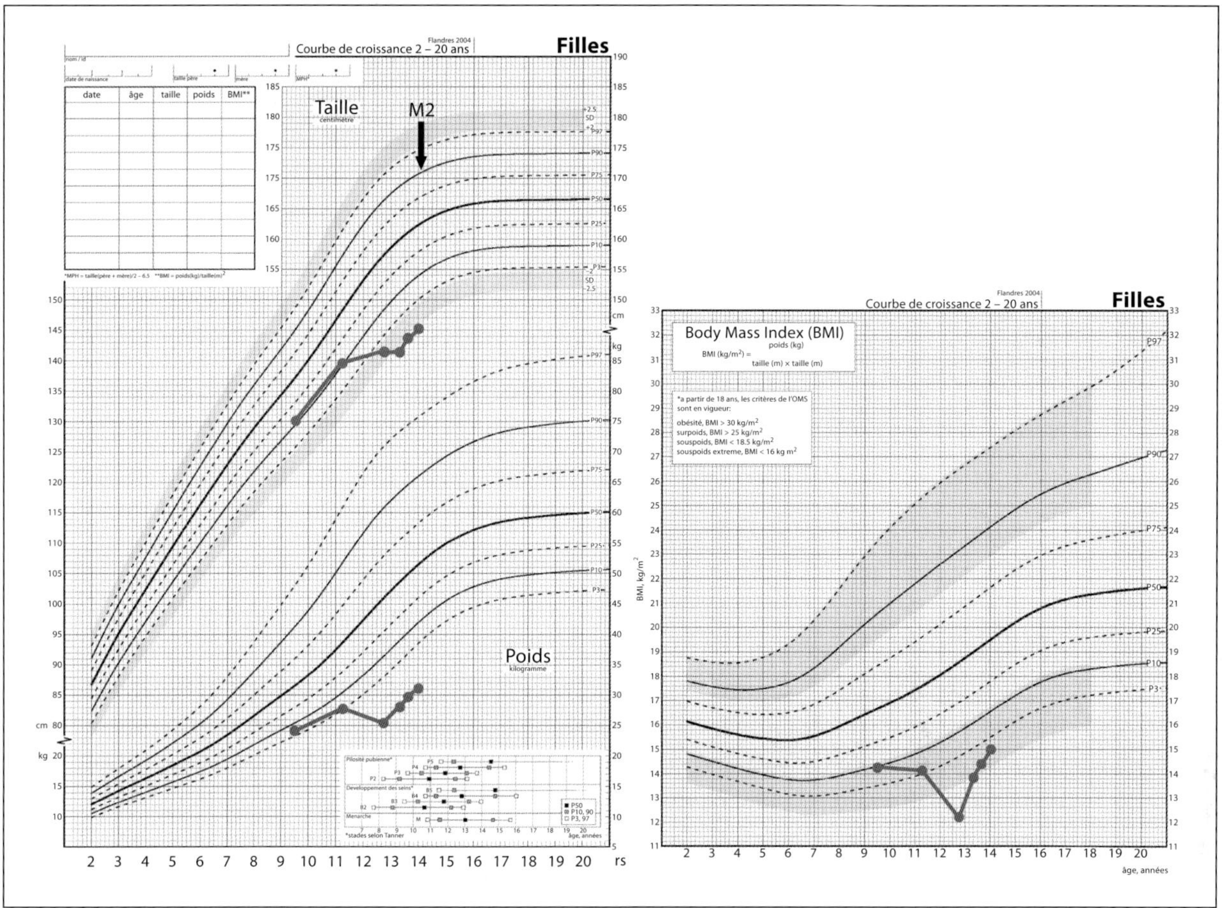

Fig. 2. Changes in height, weight and BMI in a premenarcheal adolescent girl developing AN at 10 years of age. Noteworthy, height velocity is reduced and weight loss is more obvious from the BMI curve than the weight curve.

Weight loss occurs more or less rapidly with the disease. In a still growing patient, drawing the height, weight and BMI curve is very informative as illustrated in figure 2. In a post-pubertal adolescent girl, 18 is the BMI limit of thinness. Since restriction of food intake and weight loss may be denied by the patient or underestimated due to distortion of self-image, it is important to evaluate additional signs of undernutrition including alterations of nails, hair and skin, reduced blood flow at extremities. The patient denial of thinness is fundamental for diagnosis of EDs because weight loss is acknowledged by the patient when caused by underlying somatic diseases or planned weight management in the case of dancers or gymnasts. While it is important that the patient is provided with a realistic evaluation of weight deficit and the related concerns, the physician should also express his/her awareness of the patient distortion of self-image. A BMI level considered to be life-threatening is <14 and hospital admission may be required. However, these limits need some adjustment taking into account factors such as rapidity of weight loss, mental health and neurological functioning. The mortality risk increases dramatically when BMI falls to <11.

Amenorrhea is defined as absence of menstruations during 3 or 6 consecutive months when the cycles were previously regular or irregular, respectively. Amenorrhea can occur after, together with or even before weight loss. This observation suggests that negative energy balance secondary to weight loss is not or not always the determinant of amenorrhea that could involve other mechanisms (see below).

Beyond the interconnections between the three forms of eating disorders (AN, BN, EDNOS), they can be integrated into in a larger group of more frequent disturbed eating behaviors that are linked through time and mechanisms (fig. 1). Accordingly, similar factors can predict or cause any of those minor or major forms of EDs.

Weight status can be an indication of the underlying form of ED since obesity is common in compulsive browsing and binge eating and leanness in restrictive or purgative AN [13]. Normal BMI is common in bulimic patients, irrespective of purging conducts. Among patients with a similar form of ED, however, weight or BMI can be highly variable and changes can occur in short periods of time. Thus, a normalized weight does neither justify that a previous diagnosis of ED is reconsidered nor represent a positive prognostic factor. Though adverse health effects appear to be less obvious in ED patients with normal weight, such patients may be involved in harmful conducts, like purgative behaviors, that can be pernicious because more difficult to diagnose and to treat.

Epidemiology

Because EDs are consistent with several more or less precisely defined clinical conditions, their prevalence is not easy to determine. As far as AN in late adolescent and young adult females is concerned, a prevalence of 0.5–1% is usually mentioned [14]. The incidence appears to be different among studies: 1–12/100,000/year [14]. It seemed to have increased during the 1980s with no further increase currently [8]. The mean age of occurrence of AN is around 17, between 15 and 19 years [14]. Some later forms of AN start in adulthood though they are rather consistent with the adult emergence of a latent eating disorder existing since childhood or adolescence.

Pathogenesis, Homeostatic Disturbances

Pathogenesis of EDs

Despite abundant literature, the etiology of EDs remains complex and obscure. Several factors have been proposed (psychiatric, genetic, neurophysiological, psychosocial, etc.) and it is agreed that there is not any single explanation or mechanism accounting for EDs. Rather, most authors consider that several additive or synergistic factors lead a patient to develop an ED though it is unclear which among those factors account for either predisposition to the disease or onset, aggravation or persistence. This is consistent with bio-psycho-social models.

Genetic and neurobiological factors are likely to play a role as suggested by family clustering of AN or other disorders. This prompted several authors to search for gene polymorphism or other anomalies but not any single gene has been identified so far. While genes related to serotonin synthesis, transport and metabolism appear to be involved in several studies, the current concept is a polygenic determinism. Since estrogens are known to promote the expression of different genes, such a mechanism could explain the increasing incidence of EDs at the time of puberty [15]. Neurobiological mechanisms could explain, for instance, distortion of self-image that has been associated with parietal cortex dysfunction [16]. Studies including imaging of the CNS demonstrated the possible involvement of neuropeptides or neurotransmitters, with emphasis on serotonin. For instance, Audenaert et al. [17] showed a specific regional reduction in binding capacity of the 5-HT2a receptors in low-weight AN patients compared with healthy volunteers. In addition, a physiologic response to the administration of serotonin agonists can be observed in low-weight AN patients [18]. A genetic origin of such serotonin dysregulation could also explain family susceptibility to AN, as suggested by twin and family studies [19]. Based on those data, some authors proposed serotonin supplementation in AN [20, 21].

Psychosocial factors are also probably involved. Adolescence is a critical period regarding not only physical changes, but also psychological and cognitive turmoil both individually and versus peers and family [9]. Corporal changes require adaptation, but may also lead to some distortion of body self-perception, frequently resulting in self-devaluation or low self-esteem [22, 23]. Body image is known to be a crucial factor predicting involvement in dieting, which may in turn sink into disturbed eating behaviors [5, 10, 24–26]. Some factors related to social environment were shown to be associated with EDs: problematic interpersonal connectedness at school, peer mobbing or teasing, and social, media or even medical pressure on weight control [25]. Sometimes, a single physician criticism at medical exam can leave a mark on an adolescent and induce some weight concerns. Factors related to family life conditions are also associated with EDs: parental couple conflicts, history of sexual or physical abuse [27], parental obesity or history of dieting or anorexia [24].

Hormonal factors include the hormonal storm of puberty and the effects of deviations in pubertal timing. The link between pubertal timing and EDs remains controversial [28]. While early puberty does not seem to influence body satisfaction or involvement in dieting, a slight but significant association was found with occurrence of EDs [28, 29]. In a recent study, however, girls self-rated as early or late maturers were both significantly more likely to present disturbed eating behaviors [30].

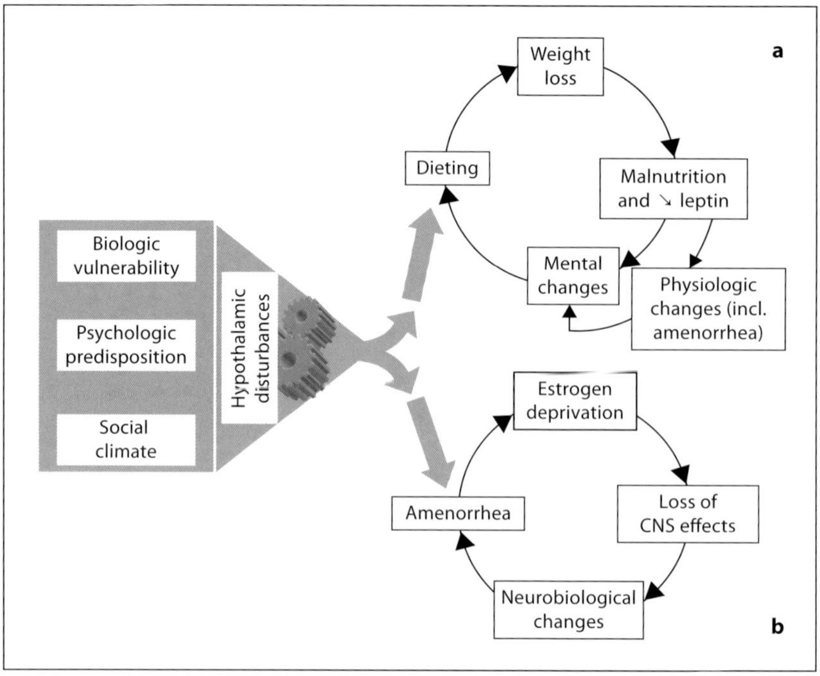

Fig. 3. Two possible mechanisms for pathogenesis of amenorrhea in anorexia nervosa.

Professional or sport practices sometimes involve strict weight control and make subjects more susceptible to EDs: fashion, esthetician, gymnast, athletes, dancer. . . [31].

Personality characteristics or psychiatric factors were shown to be predictive of AN: perfectionism, high sensitivity, empathy, competitiveness and difficulty in setting limits. Dysthymia, depression, suicidal thoughts, self-aggressiveness, obsessional compulsive disorder or borderline personality are often associated with eating disorder [1, 4, 32–35].

Pathogenesis of Amenorrhea

The functional integrity of the hypothalamic-pituitary-ovarian axis is dependent on energy availability as shown in dancers who are regularly cycling or amenorrheic depending on normal or reduced BMI, irrespective of physical activity [36]. Such a mechanism may contribute to the pathogenesis of amenorrhea in AN, as illustrated in figure 3a. Then, reduced fat mass and consequently reduced leptin is a key mechanism since the facilitatory role of leptin on the hypothalamic control of reproductive system is well established [37]. Leptin can be a final mediator independently of fat mass since recombinant leptin therapy for up to 3 months in women with hypothalamic amenorrhea restored pituitary-ovarian activity and menstrual cyclicity despite concomitant reduction in weight and fat mass [38]. Only one third of anorectic patients however start amenorrhea after a significant weight loss whereas half of them show amenorrhea from the time of onset of dieting and one sixth before [39], suggesting another mechanism (fig. 3b). It can be hypothesized that estrogen deprivation resulting from arrested pituitary ovarian activity account for the loss of the many neurobiological effects of the steroid and play some pathogenetic role. However, there is no evidence so far that estrogen replacement has any effect on the outcome of the disease though this has not been systematically studied. The time differences between onset of amenorrhea and weight loss could reflect different pathogenetic mechanisms and could explain heterogeneity in clinical presentation of the disorder.

We studied retrospectively the temporal dissociation between amenorrhea and weight loss in adolescent girls seen for EDs in our Pediatric Endocrinology/Adolescent Medicine Unit. Forty-eight percent of them presented amenorrhea before or at the beginning of weight loss. Such precocity of amenorrhea was related to higher initial weight loss, lower BMI at first visit, and preponderant in the restrictive form of ED. The persistence of menstruations was related to lower initial weight loss, higher BMI at first visit and preponderant in the purgative form of ED. The severity of ED, as reflected by several clinical parameters (weight loss velocity, duration of weight loss, lowest BMI observed, etc.), was related to the rapidity of occurrence of amenorrhea, suggesting the involvement of impaired neuroendocrine mechanisms related to disordered homeostasis, independently of energy imbalance.

Variations in ED Characteristics Depending on Age at Occurrence

In table 2 are summarized features of AN in relation to developmental stage at occurrence of the disease. As detailed in the chapter by Bourguignon and Juul [this vol.], pubic hair development in females can involve adrenal androgens that are not dependent on pituitary-ovarian activity. Thus, pubic hair could develop in an ED patient despite pituitary-ovarian inhibition.

In prepubertal premenarcheal girls, breast development can be absent or just starting. However, because initiation of the pubertal growth spurt is in fact the first clinical event of female puberty, growth stunting can be an important feature. The mechanism is complex, involving lack of energy intake and deficiency in specific nutrients (calcium, vitamin D, etc.). Among the endocrine factors, estrogen deprivation but also reduction of insulin-like growth factor-1 secretion can play a role. Recovery from AN can be associated with some increase in height velocity though a spurt comparable with that occurring physiologically is unlikely. This is because increase in age accounts normally for progressive reduction of the magnitude of the spurt and also because normalization of dietary intake, neuroendocrine and psychosocial functioning in AN is a slow and often partial process. The highest risk of insufficient bone

Table 2. Some characteristics of AN patients in relation to developmental stage at diagnosis

Prepubertal	Pubertal	Postpubertal
Premenarcheal		Postmenarcheal
Primary amenorrhea	Primary amenorrhea	Secondary amenorrhea
Stunted growth Absent puberty No breast development	Stunted growth, reduced growth spurt Arrested puberty Partial breast development	Final height (almost) attained Finalized puberty Reduced breast size
Denial ++	Denial ++	Denial +/–
Peak bone mass not achieved	Peak bone mass not achieved	Peak bone mass achieved Loss in bone density
Lower rate of full recovery	1/3 fully recovered, 1/3 partially recovered, 1/3 chronic	

mineralization and subsequent fractures can be observed in those conditions since peak bone mass is achieved during the pubertal growth spurt. Osteopenia can occur as early as after 6 months and justifies osteodensitometry to be performed in the 1st year of the disease. While osteopenia can persist for a long time [40] and is observed in 90% of AN, it can also be found in patients with EDNOS [41]. The mechanisms of osteopenia are similar to those of stunted growth. In addition, hypoleptinemia and hypercortisolism could play some role as well. Moreover, prognosis is less favorable with increased risk of chronic forms when eating disorders appear early, before puberty [42]. Further difficulties and delay in the management come from the frequent denial involving the patient, the parents and even the physician.

In pubertal premenarcheal girls, breast development has more or less occurred but is difficult to evaluate clinically due to weight loss resulting in reduced breast size. Time elapsed between onset of breast development and first clinical evidence of ED (for instance start of weight loss or altered feeding behavior) can be informative since the average interval between onset of breast and first menses is around 2 years. Due to the precocity of growth acceleration in female puberty, growth impairment in these conditions is often less than in earlier forms of EDs.

In postpubertal postmenarcheal girls, amenorrhea is secondary and breast size should have regressed after having been completed. These patients can be opposed to the very early forms since they should have experienced almost fully mature body image and functioning before starting an ED. Since about 95% of adult height is attained at the time of menarche, the consequences for growth are usually not a relevant matter of concern in such patients. However, bone mineralization can still be impaired in these conditions and warrants evaluation and management. Rationalization capacity is commonly greater in these patients with less denial.

Out-Patient vs. In-Patient Management of the Adolescent Patient with ED

In this review, we elect to discuss several somatic manifestations of EDs and address the issue whether management is possible on an out-patient basis or requires referral to an in-patient unit and based on which criteria (table 3). A prerequisite to therapy is that a diagnosis has been made as clear as possible and communicated to the patient and the close relatives. It is crucial that EDs are identified and presented as serious diseases having no single causes and overriding rational explanations and solutions. It is generally agreed that no univocal treatment does exist and that multidisciplinary management plus time are required for improvement [43].

Weight loss does usually not respond to dietary recommendations or even strict guidelines. Its management is indirect through weight limits assigned to the patient for consideration of hospital admission. The significance of the weight limit is protection against a condition that could or would become life-threatening. Weight gain objectives can also be assigned in a given period of time (weeks). Though indicative values of weight and BMI limits are given in table 3, they deserve integration with the other somatic and psychiatric components and their changes over time. In patients with weight loss exceeding 20%, refeeding must be very progressive with a supplementation in mineral nutrients because of the risk of refeeding syndrome. This involves metabolic disturbances (hypophosphoremia, hypomagnesemia, hypokalemia, hypocalcemia and hypoglycemia) and may cause a potentially lethal multivisceral failure. The daily energy intake should start with 500 kcal and increase to 1,500 within a week of time. Initial water intake should be also limited to 500 ml/day [44, 45].

Arrested puberty and amenorrhea would require estrogen alone or associated with progestin depending on the developmental stage attained. Sex steroid administration in EDs is controversial. Reappearance or occurrence of menstruations could be badly accepted by patients denying femininity and warrants open discussion with the patient before being initiated. An indication of hormonal therapy is contraception even in amenorrheic adolescents who could be sexually active. In other instances, there is no consensus about the duration of amenorrhea before treatment is proposed to the patient. Such proposal seems reasonable after 1 year of follow-up, even more when amenorrhea persists despite weight regain [44].

As discussed above, osteopenia is multifactorial and cannot be prevented by a single treatment. Because nutritional deficiency is likely a most important factor that requires a long time before getting back to normal conditions, supplementation with calcium and vitamin D is systematic. The effects of estrogen substitution are not convincing as discussed above. In patients with severe bone demineralization accounting for fractures and risk of neurological consequences when the spine is involved, biphosphonates and in-patient management should be considered.

Metabolic disturbances deserve some comments since they are especially frequent in the patients with purgative behaviors like vomiting or laxative abuse. Discrete early

Table 3. Somatic aspects in the management of anorexia nervosa

Clinical manifestations or complications	Out-patient management	Criteria for in-patient admission
Weight loss	Increase energy intake	Cachexia, weight falling below 35% of normal weight for height or BMI <14
Arrested puberty (and growth) Amenorrhea primary, secondary	Estrogen or estroprogestative replacement; after 6-12 months' evolution?	
Osteopenia	Calcium 1,000–1,500 mg/day Vitamin D min 800 U/day Estro-progestative? Biphosphonates?	Vertebrae compression Bone fracture
Dental enamel erosion due to iterative vomiting	Mouth rinsing with clear water Teeth brushing >20 min after vomiting	
Pyrosis –esophagitis – gastritis	Antiemetics Ranitidine Omeprazole Gastric plaster	Mallory-Weiss syndrome Superior mesenteric artery syndrome
Low blood pressure Moderate bradycardia	Physical effort limitation Etilefrin 5 mg/day (starting dose)	Bradycardia <40/min Systolic blood pressure <80 mm Hg QT lengthening, arrhythmia Nonobstructive cardiomyopathy
Muscle weakness, fatigue	Potassium supplements 20 to 40 mEq/day Magnesium 10 mmol/day (250 mg/day)	Severe metabolic disturbances: K <2.5 mmol/l, Na <125 mmol/l or >150 mmol/l, Mg <0.5 mmol/l, phosphorus <0.5 mmol/l, hypoglycemia <2.5 mmol/l, hypoglycaemia, renal insufficiency
Anemia	Iron supplementation if necessary	Leucocytes <2,000/mm^3 or platelets <100,000/mm^3
Constipation	Dietary counselling Osmotic laxatives, mucilages	
Motor or sensory function slowing down		Reduced speech fluency Brain damage or atrophy Seizure (hypoglycemia, water intoxication, etc.)

Table 4. Comparative features of AN and sportive lean adolescent girls with similar BMIs

	AN patient investing physical activity	Strenuously sportive lean adolescent girl
Physical activity	compulsive, restless, permanent	programmed training, competition
Energy intake	restricted	insufficient vs. energy expenditure
External factor	peers, models	coaches, peers
Weight loss	rapid, rather early	progressive with increased intensity of activity
Amenorrhea	may precede weight loss recovery of menses not systematic after weight correction	follows weight loss and resumes after weight gain
Signs of disturbed homeostasis	reduced heart rate, blood pressure and peripheral flow rate	normal heart rate, blood pressure and peripheral flow rate
Self-image	distorted	realistic
Leanness	denied	acknowledged
Effects of estrogen replacement or contraceptive pill	no significant change in general wellbeing and bone density	improvement in general well-being and bone density

signs of such behaviors can be detected: dry or scaly skin, melanodermia, breakable nails, hair loss; callus at the metacarpo-phalangeal articulations of second and third fingers due to iterative frictions during induction of vomiting; tongue inflammation and/or salivary glands hypertrophy (especially parotid gland) due to frequent compulsive binge eating. Some biological disturbances can also be found, relatively specific of AN (table 3). Severe complications involve gastrointestinal tract such as Mallory-Weiss syndrome as well as other functions such as cardiac arrhythmia secondary to electrolyte anomalies.

The Lean Exercising Adolescent

Both AN patients with hyperactive behavior and some adolescent girls involved in strenuous physical activity share amenorrhea, leanness and exercising as common features. Menstrual disturbances can involve close to 25% of lean sportive adolescent, depending on type, duration and intensity of activity as well as nutritional status [46].

In addition, biological stigmata may show similar alterations in both conditions such as hypercortisolism. This finding is consistent with chronic stress condition either physically or mentally or both. It is, however, difficult to evaluate the pathogenetic role of stress in the occurrence and the persistence of dysfunction of the energy balance and the reproductive system in those patients. In table 4 are summarized some features helping in the differentiation between adolescent girls with AN and female amenorrheic athletes. It should be noted that some subjects initially involved in strenuous physical activity can secondarily develop typical ED such as AN. Interestingly, it appears that estro-progestin treatment in female athletes result in increase in body weight and bone mineralization without affecting physical performances [47]. This is in contrast with studies in AN patients showing that use of contraceptive doses of estro-progestin does not significantly increase bone mineralization [48, 49].

Conclusions

EDs, particularly AN in female adolescents, require integration of different perspectives for pathogenesis, diagnosis and management. Age and developmental stage at occurrence of the disease determine differences in short-term consequences on growth and sexual development as well as long-term outcomes. A common feature to these patients, however, is the requirement of time for improvement, accounting possibly for similar feelings and attitudes among patients, families and even care-givers: denial or minimization, opposition or control, failure or powerlessness. Therefore, clarifying and supporting can help and global appraisal is needed together with constant re-evaluation in a network of care providers. Several conditions such as adolescents involved in strenuous physical activities, are to be separated from EDs but can predispose to EDs. This should be kept in mind to propose, when appropriate, preventive measures that could hopefully reduce the frequency of true EDs that remain serious and life-threatening conditions.

References

1 Chamay-Weber C, Narring F, Michaud PA: Partial eating disorders among adolescents: a review. J Adolesc Health 2005;37:417–427.

2 Dominé F, Berchtold A, Akré C, Michaud PA, Suris JC: Disordered eating behaviors: what about boys? J Adolesc Health 2009;44:111–117.

3 Giedd JN: The teen brain: insights from neuroimaging. J Adolesc Health 2008;42:335–343.

4 Neumark-Sztainer D, Hannan P: Weight-related behaviors among adolescent girls and boys: results from a national survey. Arch Pediatr Adolesc Med 2000;154:569–577.

5 Neumark-Sztainer D, Wall MM, Story M, Perry CL: Correlates of unhealthy weight-control behaviors among adolescents: implications for prevention programs. Health Psychology 2003;22:88–98.

6 DSM-IV – American Psychiatric Association: Diagnostic and Statistical Manual of Mental Disorders, ed 4. Washington, 1994.

7 International Statistical Classification of Diseases and Related Health Problems, revision 10. Version for 2007.

8 Godart N, Perdereau F, Jeammet P: Données épidémiologiques: anorexie chez l'adolescent. J Pédiatr Puériculture 2004;17:327–330.
9 Lewinsohn PM, Hops H, Roberts RE, Seeley JR, Andrews JA: Adolescent psychopathology. I. Prevalence and incidence of depression and other DSM-III-R disorders in high school students. J Abnorm Psychol 1993;102:133–144.
10 Patton GC, Selzer R, Coffey C, Carlin JB, Wolfe R: Onset of adolescent eating disorders: population based cohort study over 3 years. BMJ 1999;318:765–768.
11 Santonastato P, Friederici S, Favaro A: Full and partial syndromes in eating disorders: a 1-year prospective study of risk factors among female students. Psychopathology 1999;32:50–56.
12 Rome ES, et al: Children and adolescents with eating disorders: the state of the art. Pediatrics 2003;111:98–108.
13 Ferrero FP, Rouget PC: Bulimia and weight variations in a Swiss population. Int J Eating Disord 1991;10:563–569.
14 Flament MF, Ledoux S, Jeammet P: Boulimie et autres troubles du comportement alimentaire à l'adolescence: étude épidémiologique dans une population française scolarisée. Ann Med Psychol 1993;151:635–642.
15 Klump KL, Kaye WH, Strober M: The evolving genetic foundations of eating disorders. Psychiatr Clin North Am 2001;24:215–225.
16 Horne R, Van-Vactor J, Emerson S: Disturbed body image in patients with eating disorders. Am J Psychiatry 1991;148:211–215.
17 Audenaert K, et al: Decreased 5-HT2a receptor binding in patients with anorexia nervosa. J Nucl Med 2003;44:163–169.
18 Brewerton T, Jimerson D: Studies of serotonin function in anorexia nervosa. Psychiatry Res 1996;62:31–42.
19 Treasure J, Campbell I: The case for biology in the aetiology of anorexia nervosa. Psychol Med 1994;24:3–8.
20 Södersten P, Bergh C, Ammar A: Anorexia nervosa: towards a neurobiologically based therapy. Eur J Pharmacol 2003;480:67–74.
21 Kaye W, et al: Neurobiology in anorexia nervosa: clinical implications of alterations of the function of serotonin and other neuronal systems. Int J Eating Disord 2005;37:S15–S19.
22 Stice E, Presnell K, Bearman SK: Relation of early menarche to depression, eating disorders, substance abuse, and comorbid psychopathology among adolescent girls. Dev Psychol 2001;37:608–619.
23 Leon GR, Fulkerson JA, Perry CL, Keel PK, Klump KL: Three to four year prospective evaluation of personality and behavioral risk factors for later disordered eating in adolescent girls and boys. J Youth Adolesc 1999;28:181–196.
24 Stice E, Mazotti L, Krebs M, Martin S: Predictors of adolescent dieting behaviors: a longitudinal study. Psychol Addict Behav 1998;12:195–205.
25 Wang SS, Houshyar S, Prinstein MJ: Adolescent girls' and boys' weight-related health behaviors and cognitions: associations with reputation- and preference- based peer status. Health Psychol 2006;25:658–663.
26 Johnson-Sabine E, Wood K, Patton G, Mann A, Wakeling A: Abnormal eating attitudes in London schoolgirls: a prospective epidemiological study: factors associated with abnormal response on screening questionnaires. Psychol Med 1988;18:615–622.
27 Wonderlich SA, Brewerton TD, Jocic ZM, Dansky BS, Abbott DW: Relationship of childhood sexual abuse and eating disorders. J Am Acad Child Adolesc Psychiatry 1997;36:1107–1115.
28 Stice E: Risk and maintenance factors for eating pathology: a meta-analytic review. Psychol Bull 2002;128:825–848.
29 Rierdan J, Koff E: Depressive symptomatology among very early maturing girls. J Youth Adolesc 1991;20:415–425.
30 Berger U, Weitkamp K, Strauss B: Weight limits, estimations of future BMI, subjective pubertal timing and physical appearance comparisons among adolescent girls as precursors of disturbed eating behavior in a community sample. Eur Eat Disord Rev 2008;16:1–9.
31 Nichols JF, et al: Prevalence of the female athlete triad syndrome among high school athletes. Arch Pediatr Adolesc Med 2006;160:137–142.
32 Burns T, Crisp AH: Outcome in anorexia nervosa in males. Br J Psychiatry 1984;145:319–325.
33 Crisp AH, Burns T, Bhat AV: Primary anorexia nervosa in the male and female: a comparison of clinical feature and prognosis. Br J Med Psychol 1986;59:123–132.
34 Crisp AH, et al: Anorexia nervosa in males: similarities and differences to anorexia nervosa in females. Eur Eat Disord Rev 2006;14:163–167.
35 Neumark-Sztainer D, Story M, Dixon LB, Murray DM: Adolescents engaging in unhealthy weight control behaviours: are they at risk for other health compromising behaviours? Am J Publ Health 1998;86:952–955.

36 Warren MP, Ramos RH, Bronson EM: Exercise-associated amenorrhea: are altered leptin levels an early warning sign? Physician Sports Med 2002;30: 41–46.
37 Lebrethon MC, Aganina A, Fournier M, Gerard A, Parent AS, Bourguignon JP: Effects of in vivo and in vitro administration of ghrelin, leptin and neuropeptide mediators on pulsatile gonadotrophin-releasing hormone secretion from male rat hypothalamus before and after puberty. J Neuroendocrinol 2007;19:181–188.
38 Welt CK, Chan JL, Bullen J, Murphy R, Smith P, DePaoli AM, Karalis A, Mantzoros CS: Recombinant human leptin in women with hypothalamic amenorrhea. N Engl J Med 2004;351:987–997.
39 Gindoff PR: Menstrual function and its relationship to stress, exercise, and body weight. Bull NY Acad Med 1989;65:774–786.
40 Hartman D, Crisp A, Rooney B, Rackow C, Atkinson R, Patel S: Bone density of women who have recovered from anorexia nervosa. Int J Eat Disord 2000;28:107–112.
41 Golden N: Eating disorders in adolescence and their sequelae. Best Pract Res Clin Obstet Gynaecol 2003;17:57–73.
42 Godart NT, Flament MF, Lecrubier Y, Jeammet P: Anxiety disorders in anorexia nervosa and bulimia nervosa: co-morbidity and chronology of appearance. Eur J Psychiatry 2000;15:38–45.
43 Anderson AE, Hedblom JE, Hubbard FA. Multidisciplinary team treatment for patients with anorexia nervosa and their families. Int J Eat Disord 2006;2:181–192.
44 de Tournemire R, Alvin P: Prise en charge somatique dans l'anorexie mentale: recommandations médicales. Neuropsychiatr Enfance Adolesc 2001; 49:384–392.
45 Melchior JC: Le syndrome de renutrition inappropriée. Med Hyg 1996;54:850–856.
46 Nichols JF, Rauh MJ, Lawson MJ, Ji M, Barkai HS: Prevalence of the female athlete triad syndrome among highschool athletes. Arch Pediatr Adolesc Med 2006;160:137–142.
47 Rickenlund A, et al: Effects of oral contraceptives on body composition and physical performance in female athletes. J Clin Endocrinol Metab 2004;89: 4364–4370.
48 Golden NH, Lanzkowsky L, Schebendach J, Palestro CJ, Jacobson MS, Shenker IR: The effect of oestrogen-progestatin treatment on bone mineral density in anorexia nervosa. J Pediatr Adolesc Gynecol 2002;15:135–143.
49 Munoz MT, Argente J: Anorexia nervosa in female adolescents: endocrine and bone mineral density disturbances. Eur J Endocrinol 2002;147:275–286.

Dr. Françoise Dominé
Service de Pédiatrie, CHR de la Citadelle
Boulevard du 12ième de Ligne, 1
BE-4000 Liège (Belgium)
Tel. +32 4 225 61 11, E-Mail Francoise.Domine@chrcitadelle.be

Prof. Jean-Pierre Bourguignon
Service de Pédiatrie, CHU de Liège, site N.D. des Bruyères
Rue de Gaillarmont, 600
BE-4032 Chênée (Belgium)
Tel. +32 4 367 92 75, E-Mail jpbourguignon@ulg.ac.be

Sultan C (ed): Pediatric and Adolescent Gynecology. Evidence-Based Clinical Practice. 2nd, revised and extended edition. Endocr Dev. Basel, Karger, 2012, vol 22, pp 287–301

Adolescent Contraception

Dan Apter

The Sexual Health Clinic, Family Federation of Finland, Helsinki, Finland

Abstract

Sexual health for adolescents is based on three components: recognizing sexual rights, sexuality education and counseling, and confidential high-quality services. Contraception needs to include prevention of both STIs and pregnancy. The main options for adolescents are condoms backed-up by emergency contraception; and hormonal contraceptives in a longer, mutually monogamous relationship. Condoms and hormonal contraception together can be well recommended for adolescents. Condom use should not be stopped before it is reasonably certain that the partner is STI-negative. Other alternatives can be considered in special cases. Improved contraceptive methods do not automatically lead to reduced numbers of adolescent abortions. The prevention of unintended adolescent pregnancies requires four elements: a desire to use protection, a good contraceptive method, ability to obtain the contraceptive method, and ability to use it. All these components are important, and if one is missing contraception will fail. In the developed countries, we have good contraceptive methods, but improvements are still needed in the other components. When adolescent sexuality is not condemned but sexuality education and sexual health services instead are provided, it is possible to profoundly improve adolescent sexual health with comparatively small costs. Each year new groups of young people mature, requiring new efforts.

The greatest number ever of young people is now entering their reproductive age. Just based on this large number, population growth is still expected to increase in developing countries, although the number of children per couple is decreasing [1]. The use of contraception has increased markedly, also among adolescents. The demand for contraception is expected to continue to rise rapidly for the next few decades as population size continues to grow and people's aim at fertility declines to near or below replacement levels. Method choice is affected by trends in several factors, including access to different methods, user characteristics, and technology. The large majority of users rely on modern methods. There are no medical reasons to exclude any reversible method based on young age alone. Contraindications for adolescents are basically the same as for adults.

Pregnancy [2] is a leading cause of death for young women aged 15–19 years worldwide, with complications of childbirth and unsafe abortion being the major factors. For both physiological and social reasons, girls aged 15–19 years are twice as likely to die in childbirth as those in their 20s. Girls under age 15 years are five times as likely to die as those in their 20s. Thus, contraception saves lives. Effective contraception is also an essential means of reducing the burden on our environment [1].

Sexual health for adolescents is based on three fundamental components: (1) recognizing sexual rights, (2) sexuality education and counseling, and (3) confidential high-quality services. These components all need to be considered together. A holistic approach to contraceptive provision involves considering the individual's overall sexual and reproductive health needs. By informing adolescents of potential risks, benefits and uncertainties in a language that they can understand, clinicians can enable women to reach their own contraceptive choices. Access can be enhanced by service innovations such as nurse prescribing. Several means of prevention need to be considered:

1 Prevention of pregnancy – use of contraceptive methods.
2 Prevention of STIs – use of condoms and avoiding risks.
3 Prevention of bad feelings/desperation – use of sense, consideration and avoiding risk taking.

A growth milieu supporting the self-esteem of the young person together with adequate and sufficient sexuality education helps her to make choices to maintain and protect her sexual health [2].

'Studies show that money spent to delay births to adolescents and prevent HIV infections is repaid many times over in direct savings and indirect economic gains', the UNFPA report [3] says: 'Enabling young people to delay or avoid pregnancy, coupled with education and job opportunities and respect for their rights, can have enormous economic benefits for families, communities and nations and help alleviate poverty at all levels'.

Sexual Behavior

National surveys conducted in Europe show differences in the transition to younger age at first intercourse. This transition first started in the Nordic countries, and followed in most other Western Europe countries. The mean age of women at their first intercourse decreased after the 1960s by 2–3 years. During the 1980s this age remained rather stable. In some countries a further decrease occurred in the 1990s. A similar decrease started in central and Eastern Europe one generation later (20–30 years). Mean ages at first intercourse are 16–18 years for women and men in western Europe, whereas it is reported to be around 1–2 years higher for women in eastern Europe countries, as summarized by Bajos et al. [4].

Sexuality Education

Knowledge about various contraceptive methods and a desire to use protection are essential for successful contraception. Comprehensive sexuality education has been found to improve contraceptive use [5]. On the other hand, abstinence only education had no effect on the incidence of unprotected sex, number of partners, condom use, or sexual initiation [6]. Thus, the programmes need to be comprehensive in order to work. Sexuality education is described in more details in the chapter by Apter and Molina Cartes [this vol.].

Sexual Health Services

Services for adolescents can be provided in various settings, as long as certain basic principles are observed. The needs of adolescents differ from those of adults. High quality care of adolescents calls for special clinics. The clinic should have a youth-friendly atmosphere [2], where young people can feel welcome and comfortable. Unquestionable confidentiality is important. However, legislation about the rights of minors to confidentiality differs between countries. Many countries also have an age limit, age of legal consent, before which sexual intercourse is not allowed. In most legislation, it is specified that it is not allowed for an adult to have sex with a child below that age. In some countries, this specification is missing, and this has caused concerns about prescribing contraception for adolescents below the age of legal consent. Still, it is better to prescribe contraception than to have an unwanted pregnancy.

The providers must not moralize and judge the adolescents, but treat adolescents with respect indicating that young people are important. Most important is strengthening of self-esteem, contributing to a feeling that their body and their sexuality are valuable and need to be protected. In that way adolescents learn to respect and take care of themselves and others. Services should be available at an affordable price, which preferably means free of charge. The threshold to come to the clinic should be low. The adolescents should be able to drop in or get an appointment without having to wait long. School health care may provide an easy-access service, which can fulfil the requirements for a high-standard adolescent care.

Use of Contraception among Adolescents

Contraceptive prevalence and method used varies markedly [3]. With increasing availability, the percentages that have used some contraception at first intercourse have increased (fig. 1).

Condom is the most common first-used contraceptive method. With increasing age and entering a more stable relationship, adolescents switch to hormonal methods,

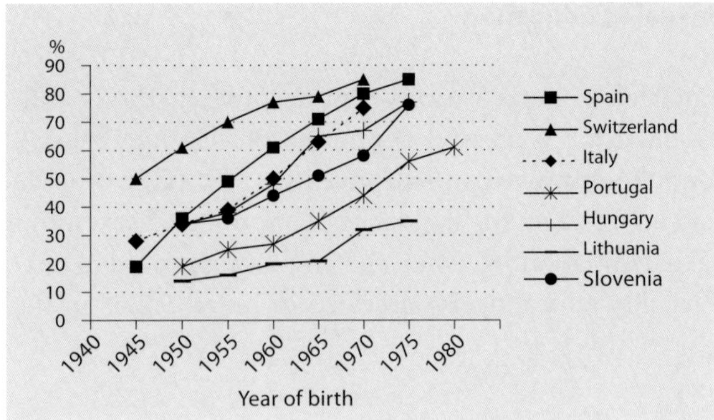

Fig. 1. Percent use of contraception at first intercourse in relation to year of birth, 1945–1980. From Bajos et al. [4].

Table 1. Recommended choices of contraception for adolescents

1	Condom + emergency contraception back up
2	Hormonal contraceptives + condom
3	Oral contraceptives or other hormonal contraception

mainly the combined oral contraceptives. Double contraception, condom for protection against STIs and combined oral contraceptives for better protection against pregnancies, is recommended (table 1), but, except in the Netherlands, not largely used. The contraceptive method used at the most recent intercourse is given in table 2 for Finland from a large school-based study [7].

The figures for abortion generally show an inverse correlation to contraceptive use. Where reliable modern methods are widely used, the need of abortion is low. In Russia, the majority of pregnancies end in abortion, which remains the primary method of birth control. In the Czech Republic, the use of hormonal contraception increased 10-fold from the early 1990s in 10 years, and abortions decreased by 60%.

What Is Needed before Prescribing?

During recent years, appropriate knowledge has been gathered and good guidance produced for prescribing contraception. The World Health Organization (WHO) has produced Medical Eligibility Criteria for Contraceptive Use (WHOMEC) [8] providing evidence-based recommendations to ensure women can select the most appropriate method of contraception without imposing unnecessary restrictions. The UK Medical Eligibility Criteria (UKMEC) was developed from the WHO document in 2005 and an updated version is available on the Faculty website [9]. Conditions

Table 2. Answers by female students in Finland 2008 to the question 'What contraceptive method did you use at your most recent intercourse', and the % having had intercourse according to school grade

	Secondary school		High school		Vocational school	
	grade 8	grade 9	grade 1	grade 2	grade 1	grade 2
Age range	14–15	15–16	16–17	17–18	16–17	17–18
Nothing, %	20	15	7	7	15	13
Condom, %	61	53	53	44	36	30
Oral contraceptive, %	11	23	31	39	40	47
Condom and oral contraceptive, %	6	8	8	9	7	8
Other method, %	1	1	1	1	1	1
Percent of all having had intercourse	14	30	36	52	69	79

Total number of responders about 100,000 [7].

Table 3. UK Medical Eligibility Criteria (UKMEC) categories

UKMEC 1	a condition for which there is no restriction for the use of the contraceptive method
UKMEC 2	a condition for which the advantages of using the method generally outweigh the theoretical or proven risks
UKMEC 3	a condition where the theoretical or proven risks usually outweigh the advantages of using the method[1]
UKMEC 4	a condition which represents an unacceptable health risk if the contraceptive method is used

[1] The provision of a method to a woman with a condition given a UKMEC category 3 requires expert clinical judgement and/or referral to a specialist contraceptive provider since use of the method is not usually recommended unless other methods are not available or not acceptable.

are divided into four categories (table 3). The WHO and UK Selected Practice Recommendations for Contraceptive Use [10, 11] recommend examinations and tests that should be performed before providing contraception (table 4). It should be observed that breast, pelvic and genital examination, cervical cytology screening and routine laboratory tests are not recommended routinely as they do not contribute substantially to combined oral contraceptive safety [12]. Particularly, fear for the pelvic examination might reduce the likelihood of young adolescents seeking services. A recording of blood pressure and BMI should be documented for all women before a first prescription of combined oral contraceptives [12]. The risk of STI should be assessed and chlamydia testing offered when appropriate.

An appropriate history should be taken. The clinician should enquire about: medical conditions (past and present), family history and drug history (prescription,

Table 4. Which examinations are needed before a first prescription of combined hormonal contraception?

1	A blood pressure recording should be documented for all women prior to a first prescription
2	BMI should be documented for all women prior to a first prescription
3	Pelvic/gynecological examination and cytology screening are not recommended

Table 5. Medical eligibility criteria for combined hormonal contraception in relation to migraine

a	Nonmigrainous headache (mild or severe)	UKMEC 1
b	Migraine	
	i Without aura, age <35 years	UKMEC 2
	ii Without aura, age ≥35 years	UKMEC 3
	iii With aura, at any age	UKMEC 4
c	Past history of migraine with aura at any age	UKMEC 3

nonprescription and herbal remedies). Knowledge of previous contraceptive use, sexual and reproductive health will help tailor advice for each individual woman. The medical history should alert the clinician to conditions or risk factors that might be a strong or absolute contraindication to combined oral contraceptive use [12]. For example, cardiovascular disease is rare in young women but potentially serious. Risk factors for cardiovascular disease (smoking, obesity, hypertension, thrombophilia, previous venous thromboembolism (VTE), hyperlipidemia)should be specifically enquired about. A woman with multiple risk factors may need to avoid combined oral contraceptives use, although individual risk factors would not necessarily contraindicate use. Various guidelines differ slightly regarding the impact of obesity. Obesity increases the risk of VTE. In the UK 2009 updated edition, BMI of 30–34 equals UKMEC 2 and BMI 35 or above equals UKMEC category 3 for combined hormonal contraception (CHC) [9]. All forms of progestin-only contraception are category 1 in relation to BMI. Age is an independent risk factor for VTE [13]. So, for women aged above 35 years with a BMI greater than 30, a more critical approach is warranted than for an adolescent. Migraine is common among adolescents and may contraindicate combined oral contraceptive use and should be enquired about. Table 5 gives examples of medical eligibility criteria in relation to migraine.

Various Contraceptive Methods

The adolescent choses to use the method she is most comfortable with, that suits her particular life situation at the moment, and that she knows well based on sufficient counseling.

Table 6. Medical eligibility criteria for combined hormonal contraception in relation to hypertension

a	Adequately controlled hypertension	UKMEC 3
b	Consistently elevated blood pressure (properly measured)	
	i Systolic >140–159 mm Hg or diastolic >90–94 mm Hg	UKMEC 3
	ii Systolic ≥160 mm Hg or diastolic ≥95 mm Hg	UKMEC 4
c	Vascular disease	UKMEC 4

Most evidence relates to combined oral contraceptives, but applicable also for ring and patch use, but not progestin only.

Condom

Condom is well-suited contraception for adolescents, because it prevents pregnancies and diminishes the risks of STIs including HIV [14] and cervical cytology changes. Young people know these benefits, but are still not using condoms regularly. Many circumstances influence condom use, like the price, difficulties in buying them, unplanned sexual experiences, alcohol and drug using and the willingness to take risks. The use of a condom may inconveniently interrupt the sexual act, because the placement of it on a penis must occur after erection has taken place, but before intercourse begins. Street survival strategies, including sexual activity for money and drug use, put street youths in situations at considerable risk for HIV infection [15].

The male condom is the most commonly used method of contraception in the age group below 18 years both for girls and boys [7]. Of sexually active men and women aged 16–19 years, 92% and 80%, respectively, had had sex using a condom in the last year [16].

The only contraindication to the use of latex condoms is for people with sensitivity or allergy to latex proteins (risks generally outweigh benefits, UKMEC Category 3 [17]. The presence of a positive skin test to latex allergens or the demonstration of specific immunoglobulin E (IgE) antibodies in serum is described as sensitivity to latex. The diagnosis of a true latex allergy is difficult. Most reactions due to latex allergy are clinically mild and localized to the penis or vulva in the form of pruritis, edema of the skin, mucous membranes or subcutaneous tissues. Symptoms usually develop 24–48 h after exposure in a sensitized person. The most serious clinical syndrome (type I hypersensitivity) can manifest with symptoms as above but the onset is quicker. People with type I latex allergy are at risk of anaphylaxis [17]. For people with sensitivity or allergy to latex proteins the use of nonsensitizing male and female polyurethane condoms is recommended. The use of a female condom has remained rather limited in most countries.

Nonoxinol-9 (N-9) is the only spermicidal agent available in many countries, including Finland and UK. Epithelial disruption in the vagina and rectum has been noted with use of N-9 [18]. The potential irritant effects of N-9 on mucosa may increase the likelihood of STI transmission including HIV. Epithelial damage is more likely with frequent use. Several studies have investigated the safety and effectiveness of N-9 and these were reviewed by WHO [18] and the Centers for Disease Control and Prevention [19]. There is no evidence that N-9 lubricated condoms provide additional protection against pregnancy or STIs compared with condoms lubricated with a nonspermicidal lubricant [18, 19]. Therefore, the use of condoms lubricated with spermicidal is not generally recommended. When using lubricant with latex condoms a non-oil-based preparation is recommended.

The true failure rate (method failure) for male condoms in the first year of use is 2% [20]. The typical use failure rate (method failure plus user failure) is around 15% [20]. A Cochrane Review of RCTs compared eight latex male condoms with four nonlatex male condoms in terms of contraceptive efficacy, rates of breakage and slippage, safety, discontinuation of use and user preference [21]. Pregnancy rates were similar for latex and nonlatex condoms.

With consistent and correct use, the method failure rate for female condoms is 5% while the typical use failure rate is 21% [20].

It is essential to learn the correct use of condoms, before they are needed. Counseling about condoms should include advice on correct use, appropriate use of lubricant, STI screening and when emergency contraception may be required.

Emergency Contraception

Emergency contraception or postcoital contraception is a method used after intercourse to prevent the beginning of a pregnancy. Thus, it is not related to abortion. Levonorgestrel only (1.5 mg) as a single dose [22] has replaced the Yuzpe method of a high-dose of ethinylestradiol (200 μg) combined with levonorgestrel (1 mg) as it has less side effects and higher efficacy. Increasing interval from intercourse to emergency contraception use lowers the efficacy [23], it should be taken as soon as possible and its efficacy is questionable after 72 h. There are no relevant contraindications to levonorgestrel emergency contraception, and it is not teratogenic. Levonorgestrel 1.5 mg is now available without prescription in most European countries. According to statistics in Finland, removing the need of prescription for emergency contraception increased its use and decreased the number of abortions among 15- to 19-year-old girls with 10% within 6 months. Otherwise, evidence is lacking of an effect at population level in reducing abortions. Promotion of its use has been restricted and the use has remained small in comparison with other contraceptive methods.

Ulipristal as a 30-mg tablet has recently become available as an alternative hormonal emergency contraception. Ulipristal acetate (also known as CDB-2914 and VA2914) is a synthetic steroid derived from 19-norprogesterone. It is a selective progesterone receptor modulator (SPRM). It is available only by prescription. The advantage is that it can be used up to 5 days. The cost is about double compared to levonorgestrel 1.5 mg, but this might vary between countries. Ulipristal has possibly more interactions with other medications, and it may weaken the effect of progestin-based continuous hormonal contraception [24]. If hormonal contraception is continued after administering ulipristal, barrier contraception should be used until the next period. In the first 3 days, its efficacy is about the same as for levonorgestrel and about 2% of the users become pregnant [25]. As placebo-controlled randomized trials have not been possible to perform, the actual preventive effect of hormonal emergency contraception is not known but seems rather low, particularly compared to other contraceptive methods.

Copper IUD can be inserted as a form of emergency contraception up to 5 days after unprotected intercourse. Particularly when it can remain in place for continuous contraception, it is a good alternative as its efficacy is much better than hormonal emergency contraception.

Emergency contraception is a good addition to condom use: if the condom breaks, there is still a further possibility to prevent pregnancy. Adolescents need to be counseled on the correct use of emergency contraception. However, the preventive efficacy of hormonal emergency contraception should not be overestimated; it is much lower than regularly used contraception. Consultation for emergency contraception should be used as an opportunity to start a continuous contraceptive method. Quick start is described below.

Combined Oral Contraception

According to the WHO guidelines, hormonal contraception can be safely used from the age of menarche onwards. Contraindications are basically the same for adolescents as for adults [8]. No intervals are needed in the use of hormonal contraception. Combined oral contraceptives work primarily by inhibiting ovulation. Ovulation is inhibited by action on the hypothalamic-pituitary-ovarian axis to reduce luteinizing hormone and follicle-stimulating hormone. The first seven pills are needed to cause inhibition of ovulation. The remaining 14 pills maintain anovulation. If used consistently and correctly combined oral contraceptives provide effective contraception. The Pearl index for combined oral contraceptives (i.e. the number of failures per 100 woman-years of exposure) is estimated at 0.3–4.0, depending on the consistency of use [12]. US studies usually report higher failure rates than European. During the usual 7 pill-free days the endometrium sheds and most women will have a withdrawal bleed. Contraceptive protection is maintained during the pill-free interval as long as pills before and after are taken consistently and correctly.

Combined oral contraceptives are widely used in adolescence. They are useful in a stable relationship. However, this can mean anything between one week to one year, and condom use should not be stopped before it is reasonable certain that the partner is STI-negative. Condoms and combined oral contraceptives together can be well recommended for adolescents. Most pills contain ethinylestradiol 20 or 30 µg. There are no clear guidelines which dose to use [26]. The 30-µg dose might provide better bleeding control in some subjects, but for most 20 μg seems enough. In cases of risk for low bone mineral density (BMD), the 30-μg pill might be better. The progestin component varies between brands and provides some specific characteristics.

What a clinician should assess before prescribing combined oral contraceptives is described above. Blood pressure measurement is essential and mandatory in all women considering combined oral contraceptive use. Women with a BP measurement consistently over 140 mm Hg systolic and/or 90 mm Hg diastolic should be advised against use of combined oral contraceptives. For females with a family history of venous thromboembolism in a first-degree relative under the age of 45 years, or with other risk factors putting her in MEC category 2–4 (obesity, migraine), a progestin only method should be considered. Epilepsy medication and other liver enzyme-inducing drugs are not very uncommon, and significantly reduce the efficacy of hormonal contraception.

There are several noncontraceptive benefits of combined oral contraceptives. Adolescents often have irregular cycles, and with combined oral contraceptives the bleedings come regularly. A randomized, double-blind placebo-controlled trial showed a significant reduction in dysmenorrhea with combined oral contraceptives [27]. The amount of bleeding usually decreases. Acne, a common condition in adolescence, significantly improves with combined oral contraceptives (summarized in ref. [12]). Some even help for PMS-like symptoms [28].

Longer continuous use is becoming increasingly popular. For example, the pill is taken continuously for 3 months, and then there is a 1-week interval allowing a withdrawal bleeding. In this way, bleedings occur four times per year. There are no particular health risks with this procedure. In situations with dysmenorrhea or other menstrual-related problems, well-being is improved. Theoretically, contraceptive efficacy would also improve, but evidence for this is still lacking. Continuous use has also been tested for up to 1 year [29]. Breakthrough bleedings occur with decreasing frequency with this rhythm.

New Routes

New ways of administering combined estrogen-progestin preparations are now available. The contraceptive vaginal ring is a good alternative for those who have difficulties in taking tablets daily, as it remains in place in the vagina for 3 weeks without the need of intervention. It has particularly good bleeding control [30] and, in our practice, has worked well for adolescents. The dermal patch is another alternative, it is changed weekly. The medical eligibility criteria are the same for the combined ring and patch as for combined oral contraceptives. Other new ways of administering hormonal contraception are being developed.

Progestin Only Contraception

The progestin-only pill needs to be taken more accurately than combined oral contraceptives and is frequently associated with poor bleeding control [8]. Therefore, its use is mainly considered when there are contraindications or problems with other methods. Obesity or hypertension for progestin-only pills and implants is MEC 1, migraine with aura MEC 2.

Adolescents have used implants extensively. First the Norplant six-implant system followed by Jadelle with two implants and Implanon with one. Contraceptive efficacy is excellent, but bleeding control is variable and nonpredictive. About a third are amenorrheic, which can be seen as an additional benefit. As a long-acting reversible contraceptive method, the implant can be a good choice.

The progestin-releasing IUD, such as Mirena, is most efficient in reducing the amount of bleeding and menstrual pain. In adolescents in whom uterine size approaches that of adults, it can be inserted easily [31]. With appropriate counseling, the amenorrheic effect is seen as an important benefit.

Hormonal injections are commonly used in some but not most European countries. Depo-medroxyprogesterone acetate (DMPA) every 3 months has been related to a tendency of weight increase and some concerns of BMD. DMPA is associated with a small reduction in BMD but this usually recovers after discontinuation [32]. Evidence for the long-term effects of DMPA on BMD in females below 18 years is lacking. Other contraceptive methods do not seem to have clinically relevant effects on BMD. MPA concentrations are not affected by epilepsy medication such as carbamazepine and other liver enzyme-inducing drugs and thus MPA is one of the few systemic hormonal contraceptive methods that can be reliably used with these medications.

Quick Start

Traditionally, hormonal contraception is advised to start on the first day of a menstrual bleeding or up to day 5 without the need of additional contraceptive protection. Quick start of contraceptives refers to starting the use of a method immediately, regardless of where the woman is in her menstrual cycle. This can be done if it is reasonably certain that she is not already pregnant. In this situation, additional contraception such as a condom is needed for the first 7 days. This rule is for starting combined hormonal contraception as well as progestin-only methods including implants and levonorgestrel IUD.

One can be reasonably sure that a woman is not pregnant if she has no signs of pregnancy (preferably checked by a pregnancy test), and has not had intercourse since the start of her last normal menses or has correctly since used a reliable method of contraception. Further details are provided elsewhere [12, 33]. Quick start increases the likelihood that the contraceptive method will indeed be started and provides client satisfaction, indirectly reducing the risk of unintended pregnancies [33].

Intrauterine Device

The ideal IUD users are women who have at least one child. However, both copper and the levonorgestrel-releasing IUD can be used in nulliparous women as well, i.e. UKMEC 1. There is no reduction in fertility associated with previous intrauterine method use. An STI might influence fertility and sexual history taking is important. The progestin-releasing IUD can be used to treat abundant bleedings also for adolescents, and it offers some protection against pelvic inflammatory disease. For the age from menarche to 20 years, the new edition of UKMEC gives category 2.

Diaphragms and Spermicides
Diaphragms, cervical caps, spermicides and sponges are usually not the first choice for adolescents because they are often uncomfortable and difficult to use, so the application is not consistent and correct. They might also increase the incidence of vaginitis, because the removal may be delayed after intercourse and postcoital hygiene is variable. Contraceptive efficacy is rather low [20], but for special situations these methods need to be available.

Rhythm Methods and Withdrawal
Adolescents often have irregular menstrual cycles making rhythm methods unreliable, and it is also difficult for adults to have periodical abstinence. For very young adolescents it is reasonable to emphasize the emotional aspects of a relationship and the desirability of sometimes saying 'no'. Withdrawal is a widely used method among adolescents, but it mainly prevents sexual pleasure, not STIs and rather poorly pregnancies.

Counseling and Follow-Up

Providing good counseling is most essential in sexual health. In taking the sexual history, the clinician learns the life situation of the adolescent, and can provide appropriate advice. Each young person should be made aware of the confidentiality of all health care team members. An adolescent aged less than 16 (might vary depending on national legislation) should also be made aware that in case coercion or abuse is suspected confidentiality might be broken and child protection will be involved. Possible health concerns and beliefs about infertility, weight gain, etc., should be addressed. Services for vulnerable young people may be delivered within the mainstream services. Prescription of contraception is done by different health care workers in different countries. Nurses or midwives can have a central role, but good contact and possibility to frequent consultations with doctors experienced in contraception is needed. Young people should be encouraged to return at any time if they develop problems with contraception. More frequent follow-ups than for adults may be appropriate [34]. Adolescents should be advised to return for follow-up in 3 months after starting hormonal contraception. Various written material can complement oral information.

Conclusions

For adolescents, contraception always needs to include the prevention of STIs as well as of pregnancies. Counseling should include all areas of risk-taking behavior: alcohol and drug use, smoking, travelling alone, situations easily leading to abuse. It is important to teach self-respect and responsibility. The contraceptive choice should be individualized considering all circumstances. The main options for adolescents are condoms backed-up by emergency contraception, and hormonal contraceptives in a longer, mutually monogamous relationship. Other alternatives can be considered in special cases.

Improved contraceptive methods do not automatically lead to reduced numbers of adolescent abortions. The prevention of unintended adolescent pregnancies requires four elements: a desire to use protection, a good contraceptive method, the ability to obtain the contraceptive method, and the ability to use it. All these components are important and if one is missing contraception will fail. In the developed countries, we have good contraceptive methods, but improvements are still needed in all the other components. Motivation to take care of oneself and others is based on many interactions, and to that we can all contribute as parents, teachers and health care providers.

The overall developments in society – gender equality, equal education opportunities for boys and girls, development of the health care system, positive attitude changes of the state and Church – all make it possible to reach good sexual health through extended provision of sufficient and reliable sexuality education, confidential services and a wide selection of contraceptive methods. When adolescent sexuality is not condemned but sexuality education and sexual health services are provided instead, it is possible to profoundly improve adolescent sexual health with comparatively small costs. Each year new groups of young people mature requiring new efforts on our parts.

References

1 UNFPA: The State of World Population 2009. http://www.unfpa.org/swp/2009/en/pdf/EN_SOWP09.pdf

2 WHO: In McIntyre P (ed): Adolescent Friendly Health Services – An Agenda for Change. Geneva, WHO, 2002.

3 UNFPA: State of the World Population 2003. Making 1 Billion Count: Investing in Adolescents' Health and Rights. www.unfpa.org: United Nations Population Fund 2003.

4 Bajos N, Guillaume A, Kontula O: Reproductive health behaviour of young Europeans. Population studies, No 42. Strasbourg, Council of Europe Publishing, 2003, vol 1.

5 Kirby DB, Laris BA, Rolleri LA: Sex and HIV education programs: their impact on sexual behaviors of young people throughout the world. J Adol Health 2007;40:206–217.

6 Underhill K, Montgomery P, Operario D: Sexual abstinence only programmes to prevent HIV infection in high income countries: systemic review. BMJ 2007;335:248–259.

7 National Institute for Health and Welfare: School Health Promotion Study. http://info.stakes.fi/kouluterveyskysely/FI/index.htm.

Table 4. Continued

Variable/category	Pregnancy		Delivery		New Born	
Height						
1.35–1.50 m	1.34	0.94–1.91	1.39	0.95–2.01	2.16 *	1.29–3.64
1.51–1.60 m	1.04	0.74–1.46	1.06	0.74–1.51	1.93 *	1.18–1.61
1.61 m and + (reference)	1		1		1	
Nutritional state (brachial perimeter)						
Normal (reference)	1		1		1	
Thinness	1.14	0.89–1.45	1.32 *	1.04–1.67	1.70 *	1.11–2.60
Obesity	1.13	0.60–2.12	1.74 *	1.14–2.67	1.70 *	1.11–2.60

Table 4 shows that the significant personal characteristics, associated with the risk of morbidity in pregnancy (RR > of 1 and $p < 0.05$) were: indifferent attitude at the onset of pregnancy and at the end of pregnancy and school level ranging between 1st and 4th grade.

The variables associated with risk of morbidity at delivery were: pregnancy resulting from rape and a nutritional level described as having lost weight or overweight according to brachial perimeter and estimation of muscle mass. The variables associated with morbidity at delivery were: a height of 1.50 or under and obesity.

Table 5 shows that the risk of pregnancy pathology is associated with the condition of 10 or more prenatal controls. The precocity of the initiation of prenatal control is also a risk factor in the newborn baby. These results are confusing, since in this experience early prenatal control is conditions greater risk of detection of pathology. This result occurs in models in which prenatal control is routine. As expected, there is a higher risk of delivery pathology and for the newborn baby in the antecedent of pregnancy and delivery pathology.

Table 6 analyses the characteristics of the progenitor of the pregnancy and the family of the adolescent. We can see that the only significant variable related to a higher risk of morbidity is being a student or being a member of the military service associated with a higher risk of pregnancy morbidity. There are no significant differences in the rest of the groups with or without evidence of pathology.

All these variables (17 during pregnancy, 18 at delivery and 19 in the newborn) were included in the multifactorial analysis, the results of which are summarized in table 7. The risk variables during pregnancy are the same as those described for student partner or military service and the attitude of the adolescent at the onset of pregnancy. In this last variable, the positive attitude is expressed as protective (β–0.90), so the negative attitude needed to appear as reciprocal to consider the risk. Two new variables appear, a significant one is the age of menarche. The more advanced the age of menarche the lower the risk of pathology (β –0.15). The age of menarche should be approximately 11 years.

Table 5. Quality of medical care and current obstetric pathology related to risk of morbidity

Variable/category	Pregnancy		Delivery		New Born	
	RR	CL	RR	CL	RR	CI
Prenatal visits						
1–3	1		1		1	
4–6	1.13	0.84–1.53	1.26	0.91–1.75	1.14	0.82–1.60
7–9	1.29	0.97–1.72	1.24	0.90–1.72	1.20	0.86–1.67
10 and +	1.37 *	1.00–1.86	1.35	0.96–1.92	1.31	0.92–1.88
Gestational age at first control						
7–15 weeks	0.93	0.63–1.37	1.07	0.71–1.63	1.55 *	1.01–2.38
16–20 weeks	1.03	0.72–1.47	1.17	0.81–1.72	1.75 *	1.17–2.61
21–25 weeks	1.09	0.76–1.54	1.20	0.82–1.77	1.57 *	1.04–2.37
26–30 weeks	1.03	0.72–1.48	1.18	0.80–1.74	1.40	0.92–2.15
31–40 (reference)	1		1		1	
Current pregnancy pathology						
No	–		1		1	
Yes	–		1.36 *	1.13–1.65	1.40 *	1.15–1.71
Current delivery pathology	–		–		1.58 *	1.30–1.92

Table 6. Partner and adolescent's family characteristics related to risk of morbidity

Variable/category	Pregnancy		Delivery		New Born	
	RR	CI	RR	CI	RR	CI
Partner activity						
Stable labor (reference)	1		1		1	
Occasional labor	1.20	0.92–1.57	0.86	0.65–1.14	1.31	0.98–1.74
Student/army service	1.53 *	1.20–1.96	1.07	0.83–1.39	1.30	0.97–1.73
No activity	1.05	0.76–1.46	1.14	0.85–1.53	1.20	0.85–1.69
Partner attitude						
Positive	1		1		1	
Negative	1.05	0.87–1.27	0.95	0.76–1.19	0.81	0.64–1.02
Indifferent	0.71	0.45–1.12	1.31	0.94–1.82	0.61	0.35–1.05
Family attitude beginning prenatal control						
Positive	1		1		1	
Negative	0.99	0.80–1.21	0.97	0.78–1.21	0.75	0.60–0.93
Indifferent	0.77	0.45–1.30	1.01	0.63–1.61	0.75	0.44–1.26
Family attitude at end prenatal control						
Positive	1		1		1	
Negative	1.09	0.91–1.31	0.94	0.77–1.16	1.00	0.81–1.25
Indifferent	0.91	0.56–1.49	1.22	0.82–1.81	1.13	0.71–1.80

Table 7. Predictive risk variables for pregnancy: delivery and newborn in pregnant adolescents

Variable	Category	Beta	SE	χ^2	p	R	Comments
Pregnancy[1]							
Partner activity	student/army service occasional work	0.978 0.467	0.257 0.277	14.51 2.86	0.0001 0.090	0.157 0.041	increases the risk increases the risk
Age of menarche	older menarche age	(–) 0.159	0.078	4.08	0.0043	(–) 0.0064	lower age is the risk
Brachial muscle area at 20 weeks	large brachial area	(–) 0.0004	0.0002	3.56	0.059	(–) 0.055	small brachial area is the risk; thinness is the risk
Adolescent attitude beginning pregnancy	positive attitude	(–) 0.904	0.553	2.67	0.102	(–) 0.036	indifferent or negative attitude is the risk factor
Delivery[2]							
Pregnancy sexual situation	seduction and rape	0.855	0.185	13.54	0.0036	0.122	in the analysis, infinite risk appears when the name of the partner is unknown
Stature	the higher stature	(–) 0.034	0.019	2.91	0.088	(–) 0.097	the risk is the lower stature
Newborn[3]							
Stature	the higher stature	(–) 0.053	0.020	6.78	0.009	(–)0.097	stature 1.50 m or less is the risk
Secondary education level	1–2 years middle	0.481	0.231	4.35	0.037	0.068	conflict of pregnant student
Partner activity	student and army service	0.384	0.230	2.80	0.094	0.040	high risk of abandonment
Delivery pathology	existence of pathology	0.419	0.218	3.69	0.055	0.058	existence of pathology

[1] Sensibility: 50.3; specificity: 74.5; correct: 63.9; false (+): 39.3; false(–): 34.3.
[2] Sensibility: 53.8; specificity: 60.2; correct: 57.5; false(+): 49.7; false(–): 36.5.
[3] Sensibility: 60.8; specificity: 55.0; correct: 57.5; false(+): 49.7; false(–): 34.8.

The other variable of significance is the nutritional state as measured by the brachial circumference before 20 weeks of pregnancy. Information shows that the larger the brachial circumference the lesser the risk of pathology during pregnancy. Nonetheless, thinness should be recorded as a factor of predictive risk. These four variables reached a specificity of 74.5%:

Table 8. Predictive risk factors regarding p value

Variable	Category	p value
Partner activity	student/army service/occasional labor	repeated p value
Stature	1.50 m or less	repeated p values
Pregnancy sexual condition	seduction or rape	0.0036
Instruction level	two years of median level	0.0370
Age of menarche	11 years old or less	0.0430
Brachial muscular area	thinness	0.059
Adolescent attitude at beginning of pregnancy	indifferent or negative	0.102

For the delivery, the model selected two variables for predicting risk of morbidity. Rape once again appears as a strong risk factor. It should be noted that in a more detailed analysis of this variable, when the aggressor is unknown to the victim, risk becomes infinite, which rarely occurs in medicine, because it becomes a certainty.

The other variable was stature. Tallness is protective (β –0.034). Small stature is a risk factor. The specificity of these two variables reached 60.2%.

The model selected four variables for the risk of morbidity in the newborn. Stature, which once again is a protection against morbidity; higher stature (β –0.05). Smaller stature is recorded as a risk factor.

The model selected a new variable, which is 1st and 2nd year secondary education. Once again the activity of the partner – student or in the military service – appears as a risk factor, a variable that is repeated in pregnancy. Delivery pathology is also a risk factor, although it is a late predictive factor. The specificity of these four variables reached 55%.

In short, the model selected a total of 10 variables, with four corresponding to pregnancy, two to delivery and four for the newborn baby. Of the latter, delivery pathology is discarded as it is a late risk predictive factor in primary and secondary levels of healthcare. There are two variables that are repeated as predictive risk factors; activity of the partner, for pregnancy and the newborn baby, and stature at delivery and in the newborn baby.

In order to design a predictive risk model to be applied at different levels of complexity, predictive risk factors were reorganized according to their p value, as can be seen in table 8.

To these factors, we can add two additional factors that were not significant in the study, but which do imply risk from a clinical point of view. These variables are: age 16 or under and being unmarried in the case of some regions or countries. Another risk factor to be considered is the apparition or existence of a prior obstetric or pregnancy related pathology, which follows the same clinical criteria applied to adult pregnant women.

Comments

After the publication of the Aubry and Nesbitt report, a series of experiments were carried out in order to apply quantitative criteria in the determination of obstetric and perinatal risk, which are very well summarized in the WHO 1977 publication. The Collaborative Perinatal Study carried out by the US Department of Health Education and Welfare, whose results were published in 1972, has also been an important contribution to the determination of risk factors. The methodology for group comparison of the latter study allows for the consideration of each factor on its own, without discriminating the relative weighting of each factor. This makes is difficult to apply findings to the selection of pregnant women using predictive risks. Other models use known or supposed risks and make unifactorial analyses to determine projections for population groups but without being able to determine individual risks.

The results of this study are based on the record of facts and conditions of a population of similar characteristics and treated in a same healthcare system. 77% of pathologies during pregnancy had an obstetric cause, with a predominance of pregnancy hypertension syndrome (28.6%), urinary tract infections (23.2%), symptoms or threat of premature labor (19.6%), and anemia (15.9%).

98% of pathologies during delivery had obstetric causes. In the Newborn's first 5 days of life, the most important pathology was icteric syndrome requiring phototherapy (29%), followed by infections and sepsis (16%), and asphyxia and respiratory distress syndrome (12%). Hemolytic disease and Rh incompatibility (11%) was considered when it required treatment.

With this information, we can conclude that the pregnant adolescent population group is a high risk group during pregnancy. The variable attitude of the adolescent towards the baby was eliminated because it was a late factor as it is asked at the end of the pregnancy when many other events have already occurred. The pregnancy and delivery pathology variables do not correspond to pregnancy so they were also disregarded.

As for delivery itself, no variable was eliminated. Three variables were eliminated in the newborn period: filiation of the adolescent, attitude of the partner on learning that the adolescent is pregnant, and attitude of the parents at the beginning of pregnancy. This criterion was adopted because inconsistencies were found when matching these factors with other variables.

We were surprised that age was not selected because it was not statistically significant although it is a clear risk variable from a clinical point of view. 85% of girls under 14 develop pathologies in any of the three periods. This phenomenon is explained because it is a continuous variable that considers year-to-year differences and for this reason differences are scarce. When this variable becomes important and is compared with adult pregnant women, it shows high levels of significance. Nonetheless, this criterion was not used to change the methodology of the multifactorial analysis designed. In this study, the pathology-free control group was also made up by adolescents. It is best to take this factor into consideration in every model as it has an indisputable clinical application. Furthermore, there are other extremely high risk variables that are associated with younger ages as is the case of sexual abuse.

The model finally selected 10 predictive risk variables of which two are repeated in some of the periods analyzed, which gives them greater predictive strength. The delivery pathology factor is a late factor in terms of predictive variables and is used routinely in the clinical context. There are only 7 predictive risk variables left. These are distributed in the three periods. But, in the applicative model they should be considered together and selected in accordance with a criterion that associated them with more than a period and with their level of signification, as expressed in table 8. On analyzing these 7 variables, we see that four are already known or used as risk factors: low stature, age of menarche, malnutrition or thinness and attitude regarding pregnancy.

Similarly, sexual abuse is an extremely high predictive risk, which is well known for its association with unwanted pregnancy and unaccepted children. But, for those countries that do not consider legal abortion, in these cases the factor becomes the highest obstetric and perinatal risk of those analyzed in this study. It was the only factor that reaches statistical infinite risk in the regression analysis when it is associated with an unknown aggressor. Education level as a risk factor is associated with lower education level, which is a confusing variable in the lower socioeconomic level. In this study risk is associated with two years of secondary school, which corresponds to a total of 9–10 years of schooling. This is explained by the serious problem posed by an unwanted pregnancy in an adolescent that attends school that results from a relationship with a sporadic partner, delay in informing the pregnancy, delated medical consultation or the existence of a pathology that cannot be hidden, sudden interruption of life plans and serious family disruptions. Apparently, in our society, pregnancy in adolescents with little schooling is associated with a social medium that has a greater cultural acceptance of the phenomenon and therefore there is an earlier medical control and greater acceptance of routine preventive measures. This factor should be considered in the context of each reality in accordance with the levels of instruction of the population treated.

A unifactorial analysis showed that the early initiation of prenatal control and the larger number of prenatal controls were a factor or greater risk. This finding is confusing, as the groups under study had adequate coverage of prenatal control, and the early control detected more pathology and is an indicator of a group presenting pathology. The same happens with the larger number of visits that is concentrated on the pathology bearing group with a higher frequency of appointments. This indicator should be carefully assessed when group comparison is carried out in an environment of high quality prenatal control.

Four of the variables selected present negative beta readings, which indicate that the risk is lower in the measure that the quality of the variable improves. So, to older age of menarche, there is less risk of pregnancy pathology; the same occurs with a larger brachial muscle area and with a positive attitude of the adolescent at the onset of pregnancy; a taller stature also reduces the risk of delivery pathologies. In these cases, the reciprocal category has been taken as a risk factor in terms of its practical application.

though she perceives her inability to do this. This is frequently reinforced by her significant figures and the professionals with whom she interacts.

(b) Little knowledge of adoption on the part of the adolescent, her family and professionals involved.

(c) Fear of anticipation of future sorrow, not only of the adolescent but also of her family.

(d) Lack of support of the professionals that give her overt orientation regarding this option.

Family Characteristics

The families of pregnant adolescents are usually defined as severely dysfunctional families both in terms of organization and composition, they are also defined as disorganized in they way in which they structure their family activities, in which they state their standards and share responsibilities.

In terms of structure, they are frequently single parent families with a high proportion of female heads of families owing to separation, paternal desertion, widowhood or because they are girls born out of wedlock.

There are often different ways of family structure in successive stages of the vital cycle of the family, which can produce enormous instability in the family's composition and organization, with the corresponding lack of role fulfillment. The natural history of the process generally begins with the marriage or initial living together of the mother, when a given number of children are born; this is followed by paternal desertion and by the mother becoming the head of the family. But in the long or short term, the mother has a new partner, and this male is expected to assume a paternal and supportive role. Nonetheless, the stability of this new relationship is usually rather fragile as it is based more on the need for survival of the family group, and ends in separation. The mother is once again alone and responsible for all her children, which have now increased in number and needs.

There are frequently negative substitute parental figures like stepfathers or mother's lover and/or alcoholic, drug addicted and or violent fathers, grandfathers, or brothers.

In general, they are families that have unsatisfied affection needs and deficient communication especially regarding sexual issues.

Parental and Family Reaction to an Adolescent Pregnancy

The above mentioned follow-up study measured parental attitudes to the pregnancy of an adolescent daughter, as appears in the following table:

Attitude	On learning about pregnancy		At the end of pregnancy	
	n	%	n	%
Positive	144	23.7	368	56.5
Indifferent	28	4.6	81	12.4
Negative	436	71.7	202	31.1
Total	608	100.0	651	100.0

Parental reaction to the news of the pregnancy of their adolescent daughter covers a range of responses which go from a high percentage of initial disapproval which can be expressed in terms of disgust, anger, verbal aggression, physical aggression and making her leave home.

But in the measure that the pregnancy advances, among a large number of parents the initial negative attitude changes to acceptance and resignation. But the percentage of parents that do not change their negative initial attitude is still worrying, as it reflects lack of support and understanding of the daughter at such critical moments. Evidence shows hat the news of the adolescent's pregnancy generates mixed feelings of anxiety, anger and pain in parents and tutors, and especially in mothers, but they must accepts the fact and get ready to receive the arrival of this grandchild into the family despite their feelings. After the birth of the baby of an adolescent mother, there may be conflictive situations within the family related to the rights and duties of rearing a child. Conflictive situations of this kind can have an adverse effect on the normal development of the child.

Social Consequences for the Adolescent Mother

Incomplete Education

The laws that protect the continuity of the education of pregnant schoolgirls are an efficient tool to encourage them to finish their education. But, school maternity generates rejection among the parents of other schoolchildren. Advanced pregnancy makes attending school more difficult and becomes even more difficult after the birth of the baby.

More Numerous Families

Women who become mothers at an earlier age have less schooling and more possibilities of having more children in the future with shorter intervals between each child. The education level achieved by the adolescent mother is strongly associated with her reproductive behavior, on the once side and to her level of awareness about health.

Difficulties in Fulfilling Their Maternal Role

These adolescent mothers have greater difficulty in raising their children. Raising a child is a difficult task even for an adult mother. Successful maternity requires a combination of skills and understanding that cannot be compared to any other responsibility in our lives. It also requires a degree of maturity which is often beyond the grasp of adolescents. This is more evident in those girls who must raise their children practically on their own, without the support of their partner, and without being able to provide for the needs of the children. Insufficient economic resources, acute stress, lack of support from the father of the child, lack of ability and training in maternity and personal problems or needs that prevent them from fulfilling the needs of the dependent child are some of the factors that can contribute to these shortcomings.

Possibility of Being Abandoned by the Partner

Pregnancy frequently changes the affective relationship with the partner who has fathered the child, and in many cases marks the end of this relationship. On telling her partner that she is pregnant, he is generally frightened by this responsibility, as paternity was not within his short-term plans. Diverse studies show that the male reacts negatively in half of the cases, withdrawing or denying his paternity, which indicates that these children will be raised without the affective and economic support of their fathers.

The future probability of these mothers increases when they have a higher degree of schooling, when they are members of a less poorer sector, when they live independently with the father of their baby, and when the father gives economic support for the upkeep of the child.

Fewer Possibilities of Having a Stable, Qualified and Well-Paid Job

Adolescent mothers are more exposed to suffer from chronic underemployment and insufficient income. The mothers and their children have a higher probability of depending on public assistance systems and remaining under the care of their families for a longer time than those women who postpone their maternity until their second decade. As should be expected, the employment participation of adolescent mothers increases with time, but the type of work they gain is related to their limited education and training. Long-term follow-up studies indicate that they have limited labor opportunities.

Greater Difficulty in Improving Their Socioeconomic Level and Less Probability of Social Advancement

The future of the pregnant adolescent is strongly marked by her economic status, by the fact that he partner has left her and the education she attains. Those adolescents that are abandoned by their partners enter the labor market later, in economic distress and with lack of training. But if they had a better education and had more training, they could have better employment opportunities and contribute more to the family income and thus increase their autonomy in family decisions, which would go in benefit of the welfare of their child.

Among the poor, early maternity is associated with the perpetuation of socioeconomic disadvantages and the inequity that women have to face at school and at work.

Lack of Protection of the Recognition of the Child

In many countries, the Civil Code covers diverse ways to establish the recognition of a child, but two are the most used: (a) the father recognizes his paternity by means of a recorded public deed or by registering the child with the Civil Registry Office, and (b) the mechanism for a mother to sue for paternity before a court of law. The alleged father is summoned to court and he must admit or deny his paternity. Once the father has admitted his paternity, the nonmatrimonial filiation link is established, together with the right and duties of each parent. But if the father denies his paternity, the case is closed and he can never be summoned to court for the same case. Other legislations admit paternity investigations through filiation testing such as ADN tests.

There is a strong association between adolescent pregnancy and recognition of the child born out of wedlock with the new filiation rules, owing to the high percentage of children born of adolescent mothers. Children of unwed mothers are greatly discriminated. This situation, in addition to being unjust, has a direct effect on that enormous proportion of mothers that accept responsibility for their children. Adolescent mothers face situations of legal lack of support, and this situating becomes even more difficult in the case of unwed mothers, when the law places them and their children in a detrimental position.

As regards alimony, the legislation has no procedural mechanisms to facilitate it. It is usual from mothers to give up on their demands owing to legal complication and the subsequent bill for food. This situation affects both children born within and outside wedlock and many legislations allow for the grandparents to be made liable for the costs in the case that the parents are unable to fulfill their duties.

In many legislations, there is a progressive acknowledgement of advantages for the child, which includes inheritance rights, social security benefits and the right to support from the father. It guarantees social protection for the child and can help her/him to develop a more positive self image. The interest and support of the father – regardless of the fact that he is married or not to the mother – is of enormous importance to the child and its development.

Measures That Can Reduce Adverse Consequences on Adolescent Mothers and Their Children

Adolescent mothers and fathers should be guided to make their own decisions regarding their child.

When They Decide to Keep the Child

When they decide to keep the child, they should be given guidance to use all the resources available in the community to fulfill their parental responsibilities.

(a) Family placement: in some specific cases, it might be necessary for the child to be placed with a family that has registered as temporary caregivers with the public system for these ends.

(b) Provide facilities for the day care of the child: crèches, day care centers and others that help the adolescent mother's reinsertion into the school system or her incorporation into the labor market.

(c) Alternative school programmes that can help the pregnant adolescent and mother to stay at school and help her to improve her scholastic achievements, together with caring for her child.

(d) Employment training programmes in which they can learn labor skills and use them for a better paid job.

(e) Give attention for the partner of the adolescent, especially if he is an adolescent. He should be taken as a subject that requires service. The adolescent father can face emotional problems that are similar to those of the adolescent mother. Paternity might generate in him conflicts and possible guilt feelings that might prevent his adjustment. He might benefit from discussing his conflicts and his responsibilities towards the child and mother.

(f) Inform the adolescent mother of the advantages of recognition of paternity, which include inheritance rights from the father, social security benefits, and right to paternal support.

(g) Educate the mother in a basic knowledge of child development and train her in discipline techniques that are appropriate for the child.

(h) Speedy access to effective contraceptive methods in order to prevent repeated and unwanted pregnancies.

When the Adolescent Mother Decides to Give Her Child for Adoption

When they decide to keep the child, she should feel that this is a responsible act to give the child a life that she cannot or does not want to give it. She should think of adoption as a responsible act of her maternity. She should receive guidance from a professional or institution that is well aware of the adoption process and can help her with it.

Suggested Reading

Aubry R: Identification of the high risk perinatal patient; in Aladjem S (ed): Perinatal Intensive Care. Springfield, Mosby, 1977.

Wiemann CM, Berenson AB, García-del Pino L, McCombs SL: Factors associated with adolescent's risk for late entry into prenatal care. Family Planning Perpect 1997;29:273–276.

Majluf N, Romero MI, Ubilla G, et al: Nivel de Salud y Atención pediátrica Preventiva: una aplicación de ingeniería de Sistemas. Santiago, Escuela de Ingeniería, Universidad Católica de Chile, 1975.

Molina R, Alarcón G, Luengo X, et al: Estudio Prospectivo de Riesgo en Adolescentes Embarazadas. Rev Ch Obst Ginecol 1988;No 1.

Molina R, Luengo X, Sandoval J, et al: Factores de Riesgo del embarazo: parto y Recién Nacido en adolescentes embrazadas. Rev Ch Obstet Ginecol Inf Adolec 1998;5:17–28.

Niswander K, Gordon M: The women and their pregnancies: the collaborative perinatal study of the National Institute of Neurological diseases and stroke. The US Department of Health, Education and Welfare. Philadelphia, Saunders, 1972.

Oficina Regional de la OMS para Europa: Simposio sobre 'Identificación de Personas de Alto Riesgo y Grupos de Población'. Copenhague, 1971 (EURO. 4911). Schlesselman.

OMS: Clasificación Internacional de Enfermedades Accidentes y Causas de Muerte. Novena Revision. Geneva, World Health Organization, 1977.

Organización Panamericana de la Salud, Organización Mundial de la Salud: La Salud del adolescente y el joven en las Américas. Publicación Científica 1985, No 489.

Singh S, Wulf D: Today's adolescents, Tomorrow's Parents: A Portrait of the Americas. New York, Alan Guttmacher Institute, 1990.

Bibliography of Social Factors Related to Adolescent Pregnancies

Anuarios de Demografía del Instituto Nacional de Estadísticas.

Buvinic M, Valenzuela J, Molina T, González E: The Fortunes of Adolescent Mothers and. Their Children: the Transmission of Poverty in Santiago, Chile. Population Dev Rev 1992;18:269–297.

Buvinic M, Valenzuela J, Molina T, González E: Poverty risk for families of chilean teenager mothers determined by woman education: father's support. Int Family Planning Persp 1993;19:75–75.

Burrows R, Muzzo S: Hijos de adolescentes; in: El adolescente chileno: características. problemas y soluciones. Editorial Universitaria, 1986.

Causby V, Nixon C, Bright J: Influences on adolescent mother-infant interactions. Adolescence 1991;26:619–630.

Compendios Estadísticos del Instituto Nacional de Estadísticas.

Código Civil Chileno.

Furstenberg FF Jr, Brooks-Gunn J, Philip Morgan S: Adolescent Mother in Later Life. New York, Cambridge University Press, 1987.

González E, et al: Actitud de la adolescente, de su pareja y de su familia frente al embarazo. Cuadernos Médico-Sociales 1984;25:112–117.

González E, et al: Características socio-económicas de adolescentes embarazadas en situación irregular. Cuadernos Médico-Sociales 1984;25:100–105.

González E: Adolescente embarazada: aspectos sociales; in: Embarazo en adolescentes. Diagnóstico 1991. Doc Sernam-Unicef 1991, pp 69–78.

González E, et al: Características Sociales y Asunción del Rol Paterno en las Parejas de las Adolescentes Embarazadas'. Contribución al II Congreso Nacional de Investigaciones Sociales y Médico-sociales Sobre Juventud, 1992.

Hardy JB, Zabin LS: Adolescent Pregnancy in an Urban Environment. Vienna, Urban & Schwarzenberg, Urban Institute, 1989.

Hayen CD: Risking the Future: Adolescent Sexuality and Childbearing. Washington, National Academy Press, 1987.

Irarrázabal I, Valenzuela JP: La ilegitimidad en Chile: Hacia un cambio en la formación de la familia? Serie Documentos de trabajo n1 188.1992, Centro de Estudios Públicos.

Mitchel F, Brindis C: Adolescent pregnancy: the responsibilities of policymakers. Health Services Res 1987;22:399–437.

Molina R, et al: Estudio Prospectivo de Factores de Riesgo en Adolescentes Embarazadas. Rev Chilena Obst Ginecol 1988;53:27–34.

Molina R, Luengo X, Guarda P, González E, Jara G: Adolescencia: sexualidad y embarazo. Serie Científica Médica n1 2, 1991.

Molina R, Luengo X, Toledo V, González E: La Adolescente Embarazada en Chile. Asociación Red para la Infancia y la Familia de América Latina y el Caribe, 1992, pp 80–105.

Molina R, Luengo X, González E: Normas para la atención de la Adolescente Embarazada; in: Manual de Medicina de la Adolescencia. OPS Washington, Serie Paltex 1992, vol 1 20, pp 486- 501.

OPS: La Salud del Adolescente y el Joven en las Américas. Publicación Científica n1, p 489.

Sexualidad y Embarazo en Adolescentes: CEAAL: Consejo de Educación de Adultos de América Latina. Centro Internacional de Investigaciones para el Desarrollo, 1989.

Smith P, Weinman M, Munford D: Social and affective factors associated with adolescent pregnancy. J School Health 1982:90–93.

La Transición de la Fecundidad en Chile, 1950–1985: Un análisis por grupos socioeconómicos y áreas geográficas. Centro Latinoamericndo de Demografía, Fascículo F/CHI. 7.

Ramiro Molina Cartes
Centro de Medicina Reproductiva y Desarrollo Integral de la Adolescencia (CEMERA), Facultad de Medicina, Universidad de Chile
8380455 Santiago (Chile)
E-Mail ramiromolina@med.uchile.cl

Sultan C (ed): Pediatric and Adolescent Gynecology. Evidence-Based Clinical Practice. 2nd, revised and extended edition. Endocr Dev. Basel, Karger, 2012, vol 22, pp 332–356

Sexuality Education: Finnish and Chilean Experiences

Dan Apter[a] · Ramiro Molina Cartes[b]

[a]The Sexual Health Clinic, Family Federation of Finland, Helsinki, Finland; [b]Centro de Medicina Reproductiva y Desarrollo Integral de la Adolescencia (CEMERA), Facultad de Medicina, Universidad de Chile, Santiago, Chile

Abstract

All children and young people have the right to age-appropriate sexuality education regardless of gender, sexual orientation, ability or faith. Sexuality education provides knowledge, skills and positive values to determine and enjoy their sexuality, have safe, fulfilling relationships if one so wishes and decides, and to take responsibility for their own and for a possible partner's sexual health and well-being. Several international programs have been developed and recently published by the Population Council, IPPF and other coworkers, by UNICEF, and by WHO Europe. This chapter will briefly describe recent global development in sexuality education, and then, as examples, experience from two countries, Finland and Chile. The experiences from these school based programs suggest an important role of sexuality education.

To write about sexuality education in a clinical book of pediatric and adolescent gynecology is very complicated. The approach should be from the clinical experience. One should also consider the approach in developed and developing countries. For that reason this chapter will recall the Symposium of the International Federation on Pediatric and Adolescent Gynecology at the XIX FIGO World Congress of Gynecology and Obstetrics hold in Cape Town, South Africa in October, 2009.

The basic differences between developing and developed countries are the fecundity rates among 15- to 19-year-olds and contraception use at the first coitus and actual contraceptive use of sexually active adolescents. There are not large differences at the age of first coitus. Many developed countries allow abortion but the majority of the developing countries do not.

What Are the Solutions to This Problem?

We will answer the question by looking at two different experiences and try to bring forward the evidence in this matter. Two approaches to these subjects will be presented. The first is a revision of sexuality education around the world and the experience in

Finland. The second is the approach to the prevention of first and repeated pregnancies in adolescents in Chile, a country with very strict abortion legislation.

Impact of Sexuality Education Programs on Adolescent Sexual and Reproductive Health

Sexual development brings along dreams and wishes of a new kind of relationship. A maturing young person is in many aspects lonely and uncertain, and thus sensitive and vulnerable. Supporting the self-esteem of the young person together with adequate and sufficient sexuality education helps her make choices to maintain and protect her sexual health. Sexual health for adolescents is based on three fundamental components:

1 Recognizing sexual rights.
2 Sexuality education and counseling.
3 Confidential high-quality services.

These components all need to be considered together. The closer sexuality education programs and sexual health services work together, the better are the results.

The term sexuality education often causes confusion, as it is not always understood what is meant by it. IPPF offers the following definition:

> 'Comprehensive sexuality education must equip young people with the knowledge, skills, attitudes and values they need to determine and enjoy their sexuality – physically and emotionally, individually and in relationships. It views sexuality holistically and within the context of emotional and social development. Information is not enough. Young people need to be given the opportunity to acquire essential life skills and develop positive attitudes and values.' [1]

Recently, in the Standards for Sexuality Education in Europe [2], sexuality education was defined as learning about the cognitive, emotional, social, interactive and physical aspects of sexuality. Sexuality education starts early in childhood and progresses through adolescence and adulthood. For children and young people, it aims at supporting and protecting sexual development. It gradually equips and empowers children and young people with information, skills and positive values to understand and enjoy their sexuality, have safe and fulfilling relationships and take responsibility for their own and other people's sexual health and well-being. It enables them to make choices which enhance the quality of their lives and contribute to a compassionate and just society. All children and young people have the right to have access to age-appropriate sexuality education. In this definition, the primary focus is on sexuality as a positive human potential and a source of satisfaction and pleasure. The clearly recognized need for knowledge and skills required to prevent sexual ill-health comes second to this overall positive approach. Furthermore, sexuality education should be based on internationally accepted human rights, in particular the right to know, which precedes prevention of ill health.

In 2009, UNESCO (together with other UN organizations) published 'Technical Guidance on Sexuality Education' in two volumes [3]. Sexuality education should equip children and young people with information, skills and positive values to determine and enjoy their sexuality, have safe fulfilling relationships if one so wishes and decides, and to take responsibility for their own and for a possible partner's sexual health and well-being. All children and young people have the right to age appropriate sexuality education regardless of gender, sexual orientation, ability or faith.

Table 1. Sexuality education must help young people to (SAFE project 2006) [3]

- Acquire accurate information
  On sexual and reproductive rights; information to dispel myths; references to resources and services
- Develop life skills
  Such as critical thinking, communication and negotiation skills, self-development skills, decision-making skills; sense of self; confidence; assertiveness; ability to take responsibility; ability to ask questions and seek help; empathy
- Nurture positive attitudes and values
  Open-mindedness; respect for self and others; positive self-worth/esteem; comfort; nonjudgmental attitude; sense of responsibility; positive attitude toward their sexual and reproductive health

A third large international program for sexuality education, It's All One Curriculum, was developed by an international working group and published by the Population Council [4].

The purpose of sexuality education to help young people as defined by the SAFE project [5] is presented in table 1.

In addition to sexuality education, sexual health services are needed to improve sexual health. Counseling is an essential part of the services. Sexual health services for adolescents can be provided in various settings, as long as certain basic principles are observed. The services should have a youth-friendly atmosphere, where young people can feel welcome and comfortable, as described by The National Adolescent-Friendly Clinic Initiative, NAFCI [6]. Unquestionable confidentiality is very important. The providers must not moralize and judge the adolescents, but have a positive attitude in changing risk behavior and treat adolescents with respect indicating that young people are important. In this way self-esteem is strengthened, and adolescents learn to respect and take care of themselves and others.

Rationale for Sexuality Education

The sexuality education provided should be well planned, continuous, and adapted to the developmental stage. Three kinds of guidance are needed:

(1) Counseling, which occurs in direct interpersonal relationship and is based on recognizing individual needs.

(2) Sexuality education is typically given in schools or other social situations, where a group of young persons of similar age listen to lectures, see educational material and can discuss. Individual needs are not possible to consider.

(3) A third approach is information campaigns about sexual health through, for example, mass media.

All young people have the right to comprehensive sexual and reproductive health information, education and services, to be active citizens, to have pleasure and confidence in their sexuality, and to be able to make their own informed choices. A comprehensive positive approach to sexuality education contributes to addressing not only the health and well-being of young people, but also their sexual and reproductive rights. According to WHO [7], countries providing extensive sexuality education have better succeeded in limiting unintended adolescent pregnancies as well as sexually transmitted infections. In some studies, it has been difficult to demonstrate an effect of individual sexuality education programs.

UNESCO commissioned a recent review of the impact of sexuality education on sexual behavior as part of the development of International Guidelines on Sexuality Education [3]. The review considered 87 studies from around the world; 29 studies were from developing countries, 47 from the United States and 11 from other developed countries. All of the programs were designed to reduce unintended pregnancy or STIs, including HIV; they were not designed to address the varied needs of young people or their right to information about many topics. The program had to be a curriculum- and group-based sex or HIV education program on sexual behavior and mediating factors <25 years anywhere in the world. The research methods had to include a reasonably strong experimental or quasi-experimental design with both intervention and comparison groups and both pre- and post-test data collection, and measure the program impact upon one or more of the following sexual behaviors: initiation of sex, frequency of sex, or number of sexual partners; use of condoms or contraception more generally; composite measures of sexual risk. 70% were implemented in schools and the remainder were implemented in community or clinic settings. Many were very modest, lasting less than 30 h or even 15 h. The review examined the impact of these programs on those sexual behaviors that directly affect pregnancy and sexual transmission of HIV and other STIs. This is an extension of earlier reviews of Kirby et al. [8]. The authors were able to show that sexuality education works. Two thirds of the programs significantly improved one or more sexual behavior. One third of the programs delayed initiation of sexual activity, two thirds had no effect, and none hastened initiation. Almost half (44%) of the programs decreased the number of sexual partners, none increased the number. Of the 46 studies measuring program impact on condom use, almost half (40%) showed increased condom use; none found decreased condom use. Thus, the evidence is strong that programs do not hasten or increase sexual behavior but, instead, some delay or decrease sexual behaviors or increase condom or contraceptive use.

Effective curricula incorporated 17 characteristics that describe the curricula development, the goals, teaching strategies, and their implementation. Programs were effective across a wide variety of countries, cultures and groups of youth. Replications of studies also indicate that programs remain effective when implemented by others in different communities, provided all the activities are implemented as intended in similar settings.

On the other hand, Underhill et al. [9] reviewed sexual abstinence-only programs to prevent HIV infection in high-income countries. 13 trials enrolling 16,000 US youths were identified, all outcomes were self-reported. No program

Table 2. How good is the evidence for effect of sex education on different outcomes?

Improved knowledge	strong
Improved skills	good
Less risk behavior	good
Contraceptive use	mixed
Pregnancy reduction	weak
STI prevention	weak

Based on presentation by Professor Judith Stephenson.

affected the incidence of unprotected sex, number of partners, condom use, or sexual initiation. Thus, the programs need to be comprehensive in order to work. Judith Stephenson, Margaret Pyke Professor of Sexual and Reproductive Health, UK, summarized our knowledge of the impact of sexuality education at FIGO in 2006 (table 2).

STIs and pregnancy occur less frequently than sexual activity, condom or contraceptive use. The distributions of the outcome measures of STI or pregnancy require that very large samples are used to measure the impact adequately. Several studies employing biological markers have failed to demonstrate significant results. A nationwide approach is described later for Finland. But the aim of sexuality education should not only be to induce behavioral changes. To increase knowledge is an aim in itself. To improve skills, like interaction and negotiation, is also important. To reflect on values and attitudes, respect for self and others, and improve self-esteem and self-confidence are essential features of sexuality education.

Introducing Sexuality Education: Example Europe

Sexuality education has been introduced at very different times in various European countries. In Sweden, sexuality education in school already became obligatory in 1955.

Introduction of mandatory sex education [5]:

1955– Sweden

1970–1980 Austria, Czech Republic, Denmark, Finland, Germany, Hungary, Iceland, Luxemburg, Norway

1990–2006 Belgium, Estonia, France, Greece, Ireland, Latvia, Netherlands, Portugal, Slovakia.

Sexuality education remains very diverse in Europe. In some countries, it is said to begin at 5–6 years of age, in others at 14–18 years. Every third country does not have specific standards available. The aims and contents are highly variable. Professional responsible for teaching might be specific teachers only, any teacher plus health professional or specific teacher plus health professional.

Across Europe, different definitions and terminology are used to refer to sexuality education, varying from 'family life education' (Hungary, Poland, Slovakia) through to 'life skills education' and 'sex and relationships education'.

In order to address the rights of young people to information about sexuality, multiple topics need to be covered. In order to promote low risk-taking among young people, both risk and protective factors that affect decision-making need to be addressed. Both of these approaches take time: nearly all the programs in schools found to have a positive effect upon long-term behavior have included 12 or more sessions, and sometimes 30 or more sessions, that last roughly 50 min.

To be maximally effective, curricula must be consistent with the community, culture, age and sexual experience of the students. Characteristics of effective programs are described in the International Guidelines on Sexuality Education of UNESCO [3], and detailed standards for sexuality education are being developed by a working group within WHO Europe [3].

Country Example: Finland

The experience from Finland reflects the impact of sexuality education and sexual health services, and particularly the importance of a good connection between these. Sexuality education became obligatory in schools in 1970. In 1972, it became the duty of local municipalities to provide counseling in contraception free of charge for the whole population. Both developed slowly, but in good cooperation. The overall development in society – gender equality, equal education opportunities for boys and girls, development of the health care system, positive attitude changes of the state and Church have all made it possible to reach the present situation through extended provision of sufficient and reliable sexuality education, confidential and high-quality services and wide selection of contraceptive methods [10].

Within The Family Federation of Finland, an approach called 'The nine stairs of sexuality' has been created based on the gradual development of sense, emotion and biology of the child (fig. 1). This has been well accepted by various faith leaders as well.

As an indicator of improving sexual health, adolescent abortion and delivery rates declined continuously to low levels in mid-1990s (fig. 2). For various reasons sexual health services were cut in the mid-1990s. At the same time, sexuality education became an optional subject which led to a deterioration of both its quality and quantity [12]. Not surprisingly, the adolescent abortion rate increased by 50% over the following 7 years (fig. 2). Annual school health surveys by Stakes (National Institute for Health and Welfare) started in the late 1990s, i.e. every even year in the eastern part of Finland, and every odd year in the western part of Finland, thus covering the whole country. The large questionnaire included questions about sexual behavior and contraceptive use. As seen in figure 3a, in the late 1990s during the time of poor sexuality education, the percentage of girls starting to have intercourse at an early age, during

Chilean Approach: Sexuality Education and the Prevention of First and Repeated of Adolescent Pregnancy

There are 5 pillars leading to prevention of the first and repeated pregnancies in adolescents.

The first pillar is the intervention on the social conditioning factors of precocious pregnancy. This measure is in the very long term.

The second pillar is the transversal, permanent, ongoing, curricular sex education by trained teachers and that includes the school community. This pillar has the evidence found in Chile as follows:

Impact of the Sex Education Program: Adolescence, Time of Decisions
A quasi experimental cohort study of cases and controls was carried out during 2 years (1994–1995), based on the implementation of a sex education program for school-attending adolescents, applied by teachers in two educational establishments (cases). The controls were three establishments in which no sex education programs were offered. The program was approved by the education authorities, the schools, the PTA centers and by Student Councils.

The teachers and administrative staff were given specific training. Two handbooks that had been tested previously were used with teachers: one for workshops with students and another for workshops with parents and caregivers. An on-site office manned by professionals was set up for 2 years to provide orientation and support to students, teachers and parents, and for referring students to the CEMERA Care Centre. Table 1 gives the characteristics of the schools that have been subjected to intervention and those that have not. The grades studied ranged from the 8th to the 11th grade, for 2 full years of cohort observation.

The information was collected from anonymous surveys carried out in each school on the same day and same time for all students. In 1993 two manuals for Teachers were produced for working with students and parents: 'Adolescence: Time of Decisions' (workshops for adolescents with 18 sessions) and 'Adolescents: Time of Decisions'. (workshops for parents — 5-session workshops). Finally, these manuals were published by Editorial Mediterraneo and are available to the public.

In January 1994, teachers received 4.5 days of training. In March, parents and caregivers were asked for written authorization which led to the 1st survey (initial survey). The first monitoring and assessment survey to assess progress was carried out in November–December 1994, and was only applied in intervened schools The second survey, together with the first follow-up, was carried out in November-December 1995, and the third survey or second follow-up took place in November-December 1996 (fig. 1).

In the course of the 2 years of intervention, different meetings were held between the CEMERA team and the intervened high schools.

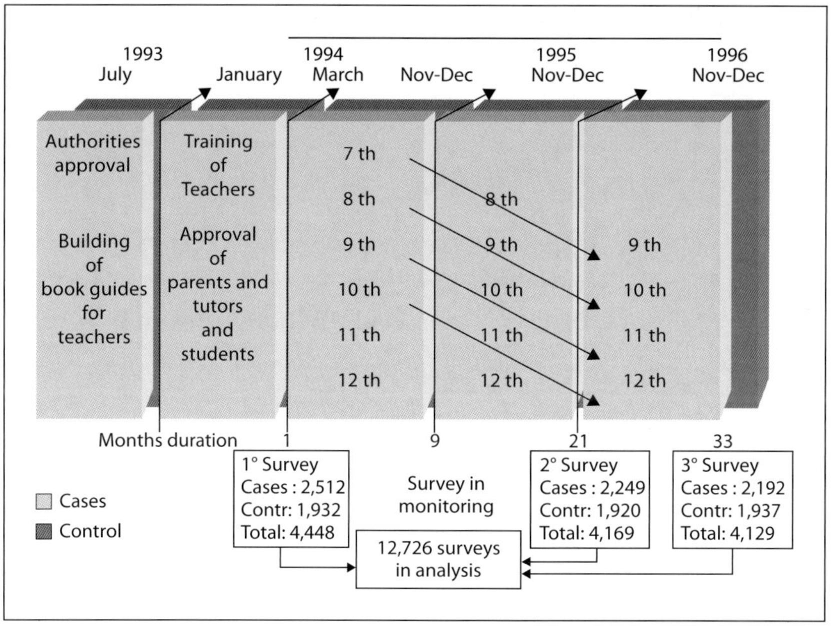

Fig. 1. Impact analysis. The surveys were anonymous. During the period in which the program was applied, there were changes in the school population, as some students graduated because they had finished school, some had changed school or abandoned the school system, to which we must add the arrival of new students coming from other schools that joined different grades. Incoming students had access to sex education, but were not given the initial or final survey. For greater security, the intermediate and final survey contained questions that made it possible to identify those that were not included in the initial survey, and ensure that they would not be taken into account in the final analysis when new students answered them despite instructions to the contrary, and would not be detected in the lists of new students in the hands of the research team. The analysis considered the total number of students who replied the initial and final survey. Therefore, the information corresponds to a group cohort subjected to intervention and assessed in a before and after pattern. The number of initial surveys is greater than the final surveys. In addition, inconsistent initial and final surveys were eliminated.

Table 1. Schools and students included in the study

Characteristics	High schools – cases						High schools – controls								
High schools involved	Darío Salas			Sta Juliana			P. Ultra			A-31			P. Balmaceda		
Years 1994–1996	94	95	96	94	95	96	94	95	96	94	95	96	94	95	96
Total number of grades	50	48	48	18	21	21	16	23	23	19	20	23	21	23	23
Number of grades intervened	45	43	43	18	21	21	nonapplicable–not intervened								

Description	Quantitative surveys				Visits to clinic and attention		Meetings	
	Initial	End	End	End	Office at high school	CEMERA	Assessment	Training
Case high school students	*	*	*	*	*	*	*	
Control high school students	*		*	*				
Delegate students							*	
Case high school teachers					*		*	*
Parents and caregivers					*	*	*	

Fig. 2. Schedule of assessments and evaluation of the controlled study.

Individual Counseling and Orientation
In the course of the 2 years, in both 'case' high schools, offices in charge of CEMERA professionals were implemented to provide individual or group attention to students and teachers, and to deal with the overall co-ordination of the project.

Clinical Attention for Adolescents
The most important component of the program was the clinical care given to adolescents at CEMERA. The requirements were for: mental health, general medicine, prevention of pregnancy, and gynecology.

Monitoring
In the course of the program, various assessment instances were developed which are summarized in figure 2.

Knowledge
The level of knowledge regarding sexuality and reproduction, contraception, STDs and AIDS was measured. The proportions of correct answers of the cohort students in 8th, 9th and 10th grades surveyed in March 1994 (before) were compared with those of the November to December 1995 group, when they were finishing the 9th, 10th and 11th grades, respectively (after). In other words, an application of a 21-month program and through three consecutive grades. The control group without sex education covered the same periods and grades. It was decided to consider 21 months in the analysis of knowledge variables in order to avoid the information bias received by mass communication media and because of the greater age of the adolescents. The

Table 2. Knowledge before and after 21 months of the application of the sex education program (% correct answers)

Knowledge of:	With program			Without program			p W/WT program
Sexuality/reproduction	before (n = 1,627)	after (n = 1,306)	delta	before (n = 883)	after (n = 1,070)	delta	
Females	57.0	72.2	15.2	54.7	61.9	7.2	<0.05
Males	51.3	67.8	16.5	46.6	55.3	8.7	<0.05
Contraception, n	1,627	1,306		1,228	1,070		
Females	66.2	81.5	15.3	64.2	73.1	8.9	<0.05
Males	65.9	79,3	13.6	63.9	71.6	7–7	<0.05
STD and AIDS, n	1,627	1,306		1,228	1,070		
Females	67.2	85.5	18.5	62.2	72.2	10.2	<0.05
Males	71.6	87.8	16.2	69.0	79.2	10.2	<0.05

statistical significances were applied to the differences between the before and after replies and between control and case replies.

Practices

Three indicators were used: initiation of sex life (intercourse), use of contraceptives by sexually active adolescents, and pregnancies and their form of termination. In the analysis of these variables, the cohorts considered were students ranging from the 7th to the 10th grade, who were surveyed at the onset of the program, after 21 months and after 33 months. In other words, four school grades.

Results

Knowledge

The schools with a sex education program (cases) show a significant increase in their levels of knowledge as compared with the controls. The differences are somewhat lower in STD and AIDS. Students from schools with no program (controls) also showed increased knowledge when making the before and after comparison (table 2)

There is a period of almost 2 years between the 'before and after'. This age difference in school-attending adolescents is very important in the acquisition of knowledge. This means that knowledge increases regardless of the existence of a sex education program.

Table 3 relates the sexual experience of youngsters and the increase of their knowledge on sexuality and reproduction. It shows that when comparing youngsters with and without prior sexual experience, knowledge increases more in those with no experience. This is given both in case and control schools.

Table 3. Change in knowledge of sexuality and reproduction in relation to previous sexual experience

Previous sexual experience	% increase in knowledge			
	with sex education program before-after difference		without sex education program before-after difference	
	females	males	females	males
With sexual experience	12.9	10.5	6.3	6.7
Without sexual experience	15.9	15.6	8.1	8.7
Difference between with and without sexual experience	+3.0	+5.1	+1.8	+2.0

Table 4. Proportion of sexual initiation in youngsters with and without sex education prior to the intervention, 21 and 33 months after the intervention

Survey time	Gender	Cases		Controls		difference Ca/Co	p
		n total	ICR	n total	IRS ISR		
Before the program	females	1,176	203 (17.3)	809	173 (21.4)	+4.1	0.02
	males	1,281	393 (30.7)	885	369 (41.7)	+11	0.00
At 21 months of program	females	1,093	307 (28.1)	923	313 (33.9)	+5.8	0.00
	males	1,131	410 (36.3)	976	443 (45.4)	+9.1	0.00
At 33 months of program	females	1,081	320 (29.6)	992	369 (37.2)	+7.6	0.00
	males	1,080	451 (41.8)	904	446 (39.4)	+7.6	0.00

Practices

Table 4 analyses the evolution of experience at the initiation of sex relations in cases and controls. Proportions are accumulative, and for this reason, the replies at 21 and 33 months accumulate the previous experience. So, for example, the females in the with sexual experience program in the initial survey answered that 17.3% had already had intercourse. 21 months later, the percentage increased to 28.1%, which owing to its cumulative nature implies that the group increased by 10.8 points in almost 2 years' of observation. It shows that both groups had increased the cumulative ratio of their coital experience. The females of the case group increased by 12.3 points in 33 months (29.6–17.3), while those of the control group increased by 15.8 points (36.2–21.4). If the prevalence of the control group (37.2%) had corresponded to students of the intervened schools, we would have expected 402 youths with sexual experience, while the figure was 320, in other words 82 adolescents (8%) did not behave as expected, according to the control group. Possibly, this 8% delay intercourse.

Table 5. Use of contraceptives in male sexually active (SA) adolescents in case and control groups

Grades	Cases, % use of contraceptives			Controls, % use of contraceptives			
Males	before	after	difference	before	after	difference	p
Total	236	284		276	364		
9th grade (SA)	19	89		20	91		
n	4	38		7	43		
%	21.1	42.7	21.6	35.0	47.3	12.3	0.001
10th grade (SA)	57	79		78	104		
n	15	47		28	47		
%	26.3	59.5	33.2	35.9	43.3	7.4	0.001
11th grade (SA)	88	104		97	98		
n	36	60		31	47		
%	40.9	57.7	16.8	32.0	48.8	16.0	n/s
12th grade (SA)	72	72		81	71		
n	30	43		33	38		
%	41.7	59.7	18.0	40.7	53.5	12.8	0.001

n = Contraceptive users.
The table shows that in all the grades in the with sexual education group, sexually active males have a higher prevalence of use of contraceptives. There is a statistical significance in all the differences, with the exception of the 9th grade, although the number of adolescents using contraceptives increases by 13 in the case group, and by only 5 students in the control group.
In all the classes in the with sexual education group, sexually active female adolescents show a higher prevalence of use of contraceptives. All the differences between the with and without sex education programs reached statistical significant levels.

Males from the case group showed an 11.1 point increase in 33 months, against 7.7 in the control groups. In spite of these differences, on applying the prevalence of the control group over the case group, 83 youngsters (7.7%) in the latter group postponed their coital experience.

Between 21 and 33 months of observation, the females from the case group increased by 1.5 points while those from the control group did so by 3.3 points. In the males, the differences in increase over the same periods are very similar. In this experience the response is clearer in females than in males. In this way, school attending females from the control schools maintain an upward difference in their sexual initiation, which is greater than that in the case schools.

Tables 5 and 6 show the use of contraceptive frequency in both groups according to grade. The differences have been calculated at 21–22 months in the same cohort group per grade. Therefore, when we show 9th grade, it is the comparison between this current level (after) and their response to use of contraceptives 21–22 months before.

Table 6. Use of contraceptives in sexually active (SA) adolescent females in cases and controls

Grades	Cases: use of contraceptives, %			Controls: use of contraceptives, %			
Females	before	after	difference	before	after	difference	p
Total	134	284		125	278		
9th grade (SA)	7	50		6	71		
n	1	30		1	21		
%	14.3	50.8	36.5	16.7	29.6	12.9	0.001
10th grade (SA)	35	68		33	93		
n	10	38		8	40		
%	28.6	55.9	27.3	24.2	43.0	18.8	0.001
11th grade (SA)	36	73		49	71		
n	12	49		15	32		
%	33.3	67.1	33.8	30.6	45.1	14.5	0.001
12th grade (SA)	56	73		37	43		
n	24	53		14	24		
%	42.9	72.6	29.7	37.8	55.8	18.0	0.001

Pregnancies

This analysis considers total pregnancies and their form of termination at 33 months of observation, and compares the before and after in the total cohort of the school population. Nothing but pregnancies reported by women were chosen, as they are taken as the most reliable information. Table 7 gives the results for the totality of sexually active females.

In the group with a sex education program, 29 pregnancies were detected in 190 school-attending female adolescents who answered the question. This figure remained the same 33–34 months later in a larger population, giving a 5.6 point fall in the pregnancy ratio. The group without a sex education program had a 0.7 point fall. Table 7 also shows the net number of pregnancies reported before – after and the difference in the ratios for each school grade.

If the ratio observed in the group WITHOUT a sex education program had been applied to the 298 students WITH a sex education program, 44 pregnancies would have been expected instead of the 29 pregnancies observed. The sex education program would have contributed to avoid 15 unwanted pregnancies.

This finding is already a breakthrough. But what was most important of all was the change in the way in which the pregnancies were terminated. The change in spontaneous abortion is not as significant. There is a fall in induced abortion and in what adolescents spontaneously refer to as 'forced abortion'. This is an abortion that has been forced by parents, caregivers or the pregnant adolescent's partner. This kind of abortion increases in the school without a sex education program and falls in the school with a sex education program. This shows that once an unwanted pregnancy occurs,

Table 7. Pregnancies reported by school attending females and their results in cases and controls: distribution by grades

Grades	Cases: use of contraceptives, %					Controls: use of contraceptives, %					
	before		after		difference	before		after		difference	p
Total females*	190		298			162		300			
Repeated pregnancy	29		29			25		44			
% pregnancies	15.3		9.7		–5.6	15.4		14.7		–0.7	0.005
By grades	SA	pregnancy	SA	pregnancy	difference	SA	pregnancy	SA	pregnancy	difference	
7th grade	3	1	6	0	–33.3	9	1	6	1	+5.5	
8th grade	6	1	17	0	–16.6	6	0	16	2	+12.5	
9th grade	35	4	58	3	–10.9	33	5	72	7	–5.5	
10th grade	30	6	70	8	–8.6	48	7	92	15	+1.7	
11th grade	46	10	74	9	–9.5	36	7	67	8	–7.5	
12th grade	46	7	73	9	–2.9	29	5	47	11	+6.2	
Result of pregnancy	before		after		difference	before		after		difference	p
Delivery	31.1		58.2		+27.5	44.0		61.9		+17.9	n.s.
Spontaneous abortion	44.8		34.5		–10.3	40.0		21.4		–18.6	n.s.
Induced abortion	20.7		6.9		–13.8	12.0		2.4		–9.6	n.s.
Forced abortion	3.4		0.0		–3.4)	4.0		14.3		+10.3	0.01

* Total number of sexually active women who answered the question: 'Yes, I have been pregnant'. ** The information according to grade includes the number of 'before' and 'after' pregnancies. SA = Sexually active.

the decision to have the baby instead of interrupting the pregnancy with an abortion is a decision that is taken significantly more frequently in those schools that had sex education.

Comments

The problem of pregnancy in adolescents has been significant in these past decades. This demand for intervention does not mean that any program can be useful. This is an initiative that is not limited to the field of reproductive health, but that promotes personal development, improves self esteem, promotes better communication, prevents risk behaviors, proposes more life targets, and helps youngsters to show responsible preventive behaviors. All this has been proposed to take into account early sex initiation and thus avoid premature pregnancies, or to give those youngsters who decide to become sexually active the opportunity to avoid an unwanted pregnancy or of becoming infected with an STI or AIDS.

This study is an analysis of some of the quantitative variables of the impact assessment of a research study that includes a control group and which has been developed in Chile using professionals in the field of education that have been specially trained with methodology recommended by the Ministry of education and materials and teaching aids tested on Chilean pupils. The results obtained confirm the findings of most of the sex education programs with control groups described in developed countries.

The 'adolescence, time of decisions' program was applied by means of a transversal insertion into a school curriculum, with the participation of teachers trained in a participative, critical, confrontational and shared education system in the school community, in other words it includes parents and caregivers. The program was based on a methodology developed on the basis of many sex education programs, on previous CEMERA experiences and on multiple focus groups with adolescents explored by the research team. The 'adolescence: time of decisions' program was designed on the basis of this information.

The study shows that the control group also acquired knowledge of sexuality and reproduction even in the absence of a sex education program. Any intervention would produce this effect, nonetheless the strategy is that the application of the sex education program contributes to the maturation of knowledge in accordance with the cultures, ideologies and realities of the student and his/her family. This knowledge is what induces a change in attitudes and practices. Knowledge as mere information has a secondary value in attitudinal change and for this reason short and sporadic interventions in schools with a lack of knowledge create superficiality, a very short-term effect and even negative effects.

Another phenomenon that allows us to analyze this research is the belief that knowledge about sexuality is acquired with sexual practice. The results of the investigation show that previous sexual experiences are not the factor that increases their knowledge, and this corresponds to those who admitted to no previous sexual experience. This fact leads us to think about the need for a real comprehensive education in which sexuality is but another component of the human being as a rational and affective being, but which is essential.

The sex education offered in schools that had been subjected to intervention acted as a modulator of sexual practices. It also showed, as in many previous studies, that sex education does not increase the prevalence of schoolchildren who initiate their sexual activities. Quite the opposite, they delay it. In other calculations to be published subsequently, it was see that the program delays the initiation of intercourse between 6 to 8 months. It also shows that a sex education program does not eliminate the initiation of juvenile sex, and does not totally stop the sexual activity of those youngsters who have already become active. All the programs with controlled assessment show the same findings. In this context, sex education programs have the objective to stimulate abstinence as much as possible, until the person can take on the responsibilities of an affective commitment and commitment with a partner and the consequences of maternity/paternity, among others.

The absence of sex education does not protect individuals from sexual initiation. On the contrary, the control group is comprised of more frequent early initiators according to comparative school level analyses. This shows that ignorance or unstructured information does not prevent sexual initiation. On the contrary, sexual behavior is more responsible in those adolescents that have received intervention who decide to initiate or continue with their sex life. This responsibility is provided by the 'use of contraceptives' indicator, which is significantly higher in schools WITH sex education.

In this area, it is necessary to insist that all sex education program should be accompanied by appropriate adolescent health care services. The experience, professionalism and confidentiality offered by the Centre of Medicine and Integral Development of the Adolescent of the Faculty of Medicine of the University of Chile has proved this. It is natural that informed and educated youngsters, and adults, are aware of their health needs and tend to satisfy them with an increase in a demand for services, which is already known.

One of the important impacts of this experience has been a reduction in the prevalence of pregnancies, with a very special emphasis on those terminated by an induced abortion or an abortion forced by parents or other relatives. This research has shown us that 'forced abortion' in adolescents, reaches dimensions we suspected, without being sure of its occurrence and magnitude; in the final survey this type of abortion reached 14% of pregnancies in schools without a sex education program. This ratio is probably more exact that that obtained in the initial survey.

This figure disappears in schools with sex education programs. Similarly, in a stressful situation such as an unexpected pregnancy, results show that the outcome of a newborn child is more frequent in schools with sex education programs. These achievements can only be proved in controlled studies, given the variety of confusing factors that exist on an epidemiological level.

A phenomenon that is observed in all the variables analyzed is the difference found in male and female schoolchildren. There is an evident gender difference that tends to place the females in a situation of greater acceptance and response to the 'adolescence, time of decisions' program. This was also observed with the analysis of the gender differences in the students of the schools under study.

After the end of the experience, CEMERA has continued to support a series of schools to prove the replicability of the educational model. The first experience in the public sector was seen in the city of Coronel, in Region VIII; both the program and training of teachers and primary level health workers has continued independently, with the support of the Municipality and Hospital of Coronel.

Another experience has been developed by the Consultorio Quinta Bella in the Municipality of Recoleta, in Santiago, which trained 60% of the teachers of the Juanita

Fernandez Solar Girls' School in the 'adolescence, time of decisions' program. Today, the program has been included in the transversal objective of the school's curricular grid. In the private sector, there are schools such as Santiago College, and Scuola Italiana in Santiago and Mackay School in Viña del Mar, that are applying adaptations of the program after offering training to their teachers.

These experiences have shown that once teachers and health carers have been trained, the model can be replicated on a local level both in training and applications.

Conclusions

This intervention study proves what has already been described by other authors as regards the impact of a sex education program in the following fields.

(1) A significant increase is produced in sexuality, reproduction, contraception and sexually transmitted diseases.

(2) The adolescents that show a greater increase in knowledge related to sexuality and reproduction are those who have not had sex at the moment of the final survey.

(3) Students with previous sexual experiences do not show a significant increase in their knowledge of sexuality and reproduction.

(4) Sexual initiation is delayed in schools that are subject to intervention, although this will be studied in greater detail when the other variables of the multifactor analysis are considered.

(5) The attitudes of the students who decide to continue with sexual relations are more responsible in the schools that have been intervened, using efficient contraceptive methods, which contribute to the prevention of pregnancies and possibly of STD.

(6) There is a significant reduction of pregnancies in schools that have been subjected to intervention.

(7) The increase of pregnancies terminated in abortions has been dramatic, especially in the case of 'forced abortions' in schools without sex education.

(8) The final conclusion shows that the findings of studies of the impact of sex education in developed countries can also be found in developing countries, when the programs applied are structured, ongoing, with properly trained teaching staff and accessible health services for the teenagers.

(9) There are important gender differences in the findings of this study, which confirm previous analyses of this aspect of the same project.

(10) This study is a scientifically validated contribution to public policies in sex education and the prevention of pregnancy in school attending adolescents.

The third pillar is the existence at primary health care of preferential services for adolescents on sexual and reproductive health including preferential maternal and child care services with antenatal, postnatal and post-abortion check-ups and monitoring for adolescent contraception.

Programs for the prevention of the second pregnancy have a greater impact when they involve health and education systems and suppliers, the family, religious and community institutions, government and non-government organizations and all the adolescents involved. These should offer a comprehensive and ongoing approach, in other words the effort must come from all the sectors and create new options and promote healthy behaviors and attitudes. To work for the non-repetition of pregnancies in adolescents is a task for society as a whole, and especially when the objective is to achieve a better future for child and mother.

The fourth pillar corresponds to a network of promotion, communication and education that is correlated through the school and family. This network facilitates the attendance to sexual and reproductive health services for adolescents, when necessary.

The fifth pillar is a proved strategy for maintaining continued schooling for school-age mothers and fathers, provision of crèche and nursery school facilities. As a way of contributing to the permanence of adolescent mothers at school, the Center for Adolescent Reproductive Medicine and Development, of the Faculty of Medicine of the University of Chile, implemented in 1995 an alternative educational model for pregnant adolescents, adolescent mothers that left school because of pregnancy or maternity. It was a long-term assessment of the social impact of this alternative education model. The following were the specific objectives that were used in the development of this model:

(1) To develop an alternative education system for pregnant adolescents and adolescent mothers with programs approved by the Ministry of Education that include regular secondary school studies and vocational training.

(2) Maintain the link between the schoolgirl-mother and child through the installation of a crèche and unconventional nursery school in the educational establishment itself.

(3) Encourage functional curriculum school programs that consider the problems of the teenage girl, through participants education systems, with the inclusion of the family.

(4) Provide integrated education and health care for the community of participating schoolchildren

(5) Assess the economic feasibility of the model.

(6) Contribute to the prevention of clandestine abortion, abandonment and child abuse, and repeated pregnancies, giving development alternatives through education.

The hypothesis to be proved was the following: 'Adolescent mothers that took part in this alternative educational program have a higher probability of attaining a better level of personal development and a real labor insertion when compared with those that did not participate in the program.' The proposed research has a fundamental importance for the replication of the model on a national level and for other countries in Latin America.

Selected Reading

Card J, Niego S, Mallari E, Farrel W: The program archive on sexuality, health and adolescence: promising 'prevention programs in a box'. Family Planning Persp 1996;28:210–220.

Di Clemente R: Development of programmes for enhancing sexual health. Lancet 2001;358:1828–1829.

East P: Do adolescent pregnancy and childbearing affect younger siblings? Family Planning Persp 1996;28:148–153.

Jain A: ¿Debería seguir siendo una prioridad la eliminación de la necesidad insatisfecha de anticoncepción? Perspectivas Internacionales en Planificación Familiar 1999 N° Especial, pp 31–36.

Jara G, Molina R, Molina T, Ferrari M: Evaluación y realización de videos docentes, como complemento de la educación sexual, reflexiva y participativa. Rev Ch Obstet Ginecol Infantil Adolesc 1995;2:74–82.

Jara G, Molina R, Molina, Molina T: Seguimiento de profesores capacitados en educación sexual. Rev Ch Obstetr Ginecolo Infantil Adolescenc 1995;2:50–56.

Jemmott J III, Jemmott SL, Braverman P, Fong G: HIV/STD risk reduction interventions for African American and Latino adolescent girls at an adolescent medicine clinic: a randomized controlled trial. Arch Pediatr Adolesc Med 2005;159:440–449.

Kirby D: Sex and HIV/AIDS education in schools. BMJ 1995;311:403.

Kirby D, et al: School-based programs to reduce sexual risk behaviour: a review of effectiveness. Publ Health Rep 1994;109:339–360.

Kirby D, Laris B, Rolleri L: Impact of sex and HIV education programs on sexual behavior of youth in developing and developed countries. Family Health International, Youth Research Working Paper Series No 2, 2006. www.fhi.org

Lobos L: La Afectividad como componente de la sexualidad; en Molina R (ed): En Salud Sexual y Reproductiva del Adolescente. Santiago, Editorial Mediterraneo, 2001.

Miller B, et al (eds): Preventing Pregnancy Model Programs and Evaluation. Newbury Park, Sage, 1992.

Ministerio de Educación de Chile: Política de Educación en Sexualidad. Para el mejoramiento de la calidad de la educación. Ministerio de Educación, 1966.

Molina R, Jara G, Toledo V, Luengo X: Enfoque y Experiencia en Educación sexual del Centro de Medicina y Desarrollo integral del adolescente. Rev Ch Obstetr Ginecol Infantil Adolesc 1996;1:17–26.

Molina R, Sandoval J, Gonzalez E: Salud Sexual y Reproductiva en la Adolescencia. Santiago Chile, Editorial Mediterraneo, 2003.

Murray N, Zabin L, Toledo V, Luengo X: Diferencias de género en factores que influyen en el inicio de relaciones sexuales en adolescentes escolares urbanos en Chile. Persp Intn Planificación Familiar 1998;(N° Especial):4–10.

National Swedish Board of Education: Instruction Concerning Interpersonal Relations. Stockholm, Ed. Liber Tyck, 1982.

ONU SIDA 1997: Impacto de la Educación en materia de salud sexual y VIH sobre el comportamiento sexual de los jóvenes: actualización de un análisis. ONUSIDA. Colección. Prácticas óptimas del ONUSIDA, 1997.

Rostosky S, Wright M, Randall B: The impact of religiosity on adolescent sexual behavior: a review of the evidence. J Adolesc Res 2004;86:677–697.

Toledo V, Luengo X, Fuentes E, et al: Adolescencia Tiempo de Decisiones. Manual para Alumnos Editorial Mediterraneo, 1998.

Toledo V, Luengo X, Fuentes E, et al: Adolescencia Tiempo de Decisiones. Manual para Padres y Apoderados. Editorial Mediterraneo, 1998.

Toledo V, Luengo X, Siraqyan , Molina R: Programa de educación sexual y Prevención del embarazo en escolares adolescentes: Intervención a nivel escolar y clínico I. Rev Ch Obstet Ginecol Infantil Adolesc 1996;3:22–25.

WHO/UNICEF: A Picture Health: A Review and Annoted Bibliography of the Health in Young People in Developing Countries, 1995.

Williams T, Schutt-Aine J, Cuca Y: Measuring family planning service quality through client satisfaction exit interviews. Int Family Planning Persp 2000; 26:63–71.

Zabin L, Hirsch M: Evaluation of Pregnancy Prevention Programs in the School Context. Massachusetts, Lexington Books, 1988.

Dan Apter
The Sexual Health Clinic, Family Federation of Finland, Helsinki
POB 849
FI–00101 Helsinki (Finland)
Tel. +358 9 22805 226, E-Mail dan.apter@vaestoliitto.fi

Sultan C (ed): Pediatric and Adolescent Gynecology. Evidence-Based Clinical Practice. 2nd, revised and extended edition. Endocr Dev. Basel, Karger, 2012, vol 22, pp 357–379

High-Risk Sexual Behaviors

Thierry Troussier · Pierre Benghozi · Marc Ganem†

Chaire de Santé Sexuelle et de Droits Humain, Université Paris Diderot, Paris, France

Abstract

Adolescence is a time of life characterized by danger because of the many changes that occur, the many ties that are severed: ties to childhood, ties to the child's body as it begins to take on an adult appearance, ties to a once-familiar body image and psyche as hormones complete the transformation to adulthood, ties to an unconscious that is struggling to restructure itself anew. The creation of the romantic couple is a danger inherent in any human society. This text was written from the professional practices of each author in a multidisciplinary approach combining the approaches of public health, risk reduction, and sexual, psychological and clinical care of adolescents. How to help anticipate the dangers is to use preventive insurance verifying that security is guaranteed before committing. Risk-taking is accepting all the challenges that boost the self with oneself and with others. The risk is therefore also the commitment in love. It is still the risk to speak, to feel, to express feelings, choices, and refusal of unwanted sex. The ability of adolescents to play and defeat the risk by learning the ethical value not only to protect themselves from contracting AIDS, but also to protect others is part of the pedagogy of risk. This pedagogy of risk, as we have seen, includes three areas: information, care and initiation into love. Adolescents must be supported in their emergence by responsible people to protect them from the dangers ahead. The support is not only to prevent them from engaging in risky behavior, but to help them better manage their anxieties and support the fragility of their families in a network approach. Not knowing how to confront the risk stifles the chance of allowing the child to grow up to be independent and helps reassure parents who may resent being removed from the empowerment of their children.

"What does 'to tame' mean?" "It's something that's been too often neglected. It means, 'to create ties'. . .."
Translation from the original French: Saint Exupéry A., 1946, Le petit prince, Paris, Gallimard

Adolescence is a time of life characterized by danger because of the many changes that occur, the many ties that are severed: ties to childhood, ties to the child's body as it begins to take on an adult appearance, ties to a once-familiar body image and psyche as hormones complete the transformation to adulthood, ties to an unconscious that is struggling to restructure itself anew. In a growing number of adolescents, this period of rupture may be expressed outwardly by risk-taking behavior as long-held notions of the safety of family, religion and school seem to disintegrate around them. Illicit drug use in the schools and universities has not only social ramifications, but also transgenerational, transcultural and even religious impact.

This chapter deals with the difficulties encountered in managing the sexual risk behavior of adolescents, who appear to have developed an adult sexuality that is in fact only in its infancy.

The massive intrusion of pornography into nearly all corners of life only adds to this highly explosive combination of risk-taking behavior and sexuality. Adolescence is fraught with danger, not least of which is the danger inherent to all human societies: that of creating a romantic couple. This very first sexualized and romantic experience (think Romeo and Juliette) often ends in distress. Yet a painful ending may be necessary for some so that they can struggle through and ultimately overcome the emotional turmoil in order to attain the physical and psychological well-being of sexually mature couples. Ideally, this first romance should be experienced with serenity, although this is rarely the case today.

Sexual risk behavior is an important topic because it is very much related to both the sickness of our consumer-driven societies and the extremely unsettling distortions between body and mind that adolescents are coping with. This chapter is based on the professional practice of two of the authors: Dr. Pierre Benghozi, who has dealt with the section on adolescent psychology and clinical management, and Dr. Thierry Troussier, who has handled the section on public health: nosolgy, epidemiology and the bases for consultations to reduce the incidence of adolescent high-risk sex.

For most therapists, the world of adolescence is and will always be mysterious, haunting and sometimes deeply disturbing. Those of us who work with adolescents constantly need to question our adult preconceptions and listen attentively from the standpoint of our own experiences of rupture.

Nosology and Changes in Terminology

The past 10 years have been marked by changes in the paradigm for risk prevention in sexual behavior. Reproductive health has shifted from an approach focused on woman as mother to a far more global approach to sexuality that encompasses risk behaviors and the contexts for sexuality [1]. In November 2009, the Lert-Pialoux report [2], at the request of the French Ministry of Health, redefined the objectives for prevention programs in France. The objectives today are to reduce the incidence of HIV and sexually transmitted diseases (STDs), mainly by targeting men engaged in homosexual sex for HIV and youth under 24 years for STDs, and to reduce the individual risks of becoming infected or of spreading infection.

The program is thus to reduce the public cost of HIV and STDs and their consequences and to diminish individual risk. These objectives are realistic, as it seems unlikely that HIV and STDs will be eradicated or that the individual risk of being infected or of transmitting infection will fall to zero. This modification in the objectives has led to changes in the paradigm for prevention, especially given the latest report from the National AIDS Council in April 2009 on the role of treatment in preventing HIV, the new HAS recommendations for testing for HIV, Chlamydia, syphilis and gonorrhea, and the sections on prevention and sexuality from the experts' report on HIV 2002 [3] and HIV 2007 [4] from DOIN, which complement the report on the reduction of sexual risk [2].

The prevention paradigm now emphasizes continuity rather than rupture. The goal is to continually adapt the strategies to prevent HIV, STDs and unwanted pregnancies in the light of the latest scientific data and to combine prevention, screening, and emergency and long-term treatment. This has medicalized risk reduction and given medical caregivers a clear role in the process of preventing HIV and STDs and encouraging contraceptive use [5].

The concept of sexual and reproductive health as defined by the WHO in 2004 [6] is not limited to the absence of illness or dysfunction and consequences like sterility, abortion or cancer. Instead, it signals a global approach to sexual health as part of an ongoing process of achieving and maintaining physical, psychological and sociocultural well-being.

This chapter takes the same approach to overall sexual health and risk reduction, which is a more explicit formulation of the 'notion of combined prevention: offer to all an easy access to the means of protection, a more robust system on which to depend, and a much greater chance of being protected and of being able to protect others' [2]. The information on the means of prevention and sexual risk reduction should not dissociate HIV, STDs and unwanted pregnancies. The refusal to dissociate these situations requires a global approach to risk without specifically targeting HIV, STDs or contraception, and instead takes into account all the cofactors that are involved in sexual and other human behaviors [7].

Epidemiology and Indicators

There is a gap between the representations of health in the minds of young people and the perceptions of health professionals. A survey from INSEE 2007 found that only 1 of 10 youths declared being in poor health and yet professionals reported poor health in 15% of youth [8]. This observation suggests the need to act first in terms of youth's representations about health and their representations about risk taking.

Becoming sexually active, which occurs at about 17 years for 50% of young people today, has remained stable for the past 30 years [9, 10]. Yet, although the age for becoming sexually active has not changed for boys during this period, it has dropped by 1 year for girls over the same time frame. The proportion of youngsters who declared more than one sexual partner in the past year is in sharp augmentation, with a rate of 31% in 2004. The mean number of partners for 15- to 19-year-olds and 20- to 24-year-olds is, respectively, 2.1 and 2.4 for men and 1.4 for women. Multiple sex partners for both male and female homosexuals is quite common, much more common than in heterosexuals. The internet has become the new way to meet people: among 18- to 19-year-olds, 35% of the girls go to internet meeting sites and 24% of the boys. Twenty-nine percent of the 20- to 24-year-olds use these sites for meeting each other and nearly 10% of these encounters end in a sexual relationship. Last, 5.4% of young men between 20 and 24 years turn to prostitution.

Use of contraceptive and preventive methods has clearly progressed in the past 20 years without a drop in the number of unwanted pregnancies and abortions, which remain quite frequent: in France, 13,192 minor girls were pregnant in 2007; in Great Britain, 39,000 minors were pregnant in 2006, and 7,300 of them were under 16 years of age.

A study by the SMEREP [11] found that less than 60% of the students living in the Isle de France region systematically used a contraceptive method: 62% used oral contraception and 55% reported using condoms. Thirty-three percent had used emergency contraception and 37% had had abortions. Sixty-two percent had never been tested for HIV/AIDS, hepatitis B, hepatitis C or STDs.

According to the COCOON study [12, 13], one third of pregnancies were unwanted and 50% ended in abortion; 200,000 abortions are performed per year and this number is rising in the young, with 14 of 1,000 women having had an abortion between 15 and 45 years. Whatever the situation, 95% of sexually active women in their reproductive years use a contraceptive method in France, whereas in many developing countries only 10% of these women use contraceptives. This discrepancy between contraception-related behavior and wanted pregnancies reminds us of the French paradox. We tend to forget the predominant role of psychological factors in adolescence (knowing how to live) and the complex factors within society regarding knowledge and knowing what to do.

Physical and sexual violence is still too frequent and is often underreported. Twenty-eight percent of the women who were childhood victims of physical violence are victims of violence in marriage, whereas only 6% of those with no history of childhood abuse are victims in adulthood [14–16]. In a meta-analysis of worldwide reports on sexual behavior published in *Lancet* 2006 [17], every minute 1 young girl under 15 years is sexually abused somewhere in the world and 10 girls are sexually mutilated. Gender inequality leads to violence against women and is the principal cause of disease.

According to the KABP survey of the ORS Ile de France for France [18], the risk of transmitting HIV and STDs is highest among those youths who take the most risks (multiple partners, drug dependency, etc.).

According to a recent publication [19], HIV is also seen in young people: 86 girls and 63 boys from 0 to 9 years and 359 girls and 202 boys from 10 to 19 years. Of those between 20 and 29 years who discover that they are HIV positive, one quarter are under 20. It is likely that contamination in these young people occurred in the first sexual relations.

Since the documentation of HIV status became mandatory in March 2003, more than 6,432 people between 20 and 29 years old have been declared (figures from December 31, 2008), which is 23% of all declarations. The majority of these young people are women: 53% from the 2008 data. Of the young HIV women declared in 2005, 77% were contaminated by heterosexual sex, 1% by drug injection and for 22% the information was not available.

It should be recalled that in 2005 [20] the 15–24 age group represented 2.8% of the HIV population (9 between 15 and 19 years and 24 between 20 and 24 years).

Young people rarely have AIDS [19]. A very low percentage of the total AIDS diagnoses involve young people, nearly 2% (December 2008). However, because of the long incubation period, the current number of AIDS cases is not an indicator adapted for evaluating HIV spread in the young. At the time of AIDS diagnosis, only about half of the young people knew they were HIV positive, which means inadequate use of screening.

Sexually transmitted diseases are too frequent in young people [19]. In the age group between 20 and 29 years, STDs are seen too frequently: 2.9% of men and 4.7% of women have been infected in the last 5 years. Viral infections predominate, with herpes responsible for 18% of the declared infections. The prevalence of human papillovirus (HPV) in 20-year-old women is 25%, and the cumulative risk rises to 60% after 5 years of sexual activity. Sixty percent of cervical cancers are caused by HPV. These prevalences were reported in the representative survey within the French Sexual Context framework in 2006. The highest prevalences were observed in the low age classes: 3.6% for women and 2.4% for the men between 18 and 24 years.

Since 2000, repeated epidemics of STDs have been observed in young homosexuals: syphilis, gonorrhea, venereal lymphogranuloma (VLG), and viral hepatitis B and C (VHB and VHC).

Worldwide, STDs are the second major cause of morbidity, according to a report in *Lancet* [17]. Young people under 24 years of age are particularly vulnerable because they are subjected to a sexuality they do not always desire, they do not have access to primary health care, or they have been rejected. Every year, 340 million cases of gonorrhea, syphilis, Chlamydia and trichomonas are diagnosed, and 110 million cases concern young people aged between 15 and 24 years. The prevalence of HPV in young women under 20 years is 25%.

Psychological Aspects of Adolescence

Risk Is Not the Same as Danger

To understand the relationship between sexual risk and sexual danger in the adolescent, it is important to consider the metamorphosis that is generally termed the adolescent crisis. Risk taking helps to structure the adolescent; putting oneself into danger is a destructive act. The adolescent operates at the borders of the extreme, at the critical threshold between risk and danger. However, there is reason to suspect that crossing this threshold is not the expression of a simple misstep.

Putting oneself into sexual danger is the symptom of a veritable breakdown in individual and familial identity. Putting oneself into danger by sexual behavior is the symptom of a familial 'envelope' that is not sufficiently strong and secure to support the processes of adolescence.

Before any description of the risk behaviors and life situations to which adolescents are exposed, it is essential to have a good understanding of the importance of respecting and supporting the work that is accomplished by risk taking in the construction of the adolescent, even though this work is often destabilizing and a source of anguish for parents. Only by understanding 'the work of risk' can we best prepare to prevent danger.

Risk can be defined as the work that is necessary to define one's own personal limits, as opposed to dangerous behaviors, which are clearly self-destructive.

Risk-taking is part of how limits are structured in the unconscious image of the body that is undergoing transformation, and it contributes to the shift in identity that occurs in adolescence.

There is even a culture of risk. For example, high-risk sports are sports that are extremely challenging, with the very real possibility of accidents. Planning a solitary crossing of the Atlantic Ocean by boat demands very careful preparation and great rigor. No one makes a bungee jump off a high bridge without making absolutely certain that all security measures are operating correctly. Before climbing a mountain, the difficulties must be evaluated, adequate means must be anticipated and planned for, and physical, mental and material preparation is needed. Managing constraints in order to overcome them is not putting oneself in danger; it is to face a risk, rise to the challenge it poses, and to thoroughly enjoy the experience of (successfully) pushing one's limits.

High-Risk Sexual Behaviors and the Threats of Danger

The same planning has a role regarding the risks inherent to sexual growth in the adolescent. It is better to know oneself and recognize the other, to prepare one's mind and body, to be well informed, to be able to choose and adapt a contraceptive method, to anticipate and plan for the most favorable affective and material conditions for sexual experiences – all this planning will prepare the adolescent for a satisfying first sexual experience. However, there are risks involved: exposing oneself to a game of seduction, confronting the avatars of the encounter, overcoming fears and anxieties about the unknown, and facing the possibility of disappointment or failure. These risks are nevertheless also sources of excitement and sexual stimulation.

Sexual experiences that occur too soon or that are ill adapted to the affective or psychological maturity of the individual could be termed 'premature'. Just as a bird might pick at green fruit, not yet ripened, an adolescent may develop a precocious hypermaturity that blocks a fully harmonious maturation. Premature sexuality in fact induces sexual dysmaturation. The psychoanalyst Sandor Ferenczi described childhood victims of sexual abuse in 'Confusion in language between the adult and child', and noted that these children and adolescents displayed eroticized behaviors toward adults. It is essential to understand these provocative and often seductive attitudes as the search for attention and affection, the need to exist in the eyes of the other, and most often the desire to be loved. These can be displayed as transgressive attitudes that are sources of voluptuousness and intense pleasure.

It is also important to distinguish between sexed identity as masculine or feminine gender and sexuality. Sex and sexuality concern for both male and female adolescents the emergence of a new sensuality, exploration, the search for erotic pleasure, and genital arousal. Puberty raises the possibility of reproduction. The mystery of erotic desire and pleasure is confounded by the desire for pregnancy and a baby. Pediatricians and gynecologists often see adolescents for the first time in gynecological consultation when they request contraception. Here sexuality is confronted by ambivalence. How do you take pleasure in your sexuality without the risk of an unwanted child? The desire for pregnancy points to anxiety about and the need to confirm the integrity of the inner life within a woman's body.

The way contraception is dealt with manifests this unconscious ambivalence; for example, by forgetting to take the pill and other failures of contraception despite a wealth of information in sex education. Oral contraception is experienced as a constraint. It may be perceived as dangerous for health [21].

Contraception is perceived as a factor of progress and liberty more for women of 25 years or older. Repeated abortions indicate the ambivalence between the desire for pregnancy and the desire for a child.

Adolescent pregnancies may represent a veritable passage to the sexual act. Pierre Benghozi in 1994 called them 'premature pregnancies': the physical and psychological immaturity of both the individual and the couple raises the critical question of how best to accompany the early interactions in perinatality in order to support the baby's favorable development. The importance of risky sexual behavior is compounded in adolescence by running away behaviors, school absenteeism, and even leaving school entirely.

In some social contexts, like the favelas of Rio de Janeiro (Terezinha Ferez Carneiro) or the ghettos of some of the big French cities, very young girls exhibit a kind of triumphant sexuality by becoming the girlfriend of a drug-dealing gang leader. These girls are in danger of becoming the object of 'gang rapes'.

Adolescents are exposed to the risk of infection if they have unprotected sex (STDs like syphilis, Chlamydia, HIV, etc.), especially when they have multiple partners or sex with strangers.

Modifications in sexual practices since the first cases of AIDS have been contaminated by the association of a life-threatening illness and the discovery of genital sexual pleasure.

A youngster who progresses to repeated sex partners and 'turning tricks', whether these are homo- or heteroerotic acts, and prostitution should be considered as suicidal.

This behavior in fact has much in common with other types of addictive behavior: drug addiction, alcoholism, and eating disorders like anorexia and bulimia. Drunkenness and the loss of self-control after substance abuse expose adolescents to the risk of being victims of abuse and sexual violence. Adolescents today are deeply affected by the digital world and the power of the internet. In addition to the real addictions arising from overconsumption, pornographic behaviors have become banal and the threat of sexual predators on meeting sites is very real.

What Leads Young People to Put Their Own Bodies in Danger, as Well as Those of Other Children and Adolescents?

In a survey carried out by a student health insurance organization [22], 8% of the students presented with disturbances severe enough to require medical management and 17% were identified as 'troubled' and presented signs and symptoms of psychological distress requiring specialized help. It should be noted that the great majority, 75%, claimed to be 'doing well'. Between the extremes of a certain standardization of their behavior and their extravagance, adolescents know how to provoke and convoke the adults around them! Worried parents wonder what is happening and consult the family doctor.

Adolescence is not an illness – it is a passage. It is a process of crisis in the natural cycle of life. Adolescence is a developmental phase in the life cycle of each individual and the family, as well. How adolescence is expressed depends greatly on the social context. From this perspective, adolescence is both a symptom and a societal indicator. It is an in-between period not only in the physical transformations of puberty but also the psychological and social transformations because it is the passage from the status of child to the status of adult.

What Are the Physical Stakes in Adolescence?

Puberty is characterized by a physical transformation, with the maturation of primary sexual characteristics and the development of secondary sexual characteristics.

The body of the adolescent boy is transformed inside and out. There are transformations that can be seen, shown or hidden. There are transformations that cannot be seen and those that are revealed. This metamorphosis is imposed, and to a great extent it is uncontrollable. It cannot be mastered, it cannot be escaped. Adolescence is the time for the first stirrings of emotional love, the first use of contraception, the first sexual experience, the first disappointments, the first 'extravagance'. This growth process can be characterized by its 'first times'. It is expressed somatically, psychologically and socially. With puberty, sexuality evolves from infantile narcissistic concerns to a new manifestation of the genital oedipal stakes. It is the period of the great firsts in life, when the sex identity is confirmed with all the turmoil and disturbance of affective and sexual life.

Sexual behaviors are essentially the theater for constructing the sexed identity. Puberty according to Philippe Gutton is a time of psychological rearrangement of the relationships with the world and oneself. The theater that is the adolescent body image is a spectacle projected onto the stage of their bedrooms: an indescribable mess or perfectly arranged dollhouse. Clothing is both an envelope for and the extension of the body. We know the expression in their eyes, the scopic impulse, and the anxiety of being intruded upon while the boundaries of this envelope around intimate territory are being constructed. This suggests the importance of a respectful attitude toward displays of modesty, but not complicity with a conspiracy of silence. Respect for physical modesty goes hand in hand with the attitude of availability, or readiness to listen to the nearly invisible traces of traumatism that the body sometimes carries.

During the narcissistic and oedipal reorganization that occurs in adolescence, the way the doctor receives the body in consultation has an essential role in the work of structuring and restructuring the adolescent's body image.

Psychological Molting and Unconscious Body Image

Adolescence was described by Pierre Benghozi in 1999 as a period of *psychological molting*. The molting stage, between two outer coverings, is the 'adolescent chrysalis'. This is reflected by the unconscious body image as what Francoise Dolto called 'the lobster complex'. As she noted, when lobsters molt, they shed their old carapace and are then for a certain time without defenses, until the new carapace is produced. She further remarked that certain adults, sensing this vulnerability in adolescents, hover close by, waiting for an opportunity to strike.

With reference to the 'Me-skin' of the psychoanalyst, *Didier Anzieu,* to change one's skin is to change the psychological envelope. This helps us to better understand why the functions of this envelope are so unsteady in this period. In the transition between two outer carapaces, two protective coverings, there is psychological vulnerability. The envelope of childhood is left and a new body image is built. The doctor is thus listening to a body in transformation and must show a readiness to accept differentiation.

Clinical Anthropology of Sexual Behaviors

In the traditional societies of Africa, adolescence is a rite of passage. The encounter of masculine and feminine is structured in the Fulani of West Africa around rituals of display that engage the entire community. Physical risk-taking is always part of the initiation rituals in these traditional societies. Adolescence is an initiation and the culture of risk, the confrontation with a challenge that must be overcome, is part of all rites of passage. The body is involved and there is always a symbolic encounter with death, usually marked by a time of separation, followed by a period of transition and then incorporation into the group of initiates – the community of adults. This is undoubtedly the importance of a ritual that can provide a framework for sexual risk behaviors. Our modern and postmodern societies do not offer the adolescent structured rituals for entering into the community of adults. Adolescence as a rite of passage is not culturally codified. We can thus interpret certain adolescent behaviors as neo-rituals manifesting the diverse ways that the young take risks as they confront the challenges that must be overcome. These may be channeled and sublimated into recreational and athletic activities like extreme sports, for example. These risks are in themselves ritualized and controlled.

Ordalic Behavior

Sexual risk behaviors can be considered as the equivalent of ordalic behaviors like Russian roulette. Charles-Nicolas illustrated these ordalic behaviors by the life-threatening behaviors of young drug addicts.

Facing a challenge is the source of intense pleasure, of thrill, which, contrary to opinion, reflects neither the clear desire to destroy oneself nor a death wish, nor the denial of death. Instead, it is as if the person were trying desperately to overcome childhood fears. And implicating the body, one's very life, in order to meet this challenge seems to have no cost. What worth does a life have when it was never desired? What value can a person have when they don't even matter to their parents? In this case, how can the will to live be more forcefully expressed than by the excitement of the sacrificial risk of gambling with one's life? The imaginary identification with the heroes who brave danger is also a way to provoke a clash between the virtual world and the reality of death. Risk behavior is an attempt to manage the psychological distress tied to early affective vulnerability. The excitement of facing danger is reassuring to those who, like Don Juan, challenge the commander and feel stronger than the phantoms that obsess them. Is it also scaring oneself in order to conquer fear? We know the tropism of teenagers toward horror films with their perverse sexual dimension. Bruno Bettelheim amply demonstrated the importance of fairy tales and their cruelty in helping children to negotiate their terrifying fantasies.

Alcohol and drug-taking greatly enhance the feeling of omnipotence by removing inhibitions and facilitating the release of impulses and by attenuating anxiety.

Risk, Shame and Guilt

There are two types of threat in the relationship with risk. One is the threat of sanction if a prohibition has been transgressed. The indicator of risk taking is thus the sentiment of guilt and the fear of the police, for example. The other threat concerns how one is seen by others. This is the risk of shame. Losing face is much more difficult to bear for the adolescent than the risk of being condemned for dangerous behavior.

Honor, pride, self-esteem, reputation: all concern the image that each one of us projects to others. Any failure to conform to the sexual behaviors that are part of the values of the group to which one belongs is a source of shame. This is particularly evident in certain areas where gangs of youth belonging to multiple cultural communities come into contact. More than others, these adolescents are sensitive to the pressure to conform and the humiliation of not rising to the challenge of risk is a threat far greater than that of gambling with one's physical integrity.

Risk in Relation to 'Crisis' and 'in Crisis': Adolescence as an Individual Affair and a Familial Affair

Pierre Benghozi sees the staging of the adolescent body as the theater for the transmission of psychological genealogy. Adolescence in this sense is the family history of genealogical lineage and ties of affiliation. From this perspective, all adolescence is familial. Adolescence reflects a transformation in the body image of the individual and the family. Three modalities are possible: the crisis of adolescence, adolescence in crisis, and catastrophic adolescence, and will depend on the family's psychological capacity to envelope these transformations. Thus, the relation to risk is not the same when it is one of the characteristics of the crisis of adolescence and when it is the reflection of an adolescent in crisis.

Risk is part of the crisis of adolescence. Adolescence is a time of construction requiring individuation and separation, dependence and autonomy. Children need a threshold of basic security in order to maintain inner tranquility so that they can then open up to relationships with others. Security is constructed in the first bonding relationship, in the early and natural interactions between mother and baby, but also in all other relationships that make up the sensorial, affective and life-fostering entourage. It begins to be built very early on but over time it is strengthened or in contrast it becomes more fragile.

Adolescence strains familial and social ties where they are most vulnerable. What is unthinkable and inadmissible in the family is transmitted from generation to generation. From this perspective, Pierre Benghozi described the adolescent's function as 'the bearer of shame' as the inheritance of the unconscious transmission of familial shame.

Part of the genealogical heritage is used to construct the adolescent's body image. The psychological body is the ventriloquist of this heritage. The body gives form to the unspoken, the secrets, the inadmissible, the unthinkable, the inexpressible, the unnamable. The body says what cannot be thought, what cannot be spoken aloud. All is in fact expressed verbally or nonverbally by worries, attitudes, behaviors, symptoms, and the stakes of affective and sexual life.

In many situations of a rupture in the genealogical lineage, violence against self or others can be seen, expressing a conflict of identity. All ruptures in lineage, such as unknown origins or rifts in the genealogical transmission, create holes in the familial genealogical envelope. This means vacant spaces in identity. Symptomatically, this may be expressed by depression. How can emptiness be managed? Addictive behaviors like anorexia-bulimia, drug addiction, sex addiction or running away behavior are risk behaviors that attempt to fill this emptiness by an excess of sensory stimulation.

How can health professional be available to teens in a nonintrusive manner, when the teens themselves sometimes do not recognize themselves? How should we show our respect for what is called a necessary crisis in juvenile identity? How can we be sure we do not overlook an adolescent 'in crisis' who manifests a profound depression with the risk of suicide by, for example, a whirlwind of activity or a broken heart after the first sexual experiences?

The Syndrome of Youthful Exposure to Sexual Danger

A particularly dark form of danger seeking is that which Pierre Benghozi calls the youthful exposure to danger syndrome. In this syndrome, the youngster is the victim of repeated aggressions which, although consciously unwanted and assumed to be the result of bad luck, reflect in fact a weakness in the individual's protection systems or even behaviors that indirectly provoke the confrontation with danger. This situation is seen in families both incestuous and incestual. The weakness in the family's safeguards is a way of using an intermediary aggressor to act out intrafamilial violence. For example, there are forms of sexual promiscuity that favor the adolescent's physical danger, with no protection for his or her intimacy. The adolescent is thus left open to all intrusions including rape. This adolescent is the victim of a situation of danger that may have been induced by the perversion of the familial context.

Running away is an example of adolescent acting out to test the strength of family ties. Running away as risk in is not in itself dangerous. Running away as danger, however, may extend to wandering the streets, putting the adolescent at major risk of street life: violence, sexual predation, AIDS, drug addiction, prostitution, etc.

Running away as danger sheds light on and brings us up to date on the impasses of shame and humiliation. Adolescents cannot share what cannot be admitted (adolescent pregnancy, homosexual desires, school failure, etc.). They are often 'shame-bearers' for the entire family. Although the sexual danger-seeking behavior of young boys or girls does not concern a particular social milieu, it always reveals relational difficulties that threaten family ties.

This family is unable to contain or elaborate conflict. We insist particularly on the situations of conjugal or familial violence in which the child is taken hostage.

Health professionals encounter chaotic families in crisis, with depressed parents, but we also see pseudo aconflictual families who present as having 'no problems'. In these cases, the family avoids confronting problems by masking them with pseudo understanding. Conflict that is not externalized implodes. One form that is important to consider is the displacement of hopelessness due to weaknesses in lineage onto neo-affiliations with clan groups, with all the abuses imaginable: dependence on sects, affiliation with groups with totalitarian ideology, and so on.

How can we be nonintrusive but available for these young people who often do not recognize their own needs? How can show our respect for what we call the necessary crisis of juvenile identity? How can we be sure not to overlook an adolescent 'in crisis', whose severe depression with its risk of suicide is revealed by a broken heart or extreme acting out?

The Bases for Prevention in Interviews Conducted by Health Professionals

A History of Dissociation between Information on Contraception and on STDs

Public health strategies were implemented in the 1960s and 1970s to promote contraceptive use and in the 1980s and 1990 to prevent HIV. Since 2000, the strategies have targeted both STDs and HIV. These juxtaposed strategies contributed partially to the failures in contraception and the prevention of STDs.

Adolescents and young adults (15–24 years) use the contraceptive pill most often, with adolescents between 15 and 19 years mostly using condoms. Although in 2005, most 15- to 24-year-olds knew about emergency contraception and knew that it was available without prescription, the maximal delay in which it can be used with efficacy was not well known among women, and even less among men. The comparison of data from the Health Barometer of 2005 and 2000 indicates a sharp increase in the use of emergency contraception over the past five years, particularly in the young, although the regular contraceptive practices were not modified in the same period, which is an encouraging sign. However, diffusion of emergency contraception was not sufficient to show a drop in the prevalence of unexpected pregnancies [23].

A study from INSERM [12, 24, 25] on the circumstances of contraceptive failure indicated a perception of no risk. Among the reasons given to explain the nonuse of contraceptive methods, 30.1% of the youth stated that they did not believe they could become pregnant, 16.9% indicated that the sexual relationship was unexpected, and 16.4% simply did not think to use a contraceptive method. Condom use was reported by girls in the month preceding pregnancy (42.1%). Among them, 13.1% indicated that they had not used a condom in the vaginal intercourse that they believed had led to the pregnancy, whereas 82.4% attributed the failure to condom tearing or slipping.

The period during which behaviors to protect against risks, notably of pregnancy, has been steadily lengthening: the mean age for the first sexual encounter for young girls and boys is about 17.5 years [10, 26]. The period between the first sexual encounter and the birth of a baby is regularly increasing, with the mean age for first-time mothers about 29.9 years in 2007, according to INSEE [8].

Contraceptive methods fail for various reasons: difficulty in obtaining clear and updated information on the available methods and the methods best adapted for adolescents (difficult intra-familial exchanges, insufficient or truncated information from peers, information based on a single biology class in school, etc.). In addition to these factors are the problems encountered by most women: the prescription is not always adapted to their social, affective and sexual lifestyles, and they may have inadequate knowledge of the ways to use emergency contraception.

Condoms are regularly and massively used but paradoxically less often in youngsters with multiple partners and young women [10, 24, 26].

Condom use for the first intercourse greatly and regularly increased between 1987and 1995. It has remained high, with 89% for women and 88% for men [10, 26]. Seventy-one percent of young people use a contraceptive method, and 21% of them use the condom for this. The condom was the contraceptive method[24] most used by young girls in the month preceding pregnancy (42.1%). Among them, 13.1% indicated that they had not used a condom for the intercourse that led to their pregnancy, whereas 82.4% attributed the failure to tearing or sliding of the condom. Nearly 80% of the respondents declared using a condom during their first sexual encounter with their last partner since 2001. Condom use in the last sexual intercourse was more frequent for men under 25 years in 2004 (70%) than in 2001 (60%) or 1994 (55%). For women, use has been stable at 42%. A high proportion of youth with multiple partners did not use a condom in the past 12 months. Condom use is far from systematic by so-called users since nearly half of the men and two thirds of the women with multiple partners reported not using one in their first encounter with a new partner. Among the men, condom use dropped steadily with the duration of the relationship. Women continued to use a condom regularly for a year, whatever the intensity of the relationship.

HIV screening is more frequent in young people (21% in women and 17% in men) than in the general population (11%) [9, 10]. The fact that the younger generations know fewer individuals that are HIV-positive (63% in 2006 vs. 94% in 1992) explains in part the lack of motivation to use condoms.

Implementing Strategies for Prevention, Screening and Management

The major role of screening and treatment in prevention and the close association of HIV, STDs and unwanted pregnancies emphasize the importance of secondary prevention (early detection, early diagnosis of STDs, emergency contraception, post-exposure HIV treatment) and give doctors a central role in prevention.

In France, prevention is one of the explicit missions of health agencies, according to the law of Hospitals, Patients, Health, Territories (Article L 6112–1). Health agencies can thus be called upon to ensure in part or in whole one or several missions of public service for screening and prevention.

Emergency contraception can be dispensed without charge by not only doctors but also pharmacists, family planning centers, and health agency nurses in special cases (Article L 5134–1 of the Public Health Code).

According to Article L 4130–1, the primary care physician is responsible for prevention and screening, as are the 'health poles' (Article L 6323–4), which may 'participate in preventive actions'.

Sex education in the schools takes into account public health issues: AIDS prevention, sexually transmitted diseases, unwanted pregnancies, sexual violence, etc., using an educational approach. The abortion and contraception law of July 4, 2001, mandated that national education must ensure at least three sessions of information and education on sexuality per year in the general curricula in elementary, junior and senior high schools. Since 2003, sex education has become a major priority for the public health partnership between the Ministries of Health and National Education [5] and recently with contracts of partnership with the Ministry of Justice (judiciary protection of youth) and with the Ministry of Agriculture and Fishing. In addition, sex education and free and anonymous contraception are available to young people in family planning centers (1,196 sites in metropolitan France). The organization of information programs for young people who have left school nevertheless remains inadequate.

Traditional agents need to be supported and informed on changes in behavior and the different ways to reduce sexual risks.

In private life, may young people say they to turn to parents, siblings, friends and acquaintances for information about sexuality. In professional realms, they turn to teachers, adolescent help lines and structures, educators and medical-psychological centers.

Objectives of Public Health Strategies

Deal with the sexual and affective life of adolescents so that we can respond to the risk taking that is a call for attention and help.

- Inform on the risks of disease transmission depending on the individual, culture, environment, and factors that encourage disease transmission.
- Help adolescents to construct their motivation around prevention behaviors.
- Promote emergency contraception.
- Propose screening in cases of risk-taking behavior regarding STDs and HIV.

The objectives of health professionals are thus to:

- Build and maintain relationships of trust with youth and their parents
- Take into account the individual's degree of autonomy.
- Start with the concerns and experiences of the young person.
- Keep the parents involved.
- Differentiate complaints that are psychological, mechanical or erotic.
- Clarify the difference between relationships that make one feel secure and trustworthy relationships.
- Promote affective and sexual well-being.

These objectives should allow the young person to:

- Find ways to meet affective and erotic needs.

Clinical Management by Medical and Psychosocial Professionals of Adolescent Health

Progress in the process of change depends on the quality of the support given to the adolescent during the period of 'molting'. The adolescent's vulnerability is complicated by the fragility of the envelope to be shed and the strength of his or her network of ties. Dr Pierre Benghozi suggests an approach that is both curative and preventive, with the perspective of a new support network built from the many health-related disciplines, with health professionals bringing a variety of skills to accompany, listen to, and care for adolescents. It is important that the role of each is clearly defined for the professionals themselves, as well as for the adolescents and their families. Each has work that is different but complementary and all are bound by the laws of confidentiality, whether working in medicine, psychology, social services, the judiciary or legal services. The school personnel, the nurse, the school psychologist and the educational administrator are at the crossroads of the intimate and the private. We are thus in favor of a psychodynamic perspective for co-constructing the network that links the various partners and provides an 'envelope' for the family in crisis.

Pediatrics: Teaching about Risk and Sexual Health
The risks and dangers of adolescent *sexuality* should be seen as societal *symptoms* of a sexual health status that should be given priority in public health policies.

The prevention of sexual dangers does not begin with adolescence. It begins even before birth by accompanying the parents over the perinatal period. Pediatricians help to coordinate this period in order to encourage the best quality in the early interactions between parents and infants. For the infant, having been 'wanted', being 'lovable', feeling loved, feeling worthy of self-love, respect and recognition: all are essential in the construction of self-esteem and the protection against exposure to sexual danger during the metamorphosis of adolescence. In Great Britain, the government considers that teaching about sexuality and personal behavior in society is important and has developed the Personal, Social and Health Education program for the schools. Jim Knight, as Minister of State for Schools, stated that this was essential to help young people to avoid early pregnancy, sexually transmitted diseases, drug use and alcohol abuse.

Pediatricians have a major role because the body is a privileged means to listen to the adolescent, to give reassurance or to reestablish physical health. The somatic approach is always in fact psycho-socio-somatic. The first consultation in pediatric gynecology has an essential function in the work of ritualizing the adolescent's passage from little girl to young woman. It is 'a rite of passage toward a recognized femininity'. As in every ritual, the body is important. In the consultation, the request to be reassured about the integrity and normality of one's body and the symptoms that are presented are the expression of a rite of passage in the adolescent's life, finding meaning in the familial and social context. The body can thus be offered sacrificially or in totemic exaltation, or by way of symbolic injury. The doctor symbolically ensures the function of the initiated, the one who has passed. The consultation itself is ritualized. Every word, every gesture, every look counts. Any person who accompanies the adolescent, the good friend, the boyfriend or girlfriend, often the mother and if possible the father, and the way they take part in the consultation, are fundamental.

To receive the body in distress, the manifestations of suffering carried by the bodies of adolescents, whether functional or somatic, is to also receive a psychological experience of unconscious shame and guilt that is unable to be mentally expressed.

All consultations, even those outside the realm of sexual concerns, are occasions for a singular encounter with the adolescent. The doctor should remain very much in his or her role of medical consultant to be most effective, because through the relationship to the body, he or she has a privileged position. The doctor can reassure worried adolescents as to the integrity of the somatic body. He or she can reassure the parents that adolescents need to confront new experiences and can best do so by being informed about the risks and dangers and the ways to avoid them. The doctor needs to be attentive to suffering, and in particular to signs of depression, a lack of self-esteem, and sometimes a real hatred of one's body that often signals that an adolescent is placing him- or herself in sexual, psychological or physical danger. For this reason, the multidisciplinary work of professionals is vital, particularly the input from child psychiatrists.

This manner of receiving the adolescent, this psycho-social-somatic attentiveness, is aided by the willingness of pediatricians to become subjectively implicated in the clinical encounter with adolescents.

What should we say about preventing dangerous sexual behaviors? How can we support choices for protection regarding contraception but also STDs and AIDS? The growth process in adolescence is reflected in the rearranging in the unconscious body image. Adolescence, a time of shedding both a personal and familial 'carapace', mobilizes the vulnerability of generational ties.

As we have seen, education about the information that is available and about screening is supported by listening carefully to these processes in play during adolescence.

Prevention can be achieved by teaching about risk from the perspective of sexual health and well-being in the global, medical-psycho-social, and legal sense, according to the World Health Organization. It concerns all doctors, educators, teachers, and parents who work in unison to support and accompany the growth process in adolescents.

Conclusions

The goal is thus not to prevent risk-taking behavior. Instead, the goal is build networks to help young people to better handle their stresses and to support their families. In member of the Executive Board of the European Federation for Psychoanalytic Psychotherapy, and founder and coordinator for the section on psychoanalytic psychotherapy for couples and families.

Dr. Marc Ganem†
Gynecologist-obstetrician, sexologist, President of the French Society for Clinical Sexology, former President of the World Association for Sexual Health (2001–2005), President of the UNESCO Chair 'Sexual Health and Human Rights'. Recently died during an international congress.

References

1 Bonnet D, Guillaume A: La santé de la reproduction: une émergence des droits individuels; in Guillaume A, Khlat M (eds): Santé et droits de la reproduction au temps du sida. Paris, Les Collections Ceped, 2004, pp 11–32.

2 Lert et Pialoux, mission RDRs: Prévention et réduction des risques dans les groupes à haut risque vis-à-vis du VIH et des IST, 27 novembre 2009.

3 Troussier T, et al: Coordonnateur du chapitre: Prévention et sexualité chez les personnes infectées par le VIH, rapport d'expert sous la direction du Pr JF Delfraissy, Prise en charge des personnes infectées par le VIH, édition 2002.

4 Troussier T: Prévention primaire du VIH liée à la sexualité, in VIH 2007, sous la direction de PM Girard, édition DOIN 2007.

5 SPILF et SFLS: Consensus formalise: prise en charge de l'infection par le VIH en médecine général et médecine de ville, Mars, 2009.

6 OMS: Sexual Health: a new focus for WHO. Prog Reprod Health Res 2004;67.

7 Troussier T: La prévention passe par la qualité de vie sexuelle et affective, la santé de l'homme, n° 379. Édition INPES, 2005.

8 Degorre A, Guyon V: Sur dix jeunes entrés en 6eme en 1995, neuf se déclarent en bonne ou très bonne santé en 2007. INSEE Première N°1261, octobre 2009.

9 Bajos N, Bozon M, Beltzer N: Sexualité, prévention et rapports sociaux de sexe au cours de la vie. Méd Sci 2008;24:24–32.

10 Bajos N, Bozon M: Sexualité, genre et santé: les apports de l'enquête Contexte de la sexualité en France; in Bajos N, Bozon M (dir): L'enquête sur la sexualité en France. Pratiques, genre et santé. Paris, Editions la Découverte, 2008, pp 579–601.

11 SMEREP: 6ème édition enquête sur la santé des étudiants en Ile de France, 2009.

12 Bajos N, Ferrand M, et le groupe GINE: De la contraception à l'avortement. Sociologie des grossesses non prévue. Paris, INSERM, 2002.

13 Bajos N, Moreau C, Leridon H, Ferrand M: Pourquoi le nombre d'avortements n'a-t-il pas baissé en France depuis 30 ans? Population Sociétés 2004;407/BEH 9/10.

14 Bajos N, Bozon M: Les agressions sexuelles en France: résignation, réprobation, révolte; in Bajos N, Bozon M (dir); L'enquête sur la sexualité en France. Pratiques, genre et santé. Paris, Editions la Découverte, 2008, pp 381–410.

15 Jaspard M, l'équipe ENVEFF: Les violences envers les femmes en France. Une enquête nationale. Paris, La Documentation Française, 2003.

16 Moreau C, Bouyer J, Gilbert F, Cocoon group, Bajos N: Social, demographic and situational factors associated with inconsistent use of oral contraceptives, Perspect Sex Reprod Health, 2006,38:190–6.

17 Wellings K, Collumbien M, Slaymaker E, Singh S, Hodges Z, Patel D, Bajos N: Sexual behaviour in context: a global perspective. Lancet 2006;368:1706–1728.

18 Enquête KABP Face au VIH-SIDA en France, ANRS-ORS Ile-de-France, 2004 (www.ors-idf.org).

19 INVS: Novembre 2009, surveillance du VIH, site www.invs.gouv.fr

20 InVS: Lutte contre le VIH/SIDA et les infections sexuellement transmissibles en France, 10 ans de surveillance 1996–2005. Rapport de l'Institut de Veille Sanitaire, 2007.

21 Panel P, et al: The satisfaction of French women with their contraception. Congress European Society of Contraception, Prague, 2008.

22 USEM: la santé des étudiants en 2009, 2009.

23 Lydié N. Léon C: Sexualité, IST et dépistage du VIH; in Guilbert P, Gautier A (dir): Baromètre santé 2005 – premiers résultats. Saint Denis, Editions INPES, 2006.

24 Moreau C, Trussell J, Rodriguez G, Bajos N, Bouyer J: Contraceptive failure rates in France: results from a population-based survey. Hum Reprod. 2007;22: 2422–2427.

25 Vilain A: Les interruptions volontaires de grossesse en 2005, DREES. Etudes et résultats, n° 624, 2008.

26 Beltzer N, Bajos N: De la contraception à la prévention: les enjeux de la négociation aux différentes étapes des trajectoires affectives et sexuelles; in Bajos N, Bozon M (dir): L'enquête sur la sexualité en France. Pratiques, genre et santé. Paris, Editions la Découverte, 2008, pp 437–59.

27 Troussier T, Tourette-Turgis C: La qualité de la vie sexuelle et affective favorise la prévention chez les personnes vivant avec le VIH. Revue Européenne de Sexologie, n° 3, 2006.

28 Drew WL, Blair M, Miner RC, Conant M: Evaluation of the virus permeability of a new condom for women. Sex Transm Dis 1990;17:110–112.

Thierry Troussier
Chaire de Santé Sexuelle et de Droits Humain
Université Paris Diderot – Paris 7
40, rue d'Alleray
FR–75015 Paris (France)
E-Mail thierry.troussier@human-earth.org

Sultan C (ed): Pediatric and Adolescent Gynecology. Evidence-Based Clinical Practice. 2nd, revised and extended edition. Endocr Dev. Basel, Karger, 2012, vol 22, pp 380–385

Culturally Sensitive Gynecologic Care in Adolescence

José Enrique Pons

Obstetrics and Gynecology, University of the Republic School of Medicine, Montevideo, Uruguay

Abstract

Culturally sensitive gynecologic care means rendering gynecologic care taking into account adolescents' needs, problems and feelings, as seen by adolescents themselves. Adolescence is a period of turmoil, where limits are being tested and risks taken. A certain degree of rebellion is necessary and normal. In contemporary societies, risk-taking behaviors seem to outnumber any previous historical period. Antagonistic depictions of 'two worlds', transforms the question into one between a culture and a counterculture. Sometimes, the perspectives are exaggerated by attitudes of superiority, leading to inadequate or punitive practices. Health providers need to confront their own prejudices, so as to understand that in their role as health workers, what adolescents ask for is help to cope with their problems in the fields that professionals are qualified for, but not to behave as policemen, judges or priests. Adolescents also need help to overcome resistance to formal environments. In order to achieve success, they have to have the opportunity to be heard and to participate in tailoring programs. These undertakings should be aimed at contributing to health promotion, encouraging self-care and reaffirming confidence in adolescents' responsibility, while generating trust in health services and professionals.

The term 'culture' has been widely discussed and criticized by sociologists, there is no unanimously accepted meaning. In this chapter, the following definition will be accepted: The sum total of ways of living built up by a group of human beings and transmitted from one generation to another. The way of transmission is a cultural trait, meaning any trait of human activity acquired in social life and transmitted by communication.

'Sensitive' also has many meanings: 'quick to understand', 'wise', 'responding to stimuli', and 'showing understanding and awareness of other people's needs, problems or feelings'.

Although it seems unnecessary to define 'gynecologic care', it must be stressed that it should be considered holistically. Culturally sensitive gynecologic care can thence be understood as rendering gynecologic care in such a way that it takes into account adolescents' needs, problems or feelings, as seen by adolescents themselves through their own cultural traits.

Usually, every member of a health care team in an Adolescent Gynecology Care Unit is properly trained to understand current problems affecting adolescents and to use all appropriate skills needed in each case. Anyone working for a long time with adolescents is perfectly aware of the need to take culture into account. Unfortunately, this awareness is challenged by two shortcomings:

1 Firstly, when culture and sensitivity are incorporated into health care (gynecologic care in this case, but the same is true for any other medical field), the main focus of the question is no longer technical medicine, but anthropology. Physicians and other health professionals are not necessarily well prepared to address anthropological problems and questions.
2 Secondly, it is usually assumed that adolescents belong to a subculture, stemming from the particular culture of a nation or a region. Consequently, health professionals are encouraged to be indulgent when adolescents show attitudes and behaviors pertaining to that particular subculture. This benevolent approach, although well intentioned, indicates a lack of understanding of the actual dimension of the gaps between adolescents' and adults' perspectives. Once and again adolescents are seen behaving inconsiderately or even aggressively during their visit to outpatient clinics for a specific health problem, while nurses and doctors patiently and tolerantly let them act improperly just taking care of their health complaints. Those professionals are convinced that they are complying with the needed attitude while aiding their patients with their complaint. This being true, it is also a demonstration that they were unable to understand that they had lost the opportunity of helping those adolescents with what might be their most urgent problem, namely being in a circle of violence, acting aggressively because they have been treated brutally.

Some evaluations of comprehensive adolescent health care have shown very high percentages of lost opportunities, irrespective of care being delivered by doctors or other health professionals [1]. Some other studies concluded that health professionals pay little attention to identifying the psychosocial determinants of health conditions, ranging from 35% of opportunities lost in the case of school or work issues to 56% in the case of income level [2]. Most importantly, health professionals do not have a clear perception of their losing opportunities. The same studies show important differences indicated by adolescents' own perception of professional neglect.

Anthropology is the study of human beings as they pertain to societies. For an anthropologist 'our' habits and customs, and those of an isolated tribe in the remotest imaginable island, are just two possible social schemes to confront and respond to common problems. As Ruth Benedict stated, an anthropologist is interested in human habits not as they are modeled by his or her own society (considering such model as the proper, correct or 'good' one) but by any individual society or tradition [3]. Yet, this is just the vision of some anthropologists. Up to these days, an imposingly strong idea persists, that civilizations evolved from the most primitive forms into their final development as occurs in so called occidental civilization. It was also Benedict who used the example of three revolutions redefining the position of human beings: (a) the Copernican, moving the Earth (and hence man) from the center of the universe, (b) the Darwinian, dethroning man, formerly 'King of the Creation', to just one more among animals, and (c) a third, still evolving and not yet fully achieved, aiming at shifting the 'occidental man' from the pole position in the evolution of civilizations to a discreet place at one end in a fan-shaped scheme.

Within smaller groups of human beings such as nations or regions, the conflict to achieve the aim of the third revolution is also operating. This is specially so within complex societies where more than one ideology, religious, social, or political, and more than one way of living coexist. This is called a cultural complex: a group of culture traits mutually interrelated and dominated by one essential trait, such as nationality.

Cultures are never crystallized; they are in a state of permanent flow and change, as new challenges demand new responses. Particular responses are not always perceived as adequate by every group within a society. Democratic societies allow the rotation of different views in the role of leading the whole group, but even within them, some cultural groups are seen as retarded in their rate of change and adjustment. This is called a cultural lag: slowness in the rate of change of one part of a culture in relation to another part, resulting in maladjustments within societies. Modern societies, more complex, multiethnic and affected by migratory waves, are good examples of this state, although it is not easy to signal which part is the 'retarded' one, since different ideologies will be ready to blame each other of maladjustment.

Sometimes, certain human groups are apparently not affected by the problems of culture complexes. Such seems to be the case in small nations with strongly predominant racial groups of population, no religious fundamentalisms, and very similar traditions countrywide. Yet, this belief prevents a clear understanding of two very special cultural gaps: adult vs. adolescent culture and middle-class vs. so-called 'culture of poverty'. This chapter focuses mainly on the first one, but keeps in mind that poverty always widens the gap.

Adolescence is quite a particular phenomenon, being the solely normal stage of human development that generates tumultuous social clashes, and the only one confronting a disproportionate amount of situations endangering health and even life. Just a snippet can be mentioned here of the impact of the media in determining some of the most negative characteristics of the 'adolescent culture', imposing a rank of consumerism to a global youth audience unnoticed of being manipulated and pushed to unhealthy or even dangerous habits for the sole profit of thirds.

Adolescence is a period of turmoil, where social experimentation and risk taking are a part of the living equation, as teenagers become conscious of their previous dependence on, and subjection to, their parents and other adults. During this stage, adolescents are testing limits and taking risks; most of them do so in rather socially acceptable ways and this struggle for establishing inner forces is absolutely normal. A certain degree of rebellion is necessary when old ties are cut loose and new links are being built [4]. But in contemporary societies, risk-taking behaviors and consequent stress-related deaths and diseases seem to outnumber any other previous historical period. The leading idea – so it is proclaimed – is freedom. As Rollo May made clear rebellion must not be mistaken for freedom [5].

As individuals move out of childhood and through adolescence, peer influence gains greater importance. Peer groups adopt certain rules of behavior claimed to be unbound to adult conventions and social regulations (considering these rules 'hypocrite' ones). Yet, they are tightly bound to new stereotypes modeled on the influence of popular celebrities (actors or actresses, sports people, youth-values' activists, and so on). Sometimes, for some groups or some individuals, rebellion becomes overt revolt and rampage, defiantly and ostentatiously adopting the most adult-rejected behaviors.

As said before, adolescent behaviors and ways of life are considered a subculture. It must be remembered that the prefix 'sub' means under. The term might mean either that it is not really a culture but rather a subordinate derivative of the main culture (indicating an inferior rank) or that it is a lower manifestation in relation to the expected standards (indicating an inferior value). A verdict about the rightness of either one of these possibilities, or deciding if they are both wrong and an alternative one is yet to be found, are not the point at this time. Be that as it may, what adults transmit to adolescents, either explicitly or obliquely, when qualifying their way of life as a subculture, is a pejorative view that can only expand the gap between the adult's world and the adolescent's world.

This antagonistic depiction of the two worlds transforms the question into one between a culture and a counterculture (quite a different condition than a subculture). For a group of adults, this counterculture is based on very dangerous countervalues. For another group, it becomes an idealistic struggle against the corruption of the adult world. Both descriptions are unrealistic. If examples can be found of individuals or groups pertaining to one or the other picture, they are exceptions and never the rule. Most adolescents are, as said before, normally rebellious. But very little help, if any, is attained by the radicalization of the presentation of the problem. It may be legitimate for anthropologists, sociologists and politics to discuss and try to solve this issue, but whatever the solutions imagined, they do not seem to lead to solutions in the short term. Meanwhile, the practical problem of the culture clash remains there.

The culture clash means in clinical practice a series of discords: different language codes that obstruct mutual understanding, different interpretation of grimaces or other nonverbal messages, and sometimes opposite ethical valuation of facts leading to the intent, on the part of health professionals, of smuggling ethically oriented affirmations as if they were biological, medical or technical truths. The reaction of adolescents to this situation is one of distrust and restraint. When poverty comes into the equation, as happens in many public hospitals, the perspectives are exaggerated by the fact that service providers very often adopt attitudes of cultural and social superiority, leading to inadequate, if not overtly punitive, practices.

It must be clearly understood that these are not 'medical' problems, as defined by the traditional, pathology-centered, medical culture. These are mainly social problems and their consequence is not illness, at least not primarily, but first and foremost risk-taking behaviors. If illnesses arise, it is as a secondary consequence (complication) of those behaviors. When risk-taking behaviors become disproportionately intense or frequent, or when they are a part of a syndrome of dangerous behaviors, they turn out to be either threatening to other people's health and life or self-destructive [6].

Severe lesions or death, being the most dramatic consequences of these problems, are an appeal to sensitivity. If attention is paid to some of the meanings of the term 'sensitive', as previously stated, it becomes clear that they demand 'quickness of understanding', to be 'wise' enough as to 'respond to stimuli', and to 'show understanding and awareness of other people's (adolescents in this case) needs, problems or feelings'.

For those working in the specific field of adolescent gynecology, it becomes mandatory to contribute to solving these problems. This includes paying attention to the difficulties that underlie health professionals understanding of adolescents' problems ('caring the caretaker') [7, 8]. Many health care professionals are scarcely prepared to address the social and behavioral etiologies underlying much adolescent morbidity [9]. The timely, comprehensive and appropriate management of these behaviors require understanding of those components [10] as well as of professionals' inner resistance to avoid moralizing or adopting punitive attitudes. These are common problems in the care process of adolescents, mainly in public hospitals, but also in many private settings. If these difficulties are neglected the underlying situation may get worse.

A 'professional superiority syndrome' has been previously defined [11], meaning that in many settings service providers are still trained as if they knew better than others do, and taught that their job is to provide not only services, but also messages, education and information that will set people (and in particular adolescents) to rights. This leads to unacceptable moralizing or judgmental attitudes. Health providers need to confront their own prejudices, so as to understand that in their role as health workers what society in general – and adolescents specifically – ask for, is help to cope with their problems in the fields that professionals are qualified for, but not to behave as policemen, judges or priests.

Approaches have to be tailored to specific problems. Successful experiences may not do equally well in different settings. Realistic approaches need to consider involvement of many levels of action, and not merely the health system. The educational sector's role is of primary importance and over the past decades many countries have recognized the value of the school setting for educating adolescents about matters related to sexual and reproductive health, and have initiated school-based education programs of varying quality and coverage [12]. But in developing countries the value of such programs is limited because of early dropping out of school. The involvement of non-formal available educational resources becomes essential.

There also exists a need to help adolescents overcome resistance to formal environments. In order to achieve success, adolescents themselves have to have the opportunity to be heard and to participate in tailoring programs. All these undertakings should be aimed at contributing to health promotion, encouraging self-care and reaffirming confidence in adolescents' responsibility, while generating trust in health services and professionals.

References

1 Ruzany MH, Szwarcwald CL: Oportunidades perdidas de atenção integral ao adolescente: resultados do estudo-piloto. Adolesc Latinoam 2000;2:26–35.

2 Ministerio de Salud Pública y Bienestar Social Paraguay: Encuesta sobre oportunidades perdidas de atención integral del adolescente. Asunción, 1998, OPS/OMS.

3 Benedict R: El hombre y la cultura. Buenos Aires, Centro Editor de América Latina, 1971.

4 Weiner IB: Normalidad durante la adolescencia; in McAnarney ER, Kreipe RE, Orr DP, Comerci GD (eds): Medicina del Adolescente. Buenos Aires, Panamericana, 1994, pp 120–124.

5 May R: El hombre en busca de si mismo. Buenos Aires, Editorial Central, 1982.

6 Irwin CE Jr: The theoretical concept of the at-risk adolescent; in Strasburger VC, Greydanus DE (eds): State of the Art Reviews: The At-Risk Adolescent. Philadelphia, Hanley & Belfus, 1990.

7 Medori A, Tato M: Algunas conceptualizaciones sobre el cuidado del cuidador; in: Salud Mental Infantil. Abordaje Comunitario. Montevideo, Universidad de la República, 2001, pp 53–57.

8 Musetti D, Garrido G, Guichon Y, Rodriguez M, Sadownik S, Cherro M: Experiences of community involvement of the Child and Adolescent Psychiatric Clinic; in Osofsky JD, Fitzgerald JE (eds): Perspectives on Infant Mental Health (Handbook of Infant Mental health). New York, Wiley, 2000, pp 328–335.

9 Lammers C, Blum RWM: International health; in Friedman SB, Fisher M, Schonberg SK, Alderman EM (eds): Comprehensive Adolescent Health Care, ed 2. St Louis, Mosby, 1998, pp 17–22.

10 Ryan SA, Irwin CE Jr: Risk behaviors; in Friedman SB, Fisher M, Schonberg SK, Alderman EM (eds). Comprehensive Adolescent Health Care, ed 2. St Louis, Mosby, 1998, pp 848–857.

11 Pons JE: Culturally sensitive gynecologic care. 16th Annual Clinical Meeting of the North American Society for Pediatric and Adolescent Gynecology: 'Issues and Answers in Pediatric and Adolescent Gynecology', Miami, 2002.

12 World Health Organization: Improving the Access of School-Going Adolescents to the Health Services They Need: A Distillation of the Findings from Action Research Projects (Phase 1, Assessment Phase) in Six Countries, Draft 1. Geneva, WHO, Department of Child and Adolescent Health and Development, 2000.

Prof. José Enrique Pons
Obstetrics and Gynecology, University of the Republic School of Medicine
Vazquez Ledesma 2889 Ap. 401
11300 Montevideo (Uruguay)
Tel. +598 27115264, E-Mail jeqpons@gmail.com

Author Index

Subject Index